Suicide Prevention

Tatiana Falcone · Jane Timmons-Mitchell
Editors

Suicide Prevention

A Practical Guide for the Practitioner

Springer

Editors
Tatiana Falcone
Epilepsy Center/ Psychiatry Department
Neurological Institute - Cleveland Clinic
Cleveland, OH
USA

Jane Timmons-Mitchell
Begun Center for Violence Prevention
Research and Education
Jack, Joseph, and Morton Mandel School of
Applied Sciences School of Medicine
Case Western Reserve University
Cleveland, OH
USA

ISBN 978-3-319-74390-5 ISBN 978-3-319-74391-2 (eBook)
https://doi.org/10.1007/978-3-319-74391-2

Library of Congress Control Number: 2018936523

Printed on acid-free paper

This Springer imprint is published by the registered company Springer International Publishing AG part of Springer Nature
The registered company address is: Gewerbestrasse 11, 6330 Cham, Switzerland

Funding for this project was made possible (in part) under grant number SM062894 from the Substance Abuse and Mental Health Services Administration (SAMHSA). The views expressed in written training materials or publications and by speakers and moderators do not necessarily reflect the views, opinions, or policies of CMHS, SAMHSA, or HHS; nor does mention of trade names, commercial practices, or organizations imply endorsement by the US Government in conjunction with the Ohio Suicide Prevention Foundation.

Acknowledgments

We acknowledge our gratitude to Seungjong Cho, M.S.W., for assistance in preparing citations for all of the chapters, and to Migle Staniskyte for assistance in compiling chapter manuscripts.

Contents

Contributors

Glenn Albright, Ph.D. Department of Psychology, Baruch College, City University of New York, New York, NY, USA

Kognito, New York, NY, USA

Jessica M. Bordenave, Psy.D. Department of Neurology, University of Wisconsin School of Medicine and Public Health, Madison, WI, USA

Ruby C. Castilla-Puentes, M.D., Dr.P.H., M.B.A. Board of Directors American Society of Hispanic Psychiatry, Medical Safety at Johnson and Johnson, Philadelphia, PA, USA

Dornsife School of Public Health, Drexel University, Philadelphia, PA, USA

Cathleen Cerny University Hospitals Cleveland Medical Center, Case Western Reserve University School of Medicine, Cleveland, OH, USA

Tatiana Falcone, M.D., M.P.H. Epilepsy Center/ Psychiatry Department, Neurological Institute - Cleveland Clinic, Cleveland, OH, USA

Meghan D.M. Fondow, Ph.D. Access Community Health Centers, Madison, WI, USA

Fernando Espi Forcen, M.D., Ph.D. Department of Psychiatry, Rush University Medical Center, Chicago, IL, USA

Kathleen N. Franco, M.D. Cleveland Clinic Lerner College of Medicine of Case Western Reserve University, Cleveland, OH, USA

Department of Psychiatry and Psychology, Cleveland Clinic, Cleveland, OH, USA

Mariela Herrera, M.D. Billings Clinic, Billings, MT, USA

Michael F. Hogan, Ph.D. National Action Alliance on Suicide Prevention, Washington, DC, USA

Case Western Reserve University School of Medicine, Cleveland, OH, USA

Lisa M. Horowitz, Ph.D., M.P.H. Intramural Research Program, National Institute of Mental Health, National Institutes of Health, Bethesda, MD, USA

Michael Ignatowski, D.O. CWRU School of Medicine, Cleveland Louis Stokes VA Medical Center, Cleveland, OH, USA

Juan R. Jaramillo, M.D. Department of Psychiatry, Owensboro Health Regional Hospital, Owensboro, KY, USA

Xavier F. Jimenez, M.D., M.A. Chronic Pain Rehabilitation Section, Center for Neurological Restoration, Cleveland Clinic Lerner College of Medicine, Neurological Institute, Cleveland Clinic, Cleveland, OH, USA

Jana E. Jones, Ph.D. Department of Neurology, University of Wisconsin School of Medicine and Public Health, Madison, WI, USA

Naveed Khokhar, M.D. Department of Psychiatry, Cleveland Clinic, Cleveland, OH, USA

Jeanne M. Lackamp, M.D. University Hospitals Cleveland Medical Center, Cleveland, OH, USA

Elizabeth C. Lanzillo, B.A. Intramural Research Program, National Institute of Mental Health, National Institutes of Health, Bethesda, MD, USA

Jennifer K. Lehmann, M.A. Case Western Reserve University, Cleveland, OH, USA

Youssef Mahfoud, M.D., F.A.P.A., F.A.S.A.M. Opioid Treatment Program, CWRU School of Medicine, Cleveland Louis Stokes VA Medical Center, Cleveland, OH, USA

Jeremiah McMillan, B.A. University of Georgia, Athens, GA, USA

Clare C. Mitchell, Ph.D. University Hospitals Cleveland Medical Center, Cleveland, OH, USA

Karolina Mlynek, M.D., M.B.A. Department of Psychiatry, Cleveland Clinic, Cleveland, OH, USA

Farah Munir University Hospitals Cleveland Medical Center, Case Western Reserve University School of Medicine, Cleveland, OH, USA

Sarah Nagle-Yang University Hospitals Cleveland Medical Center, Case Western Reserve University School of Medicine, Cleveland, OH, USA

Maryland Pao, M.D. Intramural Research Program, National Institute of Mental Health, National Institutes of Health, Bethesda, MD, USA

Alexander D. Smith, Psy.D. Access Community Health Centers, Madison, WI, USA

Christopher Sola, D.O. Department of Psychiatry, Cleveland Clinic, Cleveland, OH, USA

Migle Staniskyte, B.A. Neurologic Institute, Cleveland Clinic, Cleveland, OH, USA

Carol Swetlik, B.A. Cleveland Clinic Lerner College of Medicine of Case Western Reserve University, Cleveland, OH, USA

Jane Timmons-Mitchell, Ph.D. Begun Center for Violence Prevention Research and Education, Jack, Joseph, and Morton Mandel School of Applied Sciences, School of Medicine, Case Western Reserve University, Cleveland, OH, USA

Jaime Vengoechea, M.D. Pontificia Universidad Javeriana, Bogota, Colombia

Elizabeth A. Zeidler Schreiter, Psy.D. Access Community Health Centers, Madison, WI, USA

Introduction

Suicide remains the most serious complication of any psychiatric disorder and the suicide rates in the USA have not decreased in the last 20 years; the last available information dates to 2015, which saw 12.5 deaths per 100,000 habitants. Every year, approximately 505,507 people visit the hospital due to suicide-related injuries throughout the USA. Prevention of suicide-related deaths is a major unmet public health challenge. The challenge is further complicated by the fact that nearly 80% of suicidal patients who subsequently died by suicide denied suicide ideation during their last communication with a hospital. With this book, we hope to provide additional tools for those who meet these patients every day, in order to improve care and prevent suicide.

From the provider vantage point, it may appear that the landscape of healthcare for those presenting with issues related to suicide is changing. This would be correct, since there has been a concerted effort over the last several years to rethink and then to change the provision of usual care. Based on the prevalence of suicide in the USA, and its stable (though at times increasing) place in the top ten causes of death among the population, visionary leaders look to successes that can be disseminated.

In addition to currently available information on thinking about suicide from a healthcare perspective, this volume addresses (1) how to care for people presenting to healthcare professionals in settings that often involve suicide, and in populations at known risk for suicide, and (2) how to provide training and professional development for healthcare professionals tasked with assessing and treating these individuals. Eleven chapters focus on direct patient care, while four chapters are structured around the focus on training and professional development.

Recently, the Suicide Prevention Resource Center (SPRC), the entity funded by the US government to provide technical assistance on suicide prevention, in collaboration with the National Action Alliance for Suicide Prevention, published a report entitled "Recommended Standard Care for People with Suicide Risk: Making Health Care Suicide Safe."[1] The report addresses the following prominent areas that should be included in standard care: suicide screening and assessment; safety planning; counseling on lethal means restriction; and providing caring contacts for follow-up. A review of the 16 chapters shows the following: (1) 8 (of the 11 that are focused on patient care) discuss a process of screening and assessment consistent with the recommendation. Most of these specifically mention the PHQ-9, which is a well-validated instrument that has been used with all children, adolescents, and adults. Seven of the eight chapters mention the C-SSRS (Columbia Suicide Severity Rating Scale), which includes both screening and assessment components. Two of the chapters discuss the use of the ASQ (Asking Suicide Questions), a relatively new measure developed to assess suicide issues, that includes screening, assessment, safety planning, and lethal means restriction. (2) Safety planning is addressed according to the guidelines in 7 of the 11 chapters. It is important to note that, in this context, safety planning does not mean simply asking the person whether they agree to contract for safety. As is pointed out by two of the chapter authors, this has been shown to be an invalid and therefore contraindicated process. There are several recommended approaches to addressing safety planning, including a link to a video presentation illustrating how this can be done (Chap. 11). (3) Counseling on lethal means restriction is addressed in 7 of the 11 patient care chapters, as well as in two of the training/professional development chapters. While the ASQ provides a process to guide this discussion, another approach can be found in CALM (Counseling Against Lethal Means), a training designed for those who provide patient care. CALM has been widely implemented and is noted for its ease of use, participant enthusiasm, and supporting research. (4) Caring contacts, meaning the follow-up contact with a patient after discharge from service, is discussed in only two of the chapters. Compared with the frequent mention of the other aspects in the SPRC/Action Alliance report, this is a notable difference. It may be that, because of service design, the handoff is to the next involved service. But it may also be that providers focused on the service provision at hand could improve emphasis on connecting those at risk for suicide with follow-up services outside of the healthcare setting. Local lifeline and crisis providers are the logical partners, since they include this function as part of their scope of service.

Requirements and guidelines for training (e.g., APA residency requirements), as well as training provided, generate an additional layer of complexity for those providing care. The chapters that address medical student and residency training, and the chapter on physicians, highlight the significant challenges faced by these providers. Time, preparation, and self-doubt contribute to existential crises that can be resolved in favor of increased knowledge but that can also undermine the efforts of the healer. In addition to the chapters on training and professional development, providing additional support in the form of training and other structures is a goal of the chapter on gatekeeper training and primary care behavioral health.

It is our hope that this volume will serve as a resource to inform care and also provide a benchmark for current thinking about key areas faced by healthcare providers. Effective components of suicide prevention, early identification of high-risk individuals, and effective treatment modalities are in various stages of development. Sharing these approaches is a main goal of this book.

Notes

1. National Action Alliance for Suicide Prevention: Transforming Health Systems Initiative Work Group. (2018). Recommended standard care for people with suicide risk: Making health care suicide safe. Washington, DC: Education Development Center, Inc.

Part I

Introduction

Neurobiology of Suicide

1

Tatiana Falcone[#], Migle Staniskyte[#], Fernando Espi Forcen, and Jaime Vengoechea

Introduction

Suicide is a serious global mental health problem. Every 40 seconds a person takes their own life, meaning that at least 800,000 suicides occur worldwide every year [1]. It is the second leading cause of death among those ages 15–24 [2]. Despite major advances in identifying risk factors, little is known about how these factors may interact with each other, or what biological triggers may influence suicidal behavior, therefore making suicide very difficult to predict at an early stage.

Epidemiology

In the last 45 years, the rate of suicide has increased by 60%. In 2008, the number of deaths by suicide exceeded the number of deaths by homicide (535,000) and war (182,000) combined [1, 3]. In the USA, suicide is the number 10 cause of death. The emotional impact of suicide is hard to measure, and the estimated cost in the US health-care system is around $44 billion, yearly [1]. In one day in the USA, 117 people commit suicide [1].

[#] Equal Contribution

T. Falcone, M.D., M.P.H (✉)
Epilepsy Center/Psychiatry Department, Neurological Institute - Cleveland Clinic, Cleveland, OH, USA
e-mail: falcont1@ccf.org

M. Staniskyte, B.A.
Neurologic Institute, Cleveland Clinic, Cleveland, OH, USA
e-mail: stanism2@ccf.org

F. E. Forcen, M.D., Ph.D.
Department of Psychiatry, Rush University Medical Center, Chicago, IL, USA
e-mail: Fernando_espiforcen@rush.edu

J. Vengoechea, M.D.
Pontificia Universidad Javeriana, Bogota, Colombia
e-mail: jvengoechea@cable.net.co

T. Falcone, J. Timmons-Mitchell (eds.), *Suicide Prevention*,
https://doi.org/10.1007/978-3-319-74391-2_1

The lifetime risk of suicidal ideation is 13.5%, the lifetime risk of suicidal ideation with a plan is 3.9% and the lifetime risk of suicide attempts is 4.5% [4]. The risk of suicide attempts (SA) in males is around 1.3–3.8% per year and in women is 1.5–10% [4]. The risk of recurrence is reported from 15 to 30% according to the studies. The risk of suicide in the general population is 0.5–1%, while the risk of reattempt increases in patients with a previous attempt by 10–60 times. Certain medical conditions also impact the risk of suicide such as traumatic brain injury, the presence of psychiatric diagnosis, especially mood disorders and substance abuse disorders, and pain disorders. Patients with increased impulsivity are also at a higher risk: those who practice risky driving, those with history of intimate partner violence as a victim or perpetrator, and those with history of risky sexual behavior (sexually transmitted diseases) [5].

To date, suicide is a major public health problem. Around 80% of patients who died by suicide denied suicidal ideations during their last communication with the hospital or health-care provider [6]. Currently, effective treatments to prevent suicide are very limited. Research has focused on different psychological and neurobiological factors with the goal of understanding the ultimate question, why do people commit suicide? The neurobiological research has focused on different neurotransmitters; genetic, neuroendocrine studies; and various biological markers to predict the vulnerability to suicide [7].

Clinical Predictors of Suicidality

Over the last 20 years, research has uncovered important clinical factors for risk and protection of suicide [8]. However, it is still very difficult to predict who is at imminent risk for suicide. The strongest risk factor for suicide death is a prior year history of suicide attempts [9]. Up to 30% of patients who reported suicidal thoughts will eventually make a suicide plan [1, 3]. Most studies in this population have focused on lifetime and risk factors in the last 12 months [8]. The most reported distal risk factors are adverse childhood experiences; stressful life events; family history of suicide attempts or psychiatric pathology; history of mood disorders, anxiety disorders, or psychotic disorders; previous history of suicidal thoughts and behaviors; and recent attempt by a friend or a family member [10–13]. Other well-documented risk factors are social isolation, lethality of previous attempt, and rumination. Some of the proximal risk factors reported include psychiatric illness, chronic medical illness, psychosocial stress, and availability of means [14, 15]. It is still unclear if the long-term variables help predict suicidal behavior in the short term [7]. Some risk factors that have been identified to predict the long-term (2–10 years) risk of suicide such as hopelessness and suicidal ideation are different from the risk factors used for short-term predictions such as anxiety, insomnia, and anhedonia which are more likely to predict suicide deaths occurring within 12 months [15, 16].

It remains unclear how patients transition from having suicidal thoughts to attempting suicide. Interpersonal negative life events in the week prior to the SA have been identified as an important influencing factor in these adolescents [17, 18].

History of high-risk events in the preceding 3 months has also been identified as an important risk factor in adolescents [10]. A study from the World Mental Health Survey identified the following risk factors for suicidal behavior SB: female sex, younger age, lower education and income, unmarried status, unemployment, parent psychopathology, childhood adversities, and mental disorders. Additionally, the study revealed that disorders of impulse control and anxiety are key to predicting the transition from suicidal thought to SA [9]. According to the National Comorbidity Survey, less than half of adolescents who attempt suicide and a third of adolescents with SI have received mental health care in the last year [19]. Some of the stronger predictors of SA among adolescents in the National Comorbidity Survey replication were major depressive disorder/dysthymia, eating disorders, conduct disorder, and intermittent explosive disorder [19]. In clinical trials including adolescents with mood disorders, the stronger predictors of SB were high SI at baseline, non-suicidal self-injury, family conflict, and substance abuse [11, 12]. Despite having such extensive knowledge and multiple efforts, prediction of suicide at the individual patient level remains very difficult, even among high-risk groups [2, 8]. Because the clinical risk factors for suicide have a low predictive value to identify those individuals who will ultimately commit suicide, the field has an increased interest on the biological markers for suicide risk [20].

Neurobiology

Recently, more attention has been given to the biological mechanisms of suicide. Among various studies, the discovery of low 5-HIAA levels in the cerebrospinal fluid (CSF) of suicide attempters opened a gate to a bulk of research in this direction over the last decade. Today, most of the research studies have focused on the role of serotonin abnormalities in suicide, other possible theories are also investigated; the stress-induced response involving the hypothalamic-pituitary-adrenal axis, the locus coeruleus norepinephrine system, and the opioid endogen system and the role of inflammation are pieces that complete the puzzle in the complex neurobiological mechanism of this pathology. The field goals have changed with the information learned from genetic studies, where similar genes might be involved in different psychiatric disorders and similar specific symptoms might have common specific biological pathways. Also other environmental factors such as stress and adverse childhood experiences which can alter the neuroimmune network in youth can predispose to suicide later in life.

From some of the neurology research, we have learned that the initial changes in the brain from many of the neurological diseases can appear years (even decades) before the initial symptoms appear. In psychiatric disorders, changes in the brain appear many years before, we are observing any clinical symptoms. Early stress and inflammation can slowly impact the neurovascular unit, trigger neuroinflammation, and continue the cycle, altering the blood-brain barrier, perpetuating the neuroinflammation and the psychiatric symptoms.

One of the first articles to explain the role of inflammation in mental illness was published in 1947 at the psychosomatic medicine journal; in the paper, Harry

Freeman and Fred Elmadjian found a decreased lymphopenic response to glucose administration in subjects with psychosis vs. controls. Since the discovery of cytokines in 1957 as proteins secreted by cells that signal an inflammatory response, the role of inflammation in mental illness has been an object of study in psychiatry.

Biomarkers of Suicidality

Multiple studies have evaluated biochemical, genetic, and epigenetic changes in patients who had completed suicide [20]. The serotonin system is one of the most highly studied [21], and low levels of 5-hydroxyindoleacetic acid (5-HIAA) have been found in the cerebrospinal fluid (CSF) of patients who have committed violent attempts [22, 23]. Genetic studies reported polymorphism on the serotonin transporter and in tryptophan hydroxylase in suicidal behavior [20, 24–26]. Other studies examining gamma-amino butyric acid (GABA), dopamine, and glutamate do not appear to associate these markers with suicide [21]. However, several studies using ketamine in severely depressed patients have demonstrated decrease in suicidal ideation [5, 27–29]. The role of ketamine in suicide may suggest that these markers could still be involved in a yet unexplored role [28]. Other studies have focused on the role of the hypothalamic-pituitary-adrenal axis; despite the dexamethasone suppression test (DST) continuing to be controversial, cortisol suppression has been strongly associated with suicidal behavior. Changes in the methylation of the glucocorticoid receptor in patients exposed to childhood abuse have been observed in suicide victims [30, 31]. Multiple neurotrophic factors are also of interest, with brain-derived neurotrophic factor (BDNF) being one with the most evidence linking it to suicide, to date [32, 33].

Serotonin

Decreased levels of serotonin have been reported in suicidal patients. Some of the initial neurobiological studies of suicide evaluated the serotoninergic system, in the brain or in tissue. Perhaps serotonin is one of the most studied neurotransmitters in patients with mood disorders and suicide. It is still not clear, if some of the findings in the serotonin abnormalities are related to depression or are specific to suicide [7].

Historically, low levels of 5 hydroxiindolacetic acid (5 HIAA) were first described on the CSF of patients with serious suicide attempts [22]. Later, it was described that lower concentrations of 5-HIAA in the CSF of patients can predict suicidal behavior in the future. In a study of 92 patients with previous history of depression, and previous suicide attempts, 8 out of the 11 patients who subsequently died by suicide had lower levels of 5-HIAA in CSF in the previous year. In this group the relative risk to die by suicide was 17% compared to 7% of those who had normal levels of 5-HIAA in the CSF [34].

The investigators concluded that lower levels of 5-HIAA in the CSF of suicidal patients predicted higher risk for suicide in the future and also that patients with lower levels of 5-HIAA were more likely to attempt suicide using more violent means [22]. Several other research groups have also confirmed the same finding [35]. In a study of inpatient males at high risk for suicide, those with lower levels of 5-HIAA in the CSF were more likely to reattempt [36].

In a similar study, 211 adolescents who had attempted suicide were evaluated using psychometric scales to evaluate violence, aggression, depression, impulsivity, and anxiety. The levels of 5HT were measured in the blood and were found to be lower in the control group. Authors concluded that lower levels of 5HT combined with psychometric measures could potentially be a peripheral marker to help stratify the risk among adolescents reporting suicidal thoughts [37].

Some studies in the serotonin receptor and the serotonin transporter (SERT) have also described pre- and postsynaptic changes in the prefrontal cortex of those who had committed suicide; other groups that tried to replicate the same finding were unable to replicate the study [38]. Studies on the prefrontal cortex have demonstrated abnormal levels on the serotoninergic system on the hypothalamus of suicide victims, especially in the ventral prefrontal cortex. Some of these findings were independent of the diagnosis [39–41].

Another important point in favor of the serotonergic theory was the study on patients who had attempted suicide (especially those with high lethality attempts) and the poor response to the fenfluramine challenge, an indicator of central serotonin activity, independent of the psychiatric diagnosis [42]. Similarly, it is considered that the flat response to prolactin after a challenge with fenfluramine may be a potential marker of the abnormal serotonin levels in patients who are suicidal. Interestingly this was also independent in patients with depression, schizophrenia, personality disorders matched with the same diagnosis, and history of suicide attempts [43, 44]. Lower levels of 5-HIAA were correlated with serious suicide attempts and the severity of the suicide attempt [44, 45]. Authors concluded that the lethality of the suicide attempt was associated with lower levels of CSF 5HIAA and also that these levels can predict future suicide attempts and the risk of death by suicide [34]. Similar studies evaluating the response of prolactin to the injection of d-fenfluramine in patients with depression or personality disorders who attempted suicide reported a significant decrease in the response in those patients who had previous SA [46, 47].

Noradrenergic System and Suicide

There is some evidence of an important relationship between the levels of stress and suicidal ideation. The noradrenergic system is a key regulatory component of the stress response. Some postmortem studies have demonstrated increased mRNA expression of alpha 2A-adrenoceptors, serotonin receptors, and mu-opioid receptors in the brain of suicide victims [48] and also elevated levels of tyrosine hydroxylase in the locus coeruleus from suicide victims [49]. Some of the studies evaluating the levels of noradrenaline in the CSF of suicidal patients were not able to identify any differences [50, 51]. In a postmortem study of suicide victims with major depressive disorder MDD, there was evidence of decrease number of noradrenergic neurons in the locus coeruleus [43, 44, 52, 53]. It is hard to disentangle the effect of stress or illness as a cause for this change [43, 44, 52, 54]. The role of stress can certainly play an important part in the observed brain changes in patients who died by suicide. Other changes in the noradrenergic pathway in the prefrontal cortex, such as alteration in the cycle of the protein G, have been described in postmortem studies of suicidal patients with history of depression [55].

Dopamine

Is not clear yet if dopamine plays a crucial role in suicide, other than some of the reports of lower regulation of dopamine in the patients with MDD [54]. Initial studies were not able to demonstrate changes on the levels of dopamine in the CSF of patients who had attempted suicide compared to others who didn't [50, 51, 56]. Mann et al. reported lower levels of homovanillic acid, the principal metabolite of dopamine in patients with MDD who attempted suicide [54]. Studies evaluating the levels of dopamine in different brain regions were unable to identify any differences [57]. Perhaps in patients with history of substance abuse especially alcoholism, the role of the dopamine can confer some extra risk [39]. It has been postulated that the reward system and the dopamine D2 receptor, make individuals more vulnerable to impulsivity, compulsions, alterations in the mood and potentially could increase the risk of suicide. The dopaminergic system deserves further investigation to untangle its role in the neurobiology of suicide [58].

Acetylcholine

At present, there is no conclusive evidence that changes in the cholinergic activity have a role in suicidal behavior [58]. Postmortem studies were unable to find changes in the muscarinic receptors in the brain of patients who committed suicide [59].

Neurotrophins and BDNF

Stress as one of the important mechanisms that precipitate depression is not completely understood. Important to understand is the reason why there is a delay in the response to antidepressant medication, even when these treatments reach the brain fairly efficiently [60]. Authors have hypothesized the role of slowly developing but stable adaptations, which might include epigenetic regulation. An animal model of depression, the chronic social defeat stress, mimics many of the symptoms of MDD; at the molecular level, mice in chronic defeat stress have downregulation of the BDNF in the hippocampus; these changes induce long-lasting dimethylation at the promoter of the BDNF downregulated transcript; these changes were not reversed by antidepressant treatment [61].

Stressful events in early life might also leave lasting epigenetic marks in rats. A study comparing rats with high levels of nurturing behaviors vs. low levels of nurturing behaviors demonstrated that the rats in the second group were at a molecular disadvantage; the methylation of the nerve growth factor A (NGFI-A) was disrupting the regulation of the GR gene. Interestingly enough, cross-fostering reversed the methylation differences at this site. These studies support the role of epigenetic modifications and are important in animal models of depression [62].

The brain-derived neurotrophic factor (BDNF) is one of the members of the neurotrophin family. It belongs to the extracellular signal system. It is implicated in the neuroplasticity, neuronal proliferation, and maintenance of specific neuronal populations. BDNF and the neurotrophins are key in the modulation and synthesis of proteins [63–66]. Several studies have implicated neurotrophins and the BDNF in the pathophysiology of suicide, some trying to elucidate how changes in the BDNF expression can impact the brain plasticity and perhaps the response to SSRIs on patients with depression [58, 67]. Some animal models have evaluated the role of BDNF in the pathophysiology of suicide; animals treated with antidepressants had an increased level of BDNF. In some postmortem studies, levels of BDNF have been reported to be decreased in the brain of victims of suicide [68].

Studies have reported that treatment with antidepressants can impact the expression of BDNF and trkB in the hippocampus [68, 69]. Also, depressed patients who were treated with antidepressants had higher brain levels of BDNF postmortem [70]. In several postmortem studies in patients who died by suicide (with history of MDD), the levels of BDNF and TrkB were downregulated in different regions of the brain [71–73]. Some of these studies were conducted with adolescents, demonstrating how stress has an impact in the vulnerability to suicide and the postmortem changes in the prefrontal cortex and hippocampus of adolescents who committed suicide and had downregulation of BDNF and TrkB [73, 74].

Neuroinflammatory Markers of Suicidality: Evidence of Increased Inflammation in Patients After a Suicide Attempt?

There are at least 26 published studies of peripheral inflammatory markers in patients after a suicide attempt to date [75]. The path to inflammation can vary; it can be triggered by stress, infectious agents, or autoimmunity [76]. The role of cytokines in suicidal patients has been investigated since the early 1980s, the results look more and more compelling, but some ambiguity remains. Melancholic patients have been consistently reported as having more immunological abnormalities, like low monocyte counts and cytokine abnormalities. Due to the crucial role in the acute inflammatory reaction, the monocyte-macrophage system has received the most attention. Cytokines produced by the monocytes like IL-1Beta activate the complement system. In children and adolescents, fewer studies have also reported immunological abnormalities in suicidal patients. In a recent meta-analytic review of 300 studies, describing the relationship between psychological stress and immune system, chronic stressors (like having a chronic illness) were associated with suppression of both cellular and humoral measures [77, 78]. Chronic illness also increased the vulnerability to immune changes during the stressors.

Table 1.1 Inflammatory markers in several psychiatric conditions. Several inflammatory markers have been reported to be altered, in several psychiatric conditions, including mood disorders, psychotic disorders and suicide.

Disorder	IL 1 B	IL 6	TNF-alpha	IFN G	VEGF	Orexin	BDNF	Kyn	S100 B
MDD	X	X	X	X	X	X	X	X	X
Bipolar disorder	X	X					X	X	X
Psychosis	X	X	X		X		X	X	X
Suicide	X	X	X	X	X	X	X	X	X

In the next paragraph, we will describe the potential hypothesis on how each of the biomarkers can be related to suicidal behavior and attempts. The major biomarkers associated with suicidal ideation and behavior included in this chapter are reviewed below:

Two major meta-analyses evaluating the levels of cytokines in patients with MDD have been published recently [77, 78]. In 13 studies evaluating the levels of TNF, measurements were examined for 438 patients and 350 controls, with the overall weighted mean difference (WMD) of 3.96 pg/mL $p < 0.00001$ [63, 77, 78]. In 16 studies evaluating the levels of IL-6 of 492 depressed and 400 control subjects, depressed patients had higher concentrations of IL-6 ($p < 0.00001$) with a WMD of 1.78 pg/mL [63, 77, 78]. Studies evaluating the effect of antidepressant (SSRI) treatment on serum levels of inflammatory cytokines suggested an anti-inflammatory effect of the SSRIs. In a meta-analysis of 22 studies of MDD and levels of cytokines before and after treatment, the authors concluded that SSRI treatment reduced the levels of IL-1 and IL-6 [63, 77, 78]. The authors also postulated a possible effect on TNF after SSRIs; this effect was not seen with other antidepressants [27].

In adolescents, levels of several inflammatory markers have been identified in patients with suicidal ideation and behavior. Studies have reported alterations of IL-1B, IL-6, TNF-alpha, IFN-gamma, VEGF, S100B, orexin, BDNF, and kynurenine [26, 75, 79, 80].

Individual Inflammatory Markers

Cytokines

The role of stress is important to help us understand the psychosocial and neurobiological underpinnings of suicidal patients [81, 82]. Stress activates the inflammatory cascade, and as a result of this reaction, microglia become activated [75, 81, 83–86]. These cells produce proinflammatory cytokines such as IL-1B, IL-2, IL-6, TNF, IL-1B, and IL-6, impacting the permeability of the blood-brain barrier (BBB)

[86–88]. These increases have been identified in patients who have attempted suicide. Dysregulation of the HPA axis has been reported in some studies evaluating suicidal behavior [89]. Alteration in the HPA axis is directly related to the production of cytokines. When monocytes are activated, they can cross the BBB and activate microglia, consistent with evidence from postmortem studies of patients who have committed suicide [90–93].

IL1-B

Levels of IL1-B have been shown to potentiate the brain concentrations of serotonin and norepinephrine. This cytokine has also been associated with the activation of the HPA axis and is reported to increase the secretion of ACTH and cortisol [92, 93]. A postmortem study of teenage suicide victims reported increased expression of IL-1B in the Brodmann area 10 [94, 95].

IL-2

Lowered levels of IL-2 in plasma and CSF have been found in patients presenting with suicidal ideation and following suicidal attempts. For instance, Kim and colleagues found decreased plasma levels of IL-2 in patients meeting criteria for major depressive disorder with suicidal ideation as compared to patients with major depressive disorder without suicidal ideation [97]. Similarly, other studies have found decreased IL-2 among other findings in patients after a suicide attempt [80, 96, 97].

IL-6

Levels of IL-6 are reported to be elevated in patients with depression and those with exposure to childhood trauma and suicide. Evidence from several meta-analyses from patients with mood disorders and schizophrenia have reported increased levels of IL-6 [98]. One third of the circulating levels of IL-6 come from the adipose tissue. Smoking has also been linked to increased levels of IL-6 [99]. Three studies reported an increase in the levels of IL-6 in patients with suicide [78, 93, 100].

TNF-Alpha

Animal studies found changes on levels of TNF-alpha after treatment with antidepressants. Some theories involve the effect of antidepressants to modification of the expression of the glucocorticoid receptor. Increased levels of TNF-alpha have been reported in five studies with suicidal patients [75, 78, 95, 100], with one of them in adolescents [96].

IFN-Gamma

This cytokine has been decreased after treatment in vivo or in vitro with antidepressants [101]. Two studies reported altered levels of IFN-gamma in suicidal patients [26, 80], one of them in adolescents reported a different biological pattern compared to adults. Decreased levels of this cytokine were found in suicidal adolescents, although sample size was small [26]. IFN-gamma is one of the first steps on the kynurenic pathway [102].

C-Reactive Protein

Increased levels of high-sensitive C-reactive protein have been reported in patients with mood disorders and suicidal behavior [103].

Kynurenic/Quinolinic Acid

Inflammation increases the production of quinolinic acid (QUIN) and kynurenic acid (KYNA). The kynurenic pathway is altered in patients with mood disorder and schizophrenia [26, 102]. Some preliminary studies on youth exposed to trauma may also be implicated by this pathway. Longitudinal studies of patients undergoing treatment for mood disorders [16] have demonstrated decreased levels of kynurenic acid in patients who are improving. Evidence from postmortem studies of mood disorder patients have reported alteration in certain areas of the brain on the kynurenic pathway in a group of depressed patients. Two studies have reported alterations on the kynurenic pathway in suicide attempters [94, 102, 104, 105]. Sublette compared levels between healthy controls and depressed patients who had attempted suicide and those who had not [106]. Erhardt et al. reported levels of increased QUIN acid in the CSF of 64 medication-free suicide attempters [107]. The authors hypothesize that alteration of the KYN pathway in suicide might be related to the glutamatergic transmission, since QUIN is a NMDA receptor agonist. The fact that ketamine has shown promising results in improving suicidality in 4 small studies might suggest that the NMDA receptor could be an important pathway to further study in patients with suicidal behavior [5, 27–29].

S100B

S100B is a glial and trophic marker, located primarily on the cytoplasm of oligodendrocytes and astrocytes [108, 109]. S100B stays in the brain, unless there are alterations of the BBB. When that occurs, this protein is identified in the serum [110]. In a study on adolescents presenting with suicidal behavior, levels of S100B were increased in patients compared to controls despite a diagnosis of MDD, bipolar disorder, or schizophrenia [79]. This study was later replicated by our group using the Columbia Suicidality Screen Rating Scale (CSSR-S) as the measure for suicidal ideation in adolescents. Levels of S100B were increased in those adolescents who were at greater risk for suicide [111].

S100B levels ng/mL by BPRS Suicidality Score (Fig. 1.1)

Brain-Derived Neurotrophic Factor (BDNF)

Increase in the levels of stress causes decrease in the levels of BDNF. The lower levels of BDNF were correlated with the decreased mRNA expression of BDNF in the prefrontal cortex (Brodmann area 9 of suicidal victims) [112]. BDNF is a neurotrophin classified as a nerve growth factor, affecting growth, plasticity, and

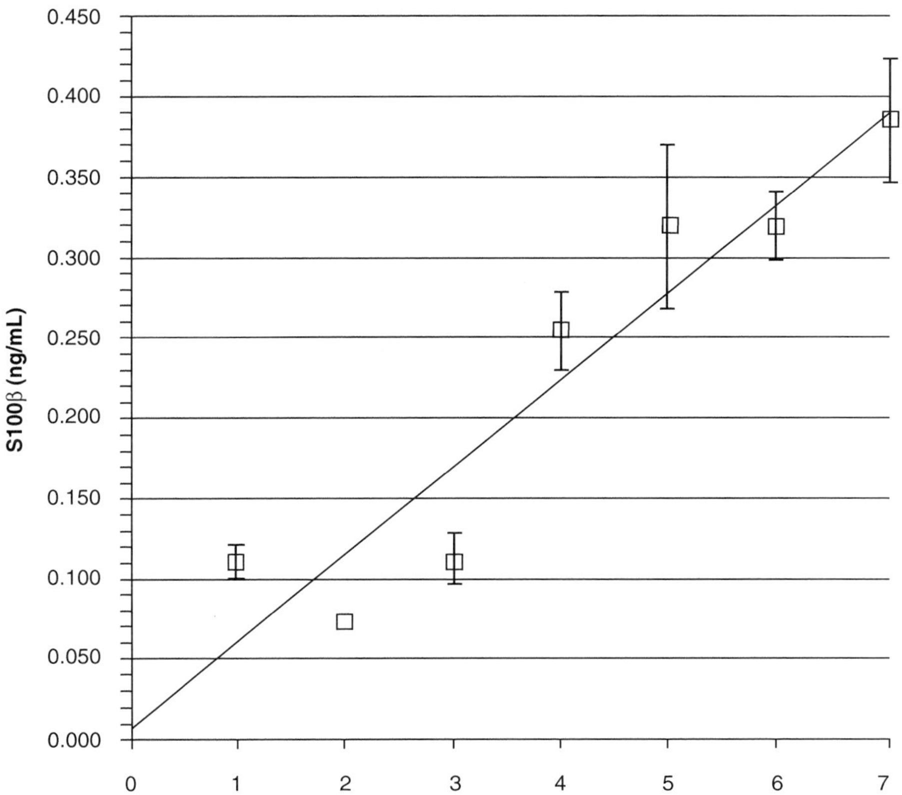

Fig. 1.1 Correlation between S100B and suicidality. Measures of S100B in a group of 64 patients with psychosis and mood disorders reveal a strong correlation between S100B levels and suicidality. Bivariate fit analysis of BPRS-C suicidal assessment (BPRS suicidality sub-score) and S100B yielded a positive correlation with a corresponding $p < 0.01$ and R^2 correlation value of 0.273. Patients with low suicidality risk are identified as having a BPRS suicidality index of 1–4; high suicidality risk has an index of 5–7. Patient groupings are displayed as a boxplot (Fig. 1.1) [79]

neurogenesis. Some suggest that suicidal behavior may be related with alterations in neural plasticity. There is evidence from postmortem studies reporting a decrease in the number of glial cells and glial density in the frontal cortex and hippocampus [88, 89]. Five studies have reported alteration in the BDNF levels of suicidal patients [79, 80, 96, 106, 107, 112, 113]. Evidence from translational studies showed that the mRNA expression of BDNF was decreased in the prefrontal cortex and hippocampus of suicide victims [94]. Independent of the diagnosis, the levels of BDNF were lower in patients who died after a suicide attempt.

Vascular Endothelial Growth Factor (VEGF)

VEGF is an angiogenic protein with an important role in neuroprotection and neurogenesis. Viikki et al. reported that patients with a VEGF polymorphism were resistant to depression treatment [114]. Two studies noted a negative correlation of VEGF plasma levels proportionate to depression severity [98, 115]. VEGF is described to be low in the plasma of suicide attempters. Additionally, VEGF is a key factor in the integrity of the BBB, and studies have reported alteration in the permeability of the BBB in patients with suicidal behavior and ideation [116].

Orexin

One of the hypothalamic neuropeptide that modulates the HPA axis, Orexin, has been linked to the regulation of sleep. Two studies have reported decreased CSF levels of Orexin in patients who attempted suicide. After patients received treatment (6 and 12 months), levels of orexin increased [97, 117].

Autoimmunity and Suicide

Several diseases that increase the body's immune response against several organs have increased risk of suicide. In multiple sclerosis the risk of suicidal ideation is up to 40%. In celiac disease there is an increased risk for mood disorders and suicide. Patients with diabetes have a 25% increase for mood disorders. Patients with epilepsy have a lifetime risk of up to 25% for suicide, and in some of the epilepsy classifications, there is clear evidence of inflammation and alteration of the BBB [118]. Steroids are commonly used to decrease the exacerbation of symptoms in several of these illnesses. Individuals suffering from lupus have a heightened risk for suicide [119].

Infections: *Toxoplasma gondii*

There are several population studies examining the association between suicidal ideation and attempts in patients who are seropositive for *Toxoplasma gondii* (30% of the population) [120–122]. Others have evaluated the antibodies for *Toxoplasma gondii* in a group of patients after a suicide attempt and compared it to a control group; the OR was 7.1 [123]. In a study of 45,000 Danish mothers, the seropositivity for *Toxoplasma gondii* increased the relative risk of suicide to 2.1 and 1.8 for violent suicides [124].

Conclusion

As shown by the studies discussed here, there is supporting evidence for a role of several neurobiological systems in the pathophysiology of suicide. The serotonin system, the dopaminergic system, and some of the neurotrophins such as BDNF are also deregulated in patients at risk for suicide. Inflammatory changes are also described as one of the issues that could be playing a role in the pathophysiology of suicide. The degree of inflammation could be related to the severity of psychiatric symptoms. In that case, those patients at higher risk of suicide could have higher levels of cytokines and other inflammatory markers. Though studies have found some patterns of inflammation, still more specific biomarkers to identify patients at higher suicide risk are lacking. It is important to integrate these findings with other neurobiological findings. Current findings about the neurobiology of the mind support a determinist and physicalist model of the mind challenging prior conceptions about free will and suicide. There are important advances in the last 50 years of the neurobiology of suicide, yet there are a lot of questions still with no answer that perhaps will continue to be explored in the years to come.

References

1. World Health Organization. Preventing suicide: a global imperative. 2014. http://apps.who.int/iris/bitstream/10665/131056/1/9789241564779_eng.pdf.
2. Nock MK, Green JG, Hwang I, McLaughlin KA, Sampson NA, Zaslavsky AM, et al. Prevalence, correlates, and treatment of lifetime suicidal behavior among adolescents: results from the National Comorbidity Survey Replication Adolescent Supplement. JAMA Psychiat. 2013;70(3):300–10. https://doi.org/10.1001/2013.jamapsychiatry.55.
3. Centers for Disease Control and Prevention. Web-based injury statistics query and reporting system (WISQARS). http://www.cdc.gov/ncipc/wisqars/.
4. Kessler RC, Borges G, Walters EE. Prevalence of and risk factors for lifetime suicide attempts in the National Comorbidity Survey. Arch Gen Psychiatry. 1999;56(7):617–26. https://doi.org/10.1001/archpsyc.56.7.617.
5. Larkin GL, Beautrais AL. A preliminary naturalistic study of low-dose ketamine for depression and suicide ideation in the emergency department. Int J Neuropsychopharmacol. 2011;14(8):1127–31. https://doi.org/10.1017/S1461145711000629.
6. Busch KA, Fawcett J, Jacobs DG. Clinical correlates of inpatient suicide. J Clin Psychiatry. 2003;64(1):14–9.
7. Maris RW. Suicide. Lancet. 2002;360:319–26.
8. Glenn CR, Nock MK. Improving the short-term prediction of suicidal behavior. Am J Prev Med. 2014;47:S176–80.
9. Borges G, Nock MK, Haro Abad JM, Hwang I, Sampson NA, Alonso J, et al. Twelve-month prevalence of and risk factors for suicide attempts in the World Health Organization World Mental Health surveys. J Clin Psychiatry. 2010;71(12):1617–28.

10. Tran T, Luo W, Phung D, Harvey R, Berk M, Kennedy RL, et al. Risk stratification using data from electronic medical records better predicts suicide risks than clinician assessments. BMC Psychiatry. 2014;14(1):76.
11. Wichers M, Maes M. The psychoneuroimmuno-pathophysiology of cytokine-induced depression in humans. Int J Neuropsychopharmcol. 2002;5(4):375–88.
12. Caplan R, Siddarth P, Gurbani S, Hanson R, Sankar R, Shields WD. Depression and anxiety disorders in pediatric epilepsy. Epilepsia. 2005;46(5):720–30.
13. Pompili M, Girardi P, Ruberto A, Tatarelli R. Suicide in the epilepsies: a meta-analytic investigation of 29 cohorts. Epilepsy Behav. 2005;7(2):305–10.
14. Ackerman JP, McBee-Strayer SM, Mendoza K, Stevens J, Sheftall AH, Campo JV, et al. Risk-sensitive decision-making deficit in adolescent suicide attempters. J Child Adolesc Psychopharmacol. 2015;25(2):109–13.
15. Ekinci O, Titus JB, Rodopman AA, Berkem M, Trevathan E. Depression and anxiety in children and adolescents with epilepsy: prevalence, risk factors, and treatment. Epilepsy Behav. 2009;14(1):8–18.
16. Asarnow JR, Porta G, Spirito A, Emslie G, Clarke G, Wagner KD, et al. Suicide attempts and nonsuicidal self-injury in the treatment of resistant depression in adolescents: findings from the TORDIA study. J Am Acad Child Adolesc Psychiatry. 2011;50(8):772–81.
17. Fawcett J, Scheftner WA, Fogg L, Clark DC, Young MA, Hedeker D, et al. Time-related predictors of suicide in major affective disorder. Am J Psychiatry. 1990;147(9):1189–94.
18. Miranda R, Shaffer D. Understanding the suicidal moment in adolescence. Ann N Y Acad Sci. 2013;1304:14–21.
19. Husky MM, Olfson M, He J, Nock MK, Swanson SA, Merikangas KR. Twelve-month suicidal symptoms and use of services among adolescents: results from the National Comorbidity Survey. Psych Serv. 2012;63(10):989–96.
20. Costanza A, D'Orta I, Perroud N, Burkhardt S, Malafosse A, Mangin P, et al. Neurobiology of suicide: do biomarkers exist? Int J Legal Med. 2014;128(1):73–82.
21. Oquendo MA, Sullivan GM, Sudol K, Baca-Garcia E, Stanley BH, Sublette ME, et al. Toward a biosignature for suicide. Am J Psychiatry. 2014;171(12):1259–77.
22. Asberg M, Traskman L, Thoren P. 5-HIAA in the cerebrospinal fluid: a biochemical suicide predictor? Arch Gen Psychiatry. 1976;33(10):1193–7.
23. Chatzittofis A, Nordstrom P, Hellstrom C, Arver S, Asberg M, Jokinen J. CSF 5-HIAA, cortisol and DHEAS levels in suicide attempters. Eur Neuropsychopharmacol. 2013;23(10):1280–7.
24. Courtet P, Picot MC, Bellivier F, Torres S, Jollant F, Michelon C, et al. Serotonin transporter gene may be involved in short-term risk of subsequent suicide attempts. Biol Psychiatry. 2014;55(1):46–51.
25. Bellivier F, Chaste P, Malafosse A. Association between the TPH gene A218C polymorphism and suicidal behavior: a meta-analysis. Am J Med Genet B Neuropsychiatr Genet. 2004;124B(1):87–91.
26. Li D, He L. Meta-analysis supports association between serotonin transporter (5-HTT) and suicidal behavior. Mol Psychiatry. 2007;12(1):47–54.
27. Price RB, Nock MK, Charney DS, Mathew SJ. Effects of intravenous ketamine on explicit and implicit measures of suicidality in treatment-resistant depression. Biol Psychiatry. 2009;66(5):522–6.
28. Diaz Granados N, Ibrahim LA, Brutsche NE, Ameli R, Henter ID, Luckenbaugh DA, et al. Rapid resolution of suicidal ideation after a single infusion of an N-methyl-D-aspartate antagonist in patients with treatment-resistant major depressive disorder. J Clin Psychiatry. 2010;71(12):1605–11.
29. Zarate CA Jr, Brutsche NE, Ibrahim L, Franco-Chaves J, Diazgranados N, Cravchik A, et al. Replication of ketamine's antidepressant efficacy in bipolar depression: a randomized controlled add-on trial. Biol Psychiatry. 2012;71(11):939–46.
30. McCrory E, De Brito SA, Viding E. Research review: the neurobiology and genetics of maltreatment and adversity. J Child Psychol Psychiatry. 2010;51(10):1079–95.

31. McGowan PO, Sasaki A, D'Alessio AC, Dymov S, Labonte B, Szyf M, et al. Epigenetic regulation of the glucocorticoid receptor in human brain associates with childhood abuse. Nat Neurosci. 2009;12(3):342–8.
32. Dwivedi Y. Brain-derived neurotrophic factor and suicide pathogenesis. Ann Med. 2010;42(2):87–96.
33. Deveci A, Aydemir O, Taskin O, Taneli F, Esen-Danaci A. Serum BDNF levels in suicide attempters related to psychosocial stressors: a comparative study with depression. Neuropsychobiology. 2007;56(2–3):93–7.
34. Nordström P, Samuelsson M, Åsberg M, Träskman-Bendz L, Åberg-Wistedt A, Nordin C, et al. CSF 5-HIAA predicts suicide risk after attempted suicide. Suicide Life Threat Behav. 1994;24(1):1–9.
35. Angst J, Degonda M, Ernst C. The Zurich Study: XV. Suicide attempts in a cohort from age 20 to 30. Eur Arch Psychiatry Clin Neurosci. 1992;242:135–41.
36. Samuelsson M, Jokinen J, Nordström AL, Nordström P. CSF 5-HIAA, suicide intent and hopelessness in the prediction of early suicide in male high-risk suicide attempters. Acta Psychiatr Scand. 2006;113(1):44–7.
37. Tyano S, Zalsman G, Ofek H, Blum I, Apter A, Wolovik L, Sher L, Sommerfeld E, Harell D, Weizman A. Plasma serotonin levels and suicidal behavior in adolescents. Eur Neuropsychopharmacol. 2006;16(1):49–57.
38. Mann JJ. A current perspective of suicide and attempted suicide. Ann Intern Med. 2002;136:302–11.
39. Bondy B, Buettner A, Zill P. Genetics of suicide. Mol Psychiatry. 2006;11:336–51.
40. Stanley M, Mann JJ. Increased serotonin-2 binding sites in frontal cortex of suicide victims. Lancet. 1983;1:214–6.
41. Mann JJ, Huang YY, Underwood MD, Kassir SA, Oppenheim S, Kelly TM, et al. A serotonin transporter gene promoter polymorphism (5-HTTLPR) and prefrontal cortical binding in major depression and suicide. Arch Gen Psychiatry. 2000;57:729–38.
42. Malone KM, Corbitt EM, Li S, Mann JJ. Prolactin response to fenfluramine and suicide attempt lethality in major depression. Br J Psychiatry. 1996;168:324–9.
43. Mann JJ. The neurobiology of suicide. Nat Med. 1988;4:25–30.
44. Van Heeringen K. The neurobiology of suicide and suicidality. Can J Psychiatr. 2003;48:292–300.
45. Mann JJ, Malone KM, Sweeney JA, Brown RP, Linnoila M, Stanley B, et al. Attempted suicide characteristics and cerebrospinal fluid amine metabolites in depressed inpatients. Neuropsychopharmacology. 1996;15(6):576–86.
46. Coccaro EF, Berman ME, Kavoussi RJ, Hauger RL. Relationship of prolactin response to d-fenfluramine to behavioral and questionnaire assessments of aggression in personality-disordered men. Biol Psychiatry. 1996;40:157–64.
47. O'Keane V, Dinan TG. Prolactin and cortisol responses to d-fenfluramine in major depression: evidence for diminished responsivity of central serotonergic function. Am J Psychiatry. 1991;148:1009–15.
48. Escribá PV, Ozaita A, García-Sevilla JA. Increased mRNA expression of [alpha] 2A-Adrenoceptors, serotonin receptors and [mu]-opioid receptors in the brains of suicide victims. Neuropsychopharmacology. 2004;29(8):1512.
49. Ordway GA, Widdowson PS, Smith KS, Halaris A. Agonist binding to α2-Adrenoceptors is elevated in the Locus Coeruleus from victims of suicide. J Neurochemistry. 1994;63(2):617–24.
50. Joiner TE Jr, Brown JS, Wingate LR. The psychology and neurobiology of suicidal behavior. Annu Rev Psychol. 2005;56:287–314.
51. Placidi GP, Oquendo MA, Malone KM, Huang YY, Ellis SP, Mann JJ. Aggressivity, suicide attempts, and depression: relationship to cerebrospinal fluid monoamine metabolite levels. Biol Psychiatry. 2001;50(10):783–91.
52. Arango V, Underwood MD, Mann JJ. Fewer pigmented locus coeruleus neurons in suicide victims: preliminary results. Biol Psychiatry. 1996;39:112–20.

53. Mann JJ, Arango V. The neurobiology of suicidal behavior. In: Jacobs DG, editor. The Harvard Medical School guide to suicide assessment and intervention. San Francisco: Jossey-Bass; 1999.
54. Mann JJ. Neurobiology of suicidal behavior. Nature. Rev Neurosci. 2003;4:819–28.
55. Valdizán EM, Díez-Alarcia R, González-Maeso J, Pilar-Cuéllar F, García-Sevilla JA, Meana JJ, et al. α2-adrenoceptor functionality in postmortem frontal cortex of depressed suicide victims. Biol Psychiatry. 2010;68:869–72.
56. Arranz B, Blennow K, Eriksson A, Maånsson JE, Marcusson J. Serotonergic, noradrenergic, and dopaminergic measures in suicide brains. Biol Psychiatry. 1997;41(10):1000–9.
57. Allard P, Norlén M. Caudate nucleus dopamine D2 receptors in depressed suicide victims. Neuropsychobiology. 2001;44(2):70–3.
58. Ernst C, Mechawar N, Turecki G. Suicide neurobiology. Prog Neurobiol. 2009;89:315–33.
59. Gonzalez-Maeso J, Rodriguez-Puertas R, Meana JJ, Garcia-Sevilla JA, Guimon J. Neurotransmitter receptor-mediated activation of G-proteins in brains of suicide victims with mood disorders: selective supersensitivity of [alpha] 2A-adrenoceptors. Mol Psychiatry. 2002;7(7):755–67.
60. Wong ML, Dong C, MaestreMesa J, Licinio J. Polymorphisms in inflammation-related genes are associated with susceptibility to major depression and antidepressant response. Mol Psychiatry. 2008;13:800–12.
61. Roth TL, Lubin FD, Funk AJ, Sweatt JD. Lasting epigenetic influence of early-life adversity on the BDNF gene. Biol Psychiatry. 2009;65(9):760.
62. Pittenger C, Duman RS. Stress, depression, and neuroplasticity: a convergence of mechanisms. Neuropsychopharmacology. 2008;33:88–109.
63. Huang EJ, Reichardt LF. Neurotrophins: roles in neuronal development and function. Annu Rev Neurosci. 2001;24:677–736.
64. Altar CA, Cai N, Bliven T, Juhasz M, Conner JM, Acheson AL, et al. Anterograde transport of brain-derived neurotrophic factor and its role in the brain. Nature. 1997;389:856–60.
65. Bartrup JT, Moorman JM, Newberry NR. BDNF enhances neuronal growth and synaptic activity in hippocampal cell cultures. Neuroreport. 1997;8:3791–4.
66. Thoenen H. Neurotrophins and neuronal plasticity. Science. 1995;270:593–8.
67. Turecki G, Ernst C, Jollant F, Labonté B, Mechawar N. The neurodevelopmental origins of suicidal behavior. Trends Neurosci. 2012;35:14–23.
68. Nibuya M, Morinobu S, Duman RS. Regulation of BDNF and trkB mRNA in rat brain by chronic electroconvulsive seizure and antidepressant drug treatments. J Neurosci. 1995;15:7539–47.
69. Nibuya M, Nestler EJ, Duman RS. Chronic anti-depressant administration increases the expression of cAMP response element-binding protein (CREB) in rat hippocampus. J Neurosci. 1996;16:2365–72.
70. Chen B, Dowlatshahi D, MacQueen GM, Wang JF, Young LT. Increased hippocampal BDNF immunoreactivity in subjects treated with antidepressant medication. Biol Psychiatry. 2001;50:260–5.
71. Dwivedi Y, Rizavi HS, Conley RR, Roberts RC, Tamminga CA, Pandey GN. Altered gene expression of brain-derived neurotrophic factor and receptor tyrosine kinase B in postmortem brain of suicide subjects. Arch Gen Psychiatry. 2003;60(8):804–15. https://doi.org/10.1001/archpsyc.60.8.804.
72. Dwivedi Y, Mondal AC, Rizavi HS, Conley RR. Suicide brain is associated with decreased expression of neurotrophins. Biol Psychiatry. 2005;58:315–24.
73. Pandey GN, Ren X, Rizavi HS, Conley RR, Roberts RC, Dwivedi Y. Brain-derived neurotrophic factor and tyrosine kinase B receptor signaling in postmortem brain of teenage suicide victims. Int J Neuropsychopharmacol. 2008;11:1047–61.
74. Pandey GN. Biological basis of suicide and suicidal behavior. Bipolar Disord. 2013;15:524–41.
75. Serafini G, Pompili M, Elena Seretti M, Stefani H, Palermo M, Coryell W, et al. The role of inflammatory cytokines in suicidal behavior: a systematic review. Eur Neuropsychopharmacol. 2013;23(12):1672–86.

76. Janelidze S, Brundin L. Inflammation in suicidality: implications for novel treatment options. Mod Trends Pharmacopsychiatri. 2013;28:188–202.
77. Capuron L, Miller A, Irwin MR. Psychoneuroimmunology of depressive disorder: mechanisms and clinical implications. Psychoneuro. 2007;1:509–30.
78. Zorrilla EP, Luborsky L, McKay JR, Rosenthal R, Houldin A, Tax A, et al. The relationship of depression and stressors to immunological assays: a meta-analytic review. Brain Behav Immun. 2001;15(3):199–226. https://doi.org/10.1006/brbi.2000.0597.
79. Falcone T, Fazio V, Lee C, Simon B, Franco K, Marchi N, et al. Serum S100B: a potential biomarker for suicidality in adolescents? PLoS One. 2010;5(6):e11089. https://doi.org/10.1371/journal.pone.0011089.
80. Janelidze S, Mattei D, Westrin A, Traskman-Bendz L, Brundin L. Cytokine levels in the blood may distinguish suicide attempters from depressed patients. Brain Behav Immun. 2011;25(2):335–9. https://doi.org/10.1016/j.bbi.2010.10.010.
81. Slopen N, Koenen KC, Kubzansky LD. Childhood adversity and immune and inflammatory biomarkers associated with cardiovascular risk in youth: a systematic review. Brain Behav Immun. 2012;26(2):239–50.
82. Segerstrom SC, Miller GE. Psychological stress and the human immune system: a meta-analytic study of 30 years of inquiry. Psychol Bull. 2004;130(4):601–30. https://doi.org/10.1037/0033-2909.130.4.601.
83. Singareddy R, Krishnamurthy VB, Vgontzas AN, Fernandez-Mendoza J, Calhoun SL, Shaffer ML, et al. Subjective and objective sleep and self-harm behaviors in young children: a general population study. Psychiatry Res. 2013;209(3):549–53.
84. Bremner JD. Does stress damage the brain? Biol Psychiatry. 1999;45(7):797–805.
85. Lucas M, O'Reilly EJ, Mirzaei F, Okereke OI, Unger L, Miller M, et al. Cigarette smoking and completed suicide: results from 3 prospective cohorts of American adults. J Affect Disord. 2013;151(3):1053–8. https://doi.org/10.1016/j.jad.2013.08.033.
86. Young SN. Elevated incidence of suicide in people living at altitude, smokers and patients with chronic obstructive pulmonary disease and asthma: possible role of hypoxia causing decreased serotonin synthesis. J Psychiatry Neurosci. 2013;38(5):130002. https://doi.org/10.1503/jpn.130002.
87. Janigro D. Are you in or out? Leukocyte, ion, and neurotransmitter permeability across the epileptic blood-brain barrier. Epilepsia. 2012;53(Suppl 1):26–34.
88. Janigro D. Blood-brain barrier, ion homeostasis and epilepsy: possible implications towards the understanding of ketogenic diet mechanisms. Epilepsy Res. 1999;37(3):223–32.
89. Oby E, Janigro D. The blood-brain barrier and epilepsy. Epilepsia. 2006;47(11):1761–74. https://doi.org/10.1111/j.1528-1167.2006.00817.x.
90. Serafini G, Girardi P, Erbuto D, Lester D, Pompili M. HPA axis and prolactin abnormalities in suicidal behavior. In: Pompili M, editor. Suicide: a global perspective; 2013. p. 246–53.
91. Motivala SJ, Sarfatti A, Olmos L, Irwin MR. Inflammatory markers and sleep disturbance in major depression. Psychosom Med. 2005;67(2):187–94. https://doi.org/10.1097/01.psy.0000149259.72488.09.
92. Rothermundt M, Arolt V, Peters M, Gutbrodt H, Fenker J, Kersting A, et al. Inflammatory markers in major depression and melancholia. J Affect Disord. 2001;63(1–3):93–102.
93. Steiner J, Bielau H, Brisch R, Danos P, Ullrich O, Mawrin C, et al. Immunological aspects in the neurobiology of suicide: elevated microglial density in schizophrenia and depression is associated with suicide. J Psychiatr Res. 2008;42(2):151–7. https://doi.org/10.1016/j.jpsychires.2006.10.013.
94. Steiner J, Gos T, Bogerts B, Bielau H, Drexhage HA, Bernstein HG. Possible impact of microglial cells and the monocyte-macrophage system on suicidal behavior. CNS Neurol Disord Drug Targets. 2013;12(7):971–9.
95. Pandey GN, Dwivedi Y. Neurobiology of teenage suicide. In: Dwivedi Y, editor. The neurobiological basis of suicide. Boca Raton: Taylor & Francis; 2012.
96. Pandey GN, Rizavi HS, Ren X, Fareed J, Hoppensteadt DA, Roberts RC, et al. Proinflammatory cytokines in the prefrontal cortex of teenage suicide victims. J Psychiatr Res. 2012;46(1):57–63. https://doi.org/10.1016/j.jpsychires.2011.08.006.

97. Kim YK, Lee HP, Won SD, Park EY, Lee HY, Lee BH, et al. Low plasma BDNF is associated with suicidal behavior in major depression. Prog Neuro-Psychopharmacol Biol Psychiatry. 2007;31(1):78–85.
98. Isung J, Mobarrez F, Nordstrom P, Asberg M, Jokinen J. Low plasma vascular endothelial growth factor (VEGF) associated with completed suicide. World J Biol Psychiatry. 2012;13(6):468–73.
99. Rothermundt M, Arolt V. Schizophrenia and immunity. In: Ader R, editor. Psychoneuroimmunology. 4th ed. Boston: Elsevier; 2007. p. 563–77.
100. Kubera M, Symbirtsev A, Basta-Kaim A, Borycz J, Roman A, Papp M, et al. Effect of chronic treatment with imipramine on interleukin 1 and interleukin 2 production by splenocytes obtained from rats subjected to a chronic mild stress model of depression. Pol J Pharmacol. 1996;48(5):503–6.
101. Himmerich H, Fulda S, Sheldrick A, Plumakers B, Rink L. IFN gamma reduction by tricyclic antidepressants. Int J Psychiatry Med. 2011;40(4): 413–24. https://doi.org/10.2190/PM.40.4e.
102. Hughes MM, Carballedo A, McLoughlin DM, Amico F, Harkin A, Frodl T, et al. Tryptophan depletion in depressed patients occurs independent of kynurenine pathway activation. Brain Behav Immun. 2012;26(6):979–87. https://doi.org/10.1016/j.bbi.2012.05.010.
103. Mitchell RH, Goldstein BI. Inflammation in children and adolescents with neuropsychiatric disorders: a systematic review. J Am Acad Child Adolesc Psychiatry. 2014;53(3):274–96.
104. Claes S, Myint AM, Domschke K, Del-Favero J, Entrich K, Engelborghs S, et al. The kynurenine pathway in major depression: haplotype analysis of three related functional candidate genes. Psychiatry Res. 2011;188(3):355–60.
105. Miura H, Ozaki N, Sawada M, Isobe K, Ohta T, Nagatsu T. A link between stress and depression: shifts in the balance between the kynurenine and serotonin pathways of tryptophan metabolism and the etiology and pathophysiology of depression. Stress. 2008;11(3):198–209.
106. Sublette ME, Galfalvy HC, Fuchs D, Lapidus M, Grunebaum MF, Oquendo MA, et al. Plasma kynurenine levels are elevated in suicide attempters with major depressive disorder. Brain Behav Immun. 2011;25(6):1272–8. https://doi.org/10.1016/j.bbi.2011.05.002.
107. Erhardt S, Lim CK, Linderholm KR, Janelidze S, Lindqvist D, Samuelsson M, et al. Connecting inflammation with glutamate agonism in suicidality. Neuropsychopharmacology. 2013;38(5):743–52. https://doi.org/10.1038/npp.2012.248.
108. Arolt V, Peters M, Erfurth A, Wiesmann M, Missler U, Rudolf S, et al. S100B and response to treatment in major depression: a pilot study. Eur Neuropsychopharmacol. 2003;13(4):235–9.
109. Andreazza AC, Cassini C, Rosa AR, Leite MC, de Almeida LM, Nardin P, et al. Serum S100B and antioxidant enzymes in bipolar patients. J Psychiatr Res. 2007;41(6):523–9. https://doi.org/10.1016/j.jpsychires.2006.07.013.
110. Marchi N, Cavaglia M, Fazio V, Bhudia S, Hallene K, Janigro D. Peripheral markers of blood-brain barrier damage. Clin Chim Acta. 2004;342(1–2):1–12. https://doi.org/10.1016/j.cccn.2003.12.008.
111. Bruce N, Janigro D, Fazio V, Franco K, Falcone T. S100B as a tool for risk assessment in suicidal youth. Proceedings of the American Academy of Child & Adolescent Psychiatry 57th Annual Meeting; 2010; New York.
112. Li Z, Qi D, Chen J, Zhang C, Yi Z, Yuan C, et al. Venlafaxine inhibits the upregulation of plasma tumor necrosis factor-alpha (TNF-alpha) in the Chinese patients with major depressive disorder: a prospective longitudinal study. Psychoneuroendocrinology. 2013;38(1):107–14.
113. Boehm J, Fischer K, Bohnert M. Putative role of TNF-alpha, interleukin-8 and ICAM-1 as indicators of an early inflammatory reaction after burn: a morphological and immunohistochemical study of lung tissue of fire victims. J Clin Pathol. 2010;63(11):967–71. https://doi.org/10.1136/jcp.2010.079863.
114. Viikki M, Anttila S, Kampman O, Illi A, Huuhka M, Setala-Soikkeli E, et al. Vascular endothelial growth factor (VEGF) polymorphism is associated with treatment resistant depression. Neurosci Lett. 2010;477(3):105–8. https://doi.org/10.1016/j.neulet.2010.04.039.

115. Isung J, Aeinehband S, Mobarrez F, Martensson B, Nordstrom P, Asberg M, et al. Low vascular endothelial growth factor and interleukin-8 in cerebrospinal fluid of suicide attempters. Transl Psychiatry. 2012;2:e196. https://doi.org/10.1038/tp.2012.123.
116. Serafini G, Pompili M, Lindqvist D, Dwivedi Y, Girardi P. The role of neuropeptides in suicidal behavior: a systematic review. Biomed Res Int. 2013;2013:687575. https://doi.org/10.1155/2013/687575.
117. Karege F, Vaudan G, Schwald M, Perroud N, La Harpe R. Neurotrophin levels in postmortem brains of suicide victims and the effects of antemortem diagnosis and psychotropic drugs. Brain Res Mol Brain Res. 2005;136(1–2):29–37. https://doi.org/10.1016/j.molbrainres.2004.12.020.
118. Marchi N, Granata T, Ghosh C, Janigro D. Blood–brain barrier dysfunction and epilepsy: pathophysiologic role and therapeutic approaches. Epilepsia. 2012;53(11):1877–86.
119. Karassa FB, Magliano M, Isenberg DA. Suicide attempts in patients with systemic lupus erythematosus. Ann Rheum Dis. 2003;62(1):58–60.
120. Arling TA, Yolken RH, Lapidus M, Langenberg P, Dickerson FB, Zimmerman SA, et al. Toxoplasma gondii antibody titers and history of suicide attempts in patients with recurrent mood disorders. J Nerv Ment Dis. 2009;3(12):905–8.
121. Okusaga O, Langenberg P, Sleemi A, Vaswani D, Giegling I, Hartmann AM, et al. Toxoplasma gondii antibody titers and history of suicide attempts in patients with schizophrenia. Schizophrenia Res. 2011;133(1):150–5.
122. Zhang Y, Träskman-Bendz L, Janelidze S, Langenberg P, Saleh A, Constantine N, et al. Toxoplasma gondii immunoglobulin G antibodies and nonfatal suicidal self-directed violence. J Clin Psychiatry. 2012;73(8):1069–76.
123. Brundin L, Erhardt S, Bryleva EY, Achtyes ED, Postolache TT. The role of inflammation in suicidal behaviour. Acta Psychiatrica. Scandinavica. 2015;132(3):192–203.
124. Cook AJ, Holliman R, Gilbert RE, Buffolano W, Zufferey J, Petersen E, et al. Sources of toxoplasma infection in pregnant women: European multicentre case-control study. BMJ. 2000;321(7254):142–7.

Mood Disorders and Suicide

2

Mariela Herrera

Introduction

Mood disorders are common among the general population. Up to 15% of the population will suffer from at least one mood disorder episode during their lifetime [1]. The Diagnostic and Statistical Manual version 5 (DSM-5) divides mood disorders in two different chapters, bipolar disorders and depressive disorders. Included in bipolar disorders are bipolar disorder type 1 and bipolar disorder type 2 and cyclothymic disorders, along with bipolar disorders due to a medical condition or substance related, and the other specified and unspecified bipolar disorder categories. As for depressive disorders, included in the DSM-5 [2] chapter are disrupted mood dysregulation disorder (DMDD), major depressive disorder (MDD), and persistent depressive disorder (PDD), along with PMDD, depressive disorders due to a medical condition or substance related, and the other specified and unspecified depressive disorder categories [3]. The 12-month and lifetime prevalence rates of MDD are 6–12%, respectively. About 90% of people who commit suicide have suffered from one or more than one mental disorder at the time of death, and between one-half and two-thirds of completed suicides occur in patients who carry a mood disorder diagnosis [4, 5]. Lifetime risk of completed suicide in patients with mood disorders is estimated to be between 5 and 6% [4]. It is important to understand the factors associated with increased risk of suicide in patients with mood disorder. The impact of suicide reaches not only the patient, but also the family of the patient and the treating providers, his community, and the society in general. This chapter presents a review of available literature to date in mood disorders and suicide, with

M. Herrera, M.D.
Billings Clinic, Billings, MT, USA
e-mail: mherrera@billingsclinic.org

T. Falcone, J. Timmons-Mitchell (eds.), *Suicide Prevention*,
https://doi.org/10.1007/978-3-319-74391-2_2

emphasis on bipolar disorders and MDD, for which more evidence-based literature is available related to suicide. It will focus on epidemiology, predominant etiological theories, risk factors and risk assessment as well as management strategies for prevention and treatment.

Epidemiology

Mood disorders are a known risk factor for suicide. In the general population, the ratio of suicide attempts to completed suicides is reported to be 30–50. For patients with mood disorder, this ratio decreases to only 5–10, showing an effect of the illness on lethality of attempts. Also, the rate of suicidal ideation to suicide attempts in the general population is at least 6 and probably higher, while among patients with mood disorder it is approximately 3. Finally, the ratio of suicidal ideation to completed suicide in the general population is about 240 while in patients with mood disorder it is about 20–25 [6].

Suicide attempts in bipolar disorders are reported to occur in 25–50% of the patients, while the percentage of patients with bipolar disorder committing suicide is estimated to be between 8 and 19% [7]. The suicide rate in bipolar disorder is 20–30 times that of the general population [8]. Suicide is the leading cause of avoidable fatalities in bipolar disorder [7].

A meta-review studying suicide risk in mental disorders found the estimated suicide risk for patient with bipolar disorder to be 17.1 (95% CI 9.8–29.5), while for depression it was 19.7 (95% CI 12.2–32.0). This was only surpassed by borderline personality disorder, which had a suicide risk estimate of 45.1 (95% CI 29.0–61.3) [4]. The risk of suicidal behavior among patients with bipolar disorder and depression is unlikely to be higher in any other psychiatric disorder [6] excluding personality disorders.

Compared to people who attempt suicide, people who complete suicide are much more often males [9, 10], used more lethal methods than overdoses, are somewhat older, and suffered from more severe psychopathology [4]. In addition, about 50% died in their first lifetime attempt [4, 7]. The percentage of individuals who attempted suicide and eventually died by suicide is up to 20% [4].

Etiological Theories

The etiology of suicide as a continuum ranging from ideation to attempted and completed suicide is complex and involves a combination of genetic, environmental, and psychological factors [1, 11]. The stress-diathesis model states that both an acutely stressful situation and a susceptibility to suicide are present for suicidal behavior to happen [12, 13].

Biological Factors

- Neurotransmitter dysregulation
  - Dysregulation in serotonin neurotransmission has been related to impulsive-aggressive behavior [1, 8] which is a known risk factor for suicide. The serotoninergic system is implicated in affective regulation, specifically the 5-HT1B receptors [8].
  - Noradrenergic dysfunction [1]
    Basal levels of monoamine metabolites have been found to be much lower in the cerebrospinal fluid of patients with unipolar depression and/or those with aggressive behavior or history of suicide attempts [14].
  - Based on recent findings evidencing the anti-suicidal effect of ketamine, the role of the glutamatergic pathways in suicide has been studied, suggesting a link between suicide and a hyper-glutamatergic state [15].
- The heritability of completed suicide is about 40% [1] but the precise genetic disposition is not fully understood yet [1]. Many factors may modify neurobiological pathways and influence the expression of genetic background [16].
- Genetic polymorphisms: The role of single polymorphism on the risk of suicidal behavior is probably very small and the impact of nongenetic factors is larger but it has been an area of research to determine which genetic factors are involved in the risk for suicide attempts [16]. There is evidence for the role of multiple loci in the genetic transmission of suicide risk [17].
  - The catechol-O-methyltransferase (COMT) gene in chromosome 22 synthesizes the COMT enzyme, which is responsible for the degradation of catecholamines. Polymorphisms in this gene result in a high or low functional activity of the enzyme and have been inconsistently associated with suicidal behavior. It might be that its association is rather indirect by increasing family types associated with suicidal behaviors such as anger, aggressive and violent temperamental traits, reward dependence, and novel to seeking/extraversion [1].
  - The brain-derived neurotrophic factor (BDNF) gene in chromosome 11 codes for a protein involved in neuronal development and synaptic plasticity. Polymorphisms in the BDNF gene have been implicated in suicidal behavior in some studies [1].
  - The mitogen-activated protein kinase 1 (MAPK1) gene in chromosome 22 codes for an enzyme involved in neuronal proliferation and differentiation and synaptic plasticity. It also plays an important function in inflammatory processes through the activation of nitric oxide and probably inflammatory cytokines. Dysregulation in the signaling pathway is involved in mood disorders and suicidal behavior. This seems to be mediated by decreased levels of extracellular signal-regulated kinase (ERK1/2) phosphorylation and/or synthesis resulting in a downregulation of the signaling cascade which affects the function within the prefrontal cortex and hippocampal regions [1].

  - The cyclic adenosine monophosphate response element-binding protein-1 (CREB1) gene in chromosome 2 encodes at prescription factor member of DNA-binding proteins, a downstream target of MAPK1 pathway. CREB-related genes may play an important role in suicide [1].
  - Single-nucleotide polymorphisms (SNPs) in the 5-hydroxytryptamine receptor (HTR) 1A gene expression have been associated with a predisposition to depression and/or suicide. The effect might be mediated by lower levels of HTR1B mRNA which is related to increased anger, hostility, and aggression, characteristics that have been associated with suicidal ideation. In particular, the rs1923885 was associated with suicidal attempts among MDD in a study involving 789 participants [14].
  - A polymorphism in the HTR2A gene was found to be associated with suicidal ideation and attempts in individuals with MDD [14].
  - Variants of the glycogen synthase kinase 3 (GSK3) ß isoenzyme gene could be associated with more impulsive behaviors among patients with bipolar disorder [8].
  - Polymorphisms in the serotonin transporter gene 5-HTTLPR have been associated with impulsiveness and suicidal behaviors [8].
  - A study of 10 "strong candidate genes" and 35 SNPs in patients with affective disorders confirmed the role of tryptophan hydroxylase (TPH) 1, TPH2, 5HTR2A, corticotropin-releasing hormone receptor (CRHR) 1, and acid phosphatase (ACP) 1 variants in the risk of suicidal behavior [16].
- Neuroanatomical correlates
  - A reduced activity in lateral prefrontal networks, as seen in depression, may contribute to a sense of hopelessness as these networks are involved in how the future is appraised. Hopeless is considered a risk factor for suicidal behavior [18]. Reduced gray matter volumes in the dorsal lateral prefrontal cortex or orbitofrontal cortex have been suggested as biological correlates of dysfunctional decision-making ability in patients with bipolar depression and a history of suicidal attempts [17].
  - Abnormalities in neural networks associated with suicide risk such as reduced orbitofrontal and ventral prefrontal cortex activity are found in patients with bipolar disorder [17].
  - Dysfunctions in frontolimbic neural network in bipolar disorder may lead to negative thoughts and feelings [18].
- Inflammatory theories
  - There is increasing evidence for the role of inflammatory abnormalities in the physiopathology of both suicidal behavior and mood disorders [8, 11]. Patients treated with cytokines were reported to be prone to experience suicidal ideation or to attempt suicide [19]. Also, research has found an increase in inflammatory markers in states associated with suicide such as aggression, impulsiveness, and depression [8] and in patients with history of suicidal ideation or suicide attempts [19].
  - A higher level of high-sensitivity C-reactive protein (CRP), a marker of low-grade systemic inflammation, was associated with a lifetime history of suicide

attempts but not with current suicidal ideation in a cross-sectional study including inpatients with depression, independently of the time between the last suicide attempt and CRP sampling [19]. The authors suggest that high level of CPR may be a trait marker of suicide attempt and not only related to the stress induced by performing a suicidal act [19].
  - Vitamin D has immune-modulating properties. A study compared vitamin D levels among patients who had attempted suicide with a variety of psychiatric disorders, non-suicidal depressed patients, and healthy controls and found vitamin D deficiency in 58% of who had attempted suicide. The mean levels of vitamin D were significantly lower in that group compared to the other two groups. In addition, there was a significantly negative association between blood levels of vitamin D and pro-inflammatory cytokines (interleukines 6 and 1ß) in the patients with psychiatric disorders, suggesting that vitamin D might be a contributing factor to the elevated pro-inflammatory cytokines reported in suicidal patients [11].
- Alterations in physiological response to stress.
  - Greater parasympathetic nerve system (PNS) reactivity in response to stress is considered a marker of the adaptive physiological stress response. Females who have attempted suicide compared to non-suicide attempters in one study showed a blunted PNS-mediated reactivity during stress, indicating a dysregulated stress response [20]. In this study, self-reported anger was greater in response to stress in suicide attempters but was similar at baseline assessment and at the post-task recovery assessment and it was inversely correlated with PNS-mediated reactivity during stress [20]. Their conclusion suggests that suicide attempt risk increases with more severe emotional reaction to stress and this is mediated by PNS-mediated emotion regulatory deficits and that PNS activity may therefore be a biomarker for suicide risk in patients with a mood disorder [20].
  - Abnormalities in the hypothalamic-pituitary-adrenal (HPA)-cortical axis stress response are also considered a risk factor for suicidal behavior [12, 13, 20]. The dysregulation in the HPA axis activity is usually measured by cortisol levels [12]. A meta-analysis of 27 studies found a significant association between cortisol and suicide attempts as a function of the patient's age. When the patient sample's mean age was below 40 years old, there was a positive association, such that higher levels of cortisol were associated with suicide attempts. When the mean age of the sample was 40 years old or above there was a negative association in which lower levels of cortisol were associated with suicide attempts [12]. Cortisol has been linked to impairments in cognitive control, decision-making, and emotional processing which are all associated to suicidal behavior [12]. The results of the study might be due to age-dependent exposure to stress over time affecting the ability to obtain an appropriate cortisol response when stressors happen [12]. Blunted cortisol reactivity to stress may represent a trait marker of suicide risk mediated by impairments in executive function increasing the vulnerability to suicide [13]. An additional study by the same authors confirmed that HPA axis activity was

markedly lower in patients who attempted suicide compared to patient with suicidal ideation, indicating a blunted cortisol responsiveness to stress as a factor associated with suicide attempt in adults [13].

- Sleep
  - Sleep disturbances are common among mood disorders and their presence predicts poor prognostic outcome for these disorders. Sleep disturbances may increase suicide risk, independent of affective episode or depressed mood [21]. Sleep complaints are considered one of the top ten warning signs of suicide based on the Substance Abuse and Mental Health Services Administration (SAMHSA) [21]. Domains of alertness including quality of sleep, amount of sleep, and presence of nightmares have been found as predictors of suicidal behaviors [22]. Insomnia may be more strongly linked to suicidal behavior than with suicidal ideation alone [23].
  - EEG sleep parameters have been proposed as a potential biomarker of suicide risk and treatment target [21]. Polysomnography sleep parameters associated with suicidal ideation among patients with MDD and bipolar disorder with treatment-resistant depression compared to participants who did not currently endorse suicidal ideation were less nonrapid eye movement (NREM) stage 4 sleep, independent of the severity of depression, and higher nocturnal wakefulness [21].

Psychological Factors

- Psychological autopsy studies of patients with mood disorders who died by suicide found an increased risk related to comorbidity, with especially strong association found for substance-use disorders (alcoholism, drug abuse, or polysubstance abuse) and cluster B or borderline personality disorders [4].
- Aggressive [4] and extremes of impulsive traits [4, 17] may predispose people to suicide, mostly in younger populations (less than 40 years) and males than in older people and females who died by suicide [4]. Hostility has also been linked to a risk for suicide attempts and death by suicide [17, 24]. Irritability traits have been associated with suicidal risk in patients with bipolar disorder [17].
- Concurrent physical illness can increase the risk for suicide in older people [4].
- Adverse life events, particularly losses and multiple stressors, appear common among suicide in patients with mood disorders [4].
- Hopelessness is a known psychological factor that increases the risk for suicide [4, 24]. In a cognitive model of suicidal acts, frequency, duration, and severity of suicide-related cognitions will determine the probability of the person engaging in a suicidal act. There is activation of a suicide schema which leads to hopelessness, paying more attention to suicide-relevant cues with an inability to disengage from them. All of these predispose to suicidal ideation. A suicidal act can strengthen suicide schemas [4].
- Anhedonia is one of the cardinal features of depression and has shown a strong association with suicidal ideation and death by suicide [24].

- Rumination about the past has also been associated with both suicidal ideation and attempts [24].
- Impaired reward processing of both positive and negative rewards has been strongly associated with suicidal behavior [24].
- Cognitive dysfunctions in attention, performance monitoring, goal selection, and working memory have associations with suicidal ideation and behavior [24]. Decision-making impairment is a cognitive trait associated with suicidal behavior and reported in patients with bipolar disorder, especially when they are suicidal [17]. Impaired decision-making processes might be linked to emotional dysfunction and constitute a neuropsychological risk factor for suicidal behaviors [8].

Social/Environmental Factors

- Worse family functioning [25] and family conflict [26] have been associated with suicide attempts in patients with bipolar disorder in different studies, including a small cross-sectional study comparing patients with bipolar disorder with and without history of suicide attempts [25]. The perceived level of family support is a characteristic of family relationships playing a role in suicidal ideation or behaviors [26]. The presence of a hostile and critical family atmosphere with highly expressed emotions can trigger an acute mood episode [26], which in turn is a high-risk state for suicide in patients with bipolar disorder.
- Social isolation has been implicated in the development of suicidal ideation [26].
- Stigmatization contributes to the development of suicidal ideation [26].
- Lack of social support, negative social experiences, not being understood or acknowledged, feeling like a burden, and reinforcing negative self-appraisals such as worthlessness were identified in a small qualitative study as social factors which triggered or worsened suicidal thoughts in patients with bipolar disorder [26].
- Social/environmental factors can also provide a protective effect against suicide when patients consider the impact of suicide on others and when they reflect on positive social experiences [26].
- Other social factors associated with suicidal behavior in patients with bipolar disorder include adversities during early life, such as childhood physical and sexual abuse, family history of suicidal behavior, a family history of mental health problems, problems with social relationships, and stressful life events such as divorcing [26].

Suicide models: Four main contemporary psychological models of suicidality specify a role for social factors in the development, maintenance, and intensification of suicidal thoughts and behaviors [26].

- The integrated motivational-volitional model of suicidal behavior: Feelings of entrapment where suicide is seen as the only solution for one's current circum-

stances determine the intention to end one's life and this intention is the proximal predictor of suicide behavior. Entrapment is triggered by defeat or humiliation appraisals. The transition from suicidal ideation to behavior is determined by pre-motivational factors (life events, personal vulnerability, environmental factors) and by specific moderators such a threat to self-moderators (social problem solving, coping), motivational moderators (burdensomeness, sense of not belonging), or volitional moderators (impulsivity, acquired capability for suicide, access to means) among others [26, 27].
- The cry of pain model: Perceptions of "no rescue" trigger and worsen suicidal ideation and behavior, with rescue factors including social support, a lack of which can lead to feelings of entrapment and suicidal ideation as a way to escape from negative life events [26].
- The interpersonal theory of suicide: A perceived low level of belongingness and of being a burden causes suicide ideation [26, 28], while the acquired capability for suicide determines whether the person with a desire to suicide has a potentially lethal attempt [28].
- The schematic appraisals model of suicide: Negative appraisals of social factors such as perceptions related to poor social support and social interactions are involved in pathways leading to the development of suicidality [26].

Risk Factors

Knowing the risk factors for suicide is important in order to establish rational prevention strategies. Since completed suicides occur in a rather low base rate [29] and it is an unpredictable and uncommon event [24], much of the research has focused on suicide ideation or suicide attempts [24, 29], with the latter being considered more closely related to completed suicides. Other proxy measures such as self-harm events or psychiatric hospitalization are also used as outcomes in suicide research [24]. Epidemiological studies suggest that there might be significantly different predictive risk factors for suicidal ideation, suicide attempts, and completed suicide [24]. Suicidal behavior is influenced by the interaction between risk and protective factors [29]. However, not all suicide risk or protective factors affect all aspects of suicidal ideation and behavior equally [24]. Central risk factors for suicide are a history of suicide attempt(s) and the presence of a mood disorder [29]. Suicidal behavior in patients with MDD of bipolar disorders tends to be state and severity dependent, being extremely rare during euthymic periods or during remission [30].

(a) Prior suicide attempt
   - This is considered one of the most robust predictors of completed suicide [31]. A study using a community sample to track mortality from 1490 patients seeking medical attention for an index self-harm or suicide attempt identified patients in the cohort who had died either due to the index suicide attempt or during a follow-up that ranged from 3 to 25 years. Five percent of

the patients died by suicide, 59% died during the index suicide attempt, and 41% died subsequently. Of those who died subsequently, 82% died within the next year [31].

(b) Family history of suicide and additional psychopathology indicate higher risks for suicide attempts and for completed suicide [10].

(c) Sociodemographic risk factors

- Adolescents and young adults, as well as females, make more frequent non-fatal suicide attempts [32].
- Advanced age and male gender are associated with completed suicide [32].
- Globally, people aged 70 years and older have the highest suicide rates [32].
- Being single or living alone are considered risks factors for completed suicide. The protective effect of marriage might be higher for men and lower among patients with psychiatric disorders. Also, impaired couple relationships, partner violence, complex attachment patterns, and separation can all increase the risk of suicidal behavior [32]. Divorce might increase the risk of suicide in males more than it does in females [32]. There also seems to be a protective effect of parenthood in females but not in males [32].
- Lower educational level, subjective or objective financial problems, unemployment, and socioeconomic inequality appear to be factors associated with suicidal behavior. The relationship between low income level and suicide appears stronger for patients with mental health problems compared to patients without any mental health diagnosis [32].
- Suicide rates have increased in manual and low-skilled occupations, which might be mediated by a poorer social environment [32].
- Being part of a social minority is associated with an increased risk for suicide attempts but mostly if the minority suffers marginalization [32].
- Religion and having reasons for living carry a protective effect against suicide [32].
- Belonging to a sexual minority group might increase the risk of suffering from mental disorders and suicidal behavior [32].
- An additive effect in suicidal risk has also been found for the combination of aggression/impulsivity and pessimism factors [7].

(d) Risk factors identified in patients with mood disorders

- Risk factors for completed suicide among subjects with mood disorders include male sex [4, 10, 33], history of a suicide attempt, family history of suicide, hopelessness, suicidal ideation, psychotic symptoms; comorbid personality disorders, anxiety disorders, and comorbid substance-use disorder [4]. Sociodemographic features associated with suicide attempts include younger age [1, 33], female gender [1, 10, 33], lower level of education, smoking habits, and patients who were not married or living with someone [1, 33]. Clinical features associated with suicide attempts include higher scores on depression scales [1, 10] and on measures of functional impairment, comorbidity with anxiety disorders (particularly panic disorder), obsessive-compulsive disorder (OCD) and post-traumatic stress disorder (PTSD), and the presence of first- and second-degree relatives with suicidal behavior [1]. Clinical factors predictive of current suicidal risk included age, gender, presence of panic disorder, comorbid PTSD, severe depressive symptoms, and higher functional disability [1].

- Risk factors for suicide behavior in bipolar disorder include prior attempts [33], family history of suicide [4, 5, 7, 10, 33], younger age [4, 33], early life adversity [4, 7, 33, 34], personality disorder [10, 33], cognitive style [7], substance use [4, 7, 33], recent life events [7, 33], comorbid psychopathology [4, 7, 10, 33], suicidal ideation [7, 33], hopelessness [7], early onset [4, 5, 7, 10, 33], severity of illness, mixed affective states [4, 33, 35], rapid cycling [4, 33], and extent and number of depressive symptoms [4, 5, 33–35]. A depressive polarity at illness onset, as compared to an elevated (hypomanic/manic) polarity, has been associated with a more than twice as high rate of suicide attempts [10, 33, 36]. Mixed features at the index episode using DSM-5 criteria were also associated with suicidal behavior in bipolar patients [33, 35]. A predominantly depressive polarity in the illness course has been associated with a higher rate of suicidal acts [33, 37]. Early adversity, such as history of childhood sexual or physical abuse, particularly more severe exposures, is strongly associated with suicide attempts in patients with bipolar disorder [4].
- Factors that increase the likelihood of death by suicide in patients with bipolar disorder include male gender, older age, polarity of current episode (depressive, mixed, manic with psychosis) [4, 10, 33], hopelessness, psychomotor agitation, comorbid anxiety disorder, first-degree family history (mood disorders, bipolar disorder, and suicide), prior suicide attempts [33], substance-use disorders among males [4], and psychosocial precipitants present within a week prior to death [33].
- The risk of suicide has been reported to be similar between bipolar disorder type 1 and type 2 [5–7, 10, 38], and is higher among those disorders compared to the risk of suicide in MDD [6]. The presence of manic-depressive mixed state recurrences [4, 6, 7] or melancholic depression [7], the percentage of days spent in depression in the prior year [4, 7], a history of antidepressant-induced affective episode, and more previous trials of antidepressants have been shown to increase the risk of suicide [7].
- Protective factors for suicide in bipolar disorder include social support, cognitive flexibility, active coping strategies, and healthy lifestyles [7].
- For patients with MDD, risk factors for suicide attempts include younger age, poor social support, severe or recurrent depression, failure to achieve remission, early age at onset, psychotic symptoms [4]—particularly during the acute episode of depression [30], melancholia, presence of a major depressive episode, comorbidity with personality disorders (especially borderline personality disorder), alcohol dependence or misuse, and chronic physical illness. A prior suicide attempt, family history of suicidal behavior, hopelessness, suicidal ideation, and aggressive impulsive traits were more specifically related to suicidal behavior. History of past suicidal behavior, recurrent or refractory depression, and comorbid alcoholism have been

found to be the most robust predictors of suicide attempt or completed suicide in MDD [4].

- Risk factors for suicidal behavior in patients with severe depression include male sex, younger age, comorbid psychiatric disorders, negative life events, not being married, having lower income, and poor social support [39]. The presence of physical illness or disability, comorbid anxiety disorder and substance misuse, and previous psychiatric admission also increase the odds of suicidal ideation and of suicide attempts [39].
- Depressive mixed states, meaning a major depressive episode along with three or more hypomanic symptoms, are frequent in bipolar disorder and also happen often in MDD, and substantially increase the risk of suicidal behaviors [5].
- In a post hoc analysis of the BRIDGE-MIX study, patients with a major depressive episode and history of suicide attempts were compared to patients with a major depressive episode without history of suicide attempts. Psychotic and atypical features, female gender, and first-degree family history of bipolar disorder were found to be more prevalent in the group of patients with history of suicide attempts [5]. Comorbid psychiatry diagnoses most strongly associated with previous history of suicide attempts were substance-use disorders and borderline personality disorder [5]. The predominance of a depressive polarity in the illness course was associated with higher number of suicide attempts and had the strongest association with a suicide attempt [5]. Patients in the suicide attempt group had a history of being treated with more than three medications concomitantly; had been prescribed all types of drugs including antipsychotics, mood stabilizers, antidepressants, and anxiolytics; and had tried ECT more frequently compared to patients in the non-suicidal attempts group. They also had more prevalent history of switches to hypomania or mania, treatment resistance, mood lability, and irritability associated with the use of antidepressants [5]. The hypomanic or manic symptoms most frequently associated with suicide attempts were risky behavior, psychomotor agitation, and impulsivity [5].
- Prospective studies in patients with bipolar disorder have established increased risk for suicidal behavior (attempted or completed suicide) in patients with a history of and increasing number of past suicidal behavior [4, 7], family history of suicide [7] or suicidal behavior, suicidal ideation, subjective rating of depression severity, percentage of days spent in depression over past year [4], younger age, high hostility scores, subjective pessimism, few reported reasons for living, hopelessness [4, 7], aggression and/or impulsivity [4] and comorbidity with borderline personality disorder [7], anxiety disorders, cigarette smoking, or alcohol dependence or abuse [4].
- Prospective studies after a depressive episode have found prior suicide attempts, recurrence of depressive episode, comorbid disorders, age, and gender to be predictive factors for a later suicide attempt [40]. Anxiety level at baseline and severity of depression 6 months after starting treatment for MDD were found to predict the emergence of suicidal ideation [41]. The

persistence of suicidal ideation was associated with residual depressive symptoms 6 months after treatment for MDD was started [41].

- A study using data from a two-wave cross-sectional retrospective survey found that, beyond previous suicide attempts, the symptom of worthlessness present during the first depressive episode was the only significant predictor of elevated risk of suicide attempt in a 3-year window after major depressive episode remission. The other variables studied during the first depressive episode included presence of suicidal ideation, marked role impairment, psychomotor retardation, and prolonged (longer than 6 months) duration, based on previous findings showing that the subset of patients with these "complicated" features had a substantial elevation of suicide attempts after the first major depressive episode. Neither of those predicted a suicide attempt after remission when controlled for past suicide attempt. The authors conclude that feelings of worthlessness should be paid particular attention to by clinicians [40].

(e) Comorbidity

- Other psychiatric diagnosis

– Trauma-related disorders

Sexual, physical, and emotional abuse and neglect all increase the risk of suicidal behavior, with especially consistent findings related to childhood sexual abuse [42].

Among patients with bipolar disorder, lifetime prevalence of post-traumatic stress disorder (PTSD) is up to 40% [43]. The co-occurrence of both diagnoses has been associated with worse course of both illnesses including an increased number of hospitalizations, increased suicide risk, more rapid cycling, lower quality of life, and a poor treatment outcome [43]. Patients with bipolar disorder and co-occurring past or present PTSD scored significantly higher for suicidal ideation in a large study that included patients seeking treatment for bipolar disorder. This study didn't detect greater rates of recent suicide attempts in patients with bipolar disorder and PTSD.

Any history of trauma in patients with bipolar disorder has been associated with greater suicidal ideation and attempts [33, 43].

The rate of comorbidity of MDD with PTSD has been reported as 48–79% and it is associated with higher rates of suicidal behavior [42]. In a study of 64 patients with MDD admitted for suicidal attempt, the subset of patients with comorbid depression and PTSD had more additional psychiatric diagnosis, a higher degree of exposure to childhood trauma, more frequent suicide attempts, and non-suicidal self-harm, and they reported significantly more interpersonal vengeful suicidal motives compared with depressed patients without PTSD [42].

It has been suggested that affective lability might be the psychological factor mediating the association between childhood traumatic experiences and more severe or complex phenotype of bipolar disorder, including more frequent suicide attempts. The anger subdomain of affective lability seems to increase vulnerability to an increased risk of suicide attempts. In particular, emotional abuse might increase internalized anger and hostility in patients with bipolar disorder [44].

- Anxiety disorders

  The lifetime prevalence of anxiety disorders in patients with bipolar disorder was reported to be 45% (95% CI 40%–51%) in a systematic review and meta-analysis. There is a threefold increase in the prevalence of anxiety disorders in patients with bipolar disorder, compared with patients without bipolar disorder. There doesn't seem to be a difference in the lifetime prevalence of anxiety between patients with bipolar disorder type I and patients with bipolar disorder type II [9].

  For patients with bipolar disorder, the presence of a co-occurring anxiety disorder in their lifetime was associated with an increased risk for suicide attempts [9, 33, 43].

  In patients with MDD, the presence of anxiety symptoms is associated with a worse clinical course, poorer treatment response, and higher risk of recurrence and suicide [41].

- Attention-deficit hyperactivity disorder (ADHD)

  The lifetime prevalence of ADHD in patients with bipolar disorder has been reported as 14.7% in male patients and 5.8% in female patients [45].

  Patients with ADHD have an earlier onset and a more severe course of bipolar disorder, experience a lower quality of life, and were more frequently depressed than patients without ADHD [45]. They also have more common comorbidities with anxiety, borderline personality symptoms, and alcohol- and drug-use disorders than those with bipolar disorder without ADHD [45].

  The role of ADHD in suicidality in 500 adolescents and young adults with bipolar disorder was evaluated in a longitudinal study, compared with 1500 patients with bipolar disorder only. They found that ADHD was an independent risk factor for attempted suicide in this population. Potential explanations for this finding included a higher presence of comorbid disorders, impulsivity which is frequently a characteristic of ADHD, and poorer medication adherence due to inattention [45].

- Substance-use disorder

  The presence of alcohol- and substance-use disorders carries very high rates of suicidal ideation and behavior [24], independent of bipolar disorder status [46]. Comorbidity with alcohol- and substance-use disorder increases the risk for suicide attempts and suicide deaths in patients with mood disorders [10, 33].

  In a large epidemiological study involving patients with bipolar disorder, 54% also had a comorbid alcohol-use disorder [47]. Up to 72% of patients with bipolar disorder have lifetime abuse or dependence on one or more substances [46]. The prevalence of substance-use disorder in patients with bipolar disorder is reported to be as high as 44%, with cannabis being the most frequently abused substance in their lifetime [46]. Patients with comorbid alcohol-use disorder were at greater risk for suicide attempt than those without alcohol-use disorder (OR = 2.25; 95% CI, 1.61–3.14) [47]. The presence of nicotine dependence and drug-use disorder didn't increase the risk for suicide in one study [48].

A systematic review and meta-analysis found a significant association between alcohol-use disorders in general as well as alcohol abuse and alcohol dependence and a history of suicide attempts in patients with bipolar disorder (OR = 1.72, OR = 1.64, and OR = 1.70, respectively) compared to patients with bipolar disorder who didn't present these comorbidities. It also found an increased risk for suicide attempts in patients with bipolar disorder and substance-use disorders as compared to patients without this comorbidity (OR = 1.77, 95% CI = 1.49–2.10, $p < 0.01$, z = 6.46). In patients with bipolar disorder misusing cannabis, the OR for suicide attempts was 1.44 (95%CI = 1.07–1.94, $p = 0.02$, z = 2.40) [46].

Potential explanations for the association between bipolar disorder and substance/alcohol-use disorders include the fact that both carry a high risk of suicide independently of the presence of the other disorder as comorbidity. Also, poor coping skills and inadequate social support might be more common in patients with comorbid alcohol- or substance-use disorders, and these can also increase the risk for suicide in patients with bipolar disorder. There might also be a genetic factor having an impact in this association, based on reported family clusters of bipolar disorder, alcohol-use disorder, and attempted suicide, potentially mediated by the phenotype of impulsivity, hostility, and/or aggression [46]. People with bipolar disorder and alcohol/substance use-disorder might be more prone to mood instability, which in turn increases the likelihood of suicidal ideation or attempts [46].

- Personality disorders

30–40% of patients who commit suicide have a personality disorder. The majority of suicides occur in patients with comorbid mood and personality disorders. The presence of a personality disorder comorbid with a mood disorder increases the patient's risk of suicide attempt to approximately twofold [49].

The most consistent predictors for a suicide attempt have been borderline personality disorder comorbid with MDD, bipolar disorder with current major depressive episode, and both MDD and bipolar disorder with current MDE or dysthymia [49]. Suicide attempts are particularly associated with a comorbid cluster B/borderline personality disorder [10, 33].

The prevalence of borderline personality disorder in patients with bipolar disorder ranges between 0 and 52%, with a mean of 22% [50]. Patients with bipolar disorder and comorbid borderline personality disorder have higher suicidality compared to bipolar disorder alone [10, 38, 50]. This association might be explained by the facts that borderline personality disorder carries a cumulative burden of impairment, is most likely to be inappropriately recognized or treated, and can increase noncompliance with treatment [50]. Among symptoms of borderline personality disorder, unstable relationships and impulsivity were found to be independent predictors for suicidality [50]. The co-occurrence of bipolar disorder and borderline personality disorder seems to confer an additive risk of suicide, although borderline personality disorder might have a greater influence than that of bipolar disorder [38].

Other personality disorders have been associated with increased risk for suicide attempts at follow-up including those in the cluster C in general, dependent, avoidant, paranoid, schizoid, schizotypal, or any personality disorder with MDD or major depressive episode in patients with bipolar disorder [49].

The relationship with suicide in comorbid mood and personality disorders has been found to be mediated by a higher propensity to spend time in major depressive episodes seen in patients with comorbid personality disorders [49]. The proportion of time spent in major depressive episodes is a key predictor of accumulated risk for suicidal behavior [49], especially in patients with borderline personality disorder. However, there also seems to be a direct effect from the presence of personality disorders modifying the risk of suicide attempt in patients with mood disorders, especially in patients with cluster C personality disorders [49]. In particular, avoidant and dependent, but not obsessive-compulsive personality, disorders are linked to an increased rate of new suicide attempts [49].

Increased suicide attempts in patients with cluster A personality disorders are probably mediated by increased time depressed, poor social support, and direct effects of the personality disorder when depressed [49].

- Medical conditions: Medical illness is a significant factor in about 50% of suicides in people older than 50 years old [51].

– Chronic illnesses that carry an increased risk of suicide include cancer, diabetes mellitus, stroke and neurological conditions, and cardiovascular disease [51]. Pain disorders have been highly correlated with suicidal ideation and behavior [24].

– Cardiovascular disease

Cardiovascular disease is associated with depression and patients with heart disease have a higher prevalence of psychological distress as compared to patients without heart disease [51]. The presence of depression seems to be the key mediator of suicidal ideation in individuals with cardiovascular disease [51].

Several factors, other than this association between cardiovascular disease and depression, could contribute to increased risk of suicide in patients with cardiovascular disease including its association with physical disability and decreased function leading to psychological distress with a sense of loss, frustration, anger, hopelessness, and negative expectation about the future. Medications could also negatively impact depression [51].

In people who committed suicide, people with cardiovascular disorder and depression were more likely to have had a past suicide attempt and to have experienced a mental or financial stressor in the past year as compared to people with cardiovascular disease without depression. The majority of those with cardiovascular disease who died from suicide were male. Males with cardiovascular disease and depression died from a suicide significantly more commonly by shooting compared to females who mostly died from self-poisoning. Hanging was also more common among males than females [51].

Risk Assessment

Although it is difficult to predict suicide in an individual level [52], guidelines recommend that every encounter with a patient with depression should include an assessment of suicide risk [52]. Clinicians should assess risk for suicide with a consideration for predisposing risk factors and precipitant risk factors.

Acute events or warning signs would be considered precipitants and are relevant for suicide prevention by clinicians or family members [7]. The most concerning ones which should prompt emergent assessment include patients threatening self-harm, seeking access to means to self-harm, making a trust, or making comments about death. Other warning signs that should prompt professional assessment include hopelessness, anger, engagement in risky behaviors, increase in substance use, social isolation [7], anxiety [7, 29, 41], insomnia, dramatic mood swings, and lack of purpose in life [7]. The predictive value of passive suicidal ideation, meaning thoughts of not wanting to be alive, is probably lower than that of active suicidal ideation, where there is planning and preparing for a suicide attempt, and this intent to die should be taken into account [6]. Other proximal clinical risk factors include the severity of depressive symptoms, comorbid cluster B traits, and substance abuse [29].

Chronic factors that act as predisposing risk factors should also be taken into consideration when performing a suicide risk assessment as their presence may lead to a suicide death sometime in the patient's lifetime [48]. The strongest predictor of a suicide attempt is the history of suicide attempt [7, 52]. Up to 20% of patients who attempt suicide will eventually die by suicide [4]. However, only about 50% of people who complete suicide had a prior attempt [4]. Other longer term risk factors identified in patients with bipolar disorder include high-risk behavior and increased psychomotor agitation [48]. A mental health diagnosis is a strong predictor of suicidal behavior but its specificity is low as the majority of people who experienced mental illness do not die by suicide [26].

Efforts have been made to identify the clinical features that lead to suicidal ideation given that suicidal ideation is a strong predictor of suicide attempts. Depression symptom severity has been identified as a strong predictor of suicidal ideation [53]. In MDD, symptoms of poor sleep, reduced appetite, and guilt have been associated with suicidal ideation [53].

Using data from the systematic treatment enhancement program for bipolar disorder (STEP-BD), a study evaluated potential acute risk factors that were present in the 6 months before suicidal behavior in a sample of 103 outpatients with bipolar disorder who attempted suicide or died by suicide during the trial, compared with patients who didn't attempt or die by suicide. The strongest relationship for subsequent suicidal behavior was found for suicidal ideation which was elevated for up to 4 months before the event. Loss of interest was also moderately elevated before suicidal behavior. To a lesser extent, anxiety also emerged as an acute risk factor for suicide [48]. Another study by the same authors and also using data from the STEP-BD study aimed at assessing which specific mood symptoms precipitated the onset or worsening of suicidal ideation in adults with and without a history of a suicide attempt. Symptoms of guilt, reduced self-esteem, psychomotor retardation and agitation, increase in appetite, and distractibility predicted more severe levels of subsequent suicidal ideation at the next visit. In patients with a history of a suicide attempt, symptoms that predicted subsequent suicidal ideation more strongly included problems with concentration, distractibility, sleep loss, and decreased need for sleep. Elevated self-esteem was found to protect against subsequent suicidal ideation only in individuals without a history of a suicide attempt. The authors mention that, overall, effect sizes were small, consistent with the fact that relatively few strong proximal additive risk factors of suicide are known and that the predictive value of more distal predictors is relatively weak [53]. Cross-sectional studies in bipolar disorder have identified attenuated self-esteem and elevated psychomotor agitation as correlates of suicidal ideation [53].

But, how can we know which patients with suicidal ideation will attempt suicide? Only about one-third of patients who think about suicide make an attempt during their lifetimes [27] meaning that the majority of patients who have suicidal ideation never make a suicide attempt or die by suicide [24]. Another route of research focuses on this question by assessing the development of suicidal ideation and its progression to potentially lethal attempts as distinct processes with different explanations or predictions. For this, it uses an ideation-to-action framework [28] instead of focusing on traditional risk factors for suicide, which tend to predict suicide ideation but aren't necessarily strongly and specifically related to suicide attempts. This research has shown that factors associated with decreased fear of pain, injury and death, knowledge about and access to lethal means, and experience with self-inflicted injury increase the patient's capability to attempt suicide [28]. Other factors found more commonly among patients who attempt suicide than patients with suicidal ideation have included recent stressful life events, lower self-forgiveness, psychotic symptoms, lower executive functioning skills, and emotional abuse [28]. A depressive diagnosis, the severity of depression, PTSD, drug abuse, and history of sexual abuse have showed small-to-moderate effects in differentiating patients with suicide ideation from patients who attempt suicide [27]. The presence of borderline personality disorder symptoms, a lack of meaning in life, hopelessness, and non-suicidal self-injury were most commonly found in patients with a recent suicide attempt (over the last year) than in patients with recent suicide ideation, but this sample consisted mainly of female patients with eating disorders [27].

Along those lines, an observational retrospective study compared multiple potential risk factors from multiple domains for suicidal behavior and investigated differences between risk factors for suicidal ideation and single or repeated suicide attempts among patients with mood disorders [29]. Depressive symptomatology and hopelessness were identified as salient predictors for suicidal ideation, while severity of mood disorder, especially with psychotic symptoms, comorbid borderline personality traits, and comorbid alcohol-use disorder were predictors of suicide attempts. Other risk factors for pure suicidal ideation without suicide attempts were younger age, diagnoses of depressive disorder without psychotic symptoms, bipolar disorder type 2 or NOS, and history of childhood physical abuse. Other risk factors associated with repeated suicide attempts included female gender, younger age, bipolar disorder type 2 or NOS, and childhood physical abuse [29].

Risk factors for suicide have also been divided into modifiable and non-modifiable risk factors [52]. This division is important since we can't change a patient's history so for clinical practice some factors will be more relevant when formulating prevention and management plans [7]. Modifiable risk factors for suicide during a major depressive episode include active suicidal ideation, hopelessness [52], psychotic symptoms [28, 30, 52], anxiety [41, 52], impulsivity [52], stressful life events [28, 52] and victimization, substance-use disorders (especially alcohol-use disorder), post-traumatic stress disorder, comorbid personality disorders (especially cluster B personality disorders), presence of medical conditions that involve chronic pain, and cancer [52]. Non-modifiable risk factors for suicide in MDD include older men, past suicide attempt, history of self-harm behavior, belonging to a sexual minority, family history of suicide, and history of legal problems [52].

There are suicide risk assessment tools that can be useful for a systematic assessment and documentation but are not particularly reliable in predicting future suicide attempts [52]. Assessment of suicidal ideation is not the same as assessment of suicide attempts [24]. Examples of scales for assessment of suicidal ideation include SADPERSONS, Columbia Suicide Severity Rating Scale (C-SSRS), and Chronological Assessment of Suicide Risk interview guide [52]. The Scale for Suicidal Ideation (SSI) might be more appropriate for high-risk settings [4]. The Suicide Status Form (SSF) was also developed for the direct assessment of suicidal thoughts [48]. The Beck Scale for Suicidal Ideation is a patient-administered version of the SSI [24].

Finally, moving to a more individualized risk stratification approach where a patient who presents in an office and is found to have a high risk of attempting suicide can identify patients who would benefit from preventive strategies or from using drugs with anti-suicidal effect [54]. Research is growing in trying to find algorithms that might help determining individual patients likely to commit suicide [54].

Another encouraging approach is a diagnostic-specific approach for understanding suicide attempts and deaths in patients with bipolar disorder. It considers three types of information when assessing risk for suicide. The first one includes general factors related to suicide attempts and deaths. The second one includes general factors related to suicide attempts and deaths that are influenced by the presence of bipolar disorder. The third one includes factors that are specific to bipolar disorder [33].

Management

Prevention and Treatment

(a) Improved attention and management of depression in primary health care [4]:
  - Studies in primary care setting suggested that suicidal behaviors tend to occur during major depressive episodes of complicated high-risk patients [22, 40], but their suicidal intention or acts were commonly unrecognized. Up to two-thirds of suicide victims and suicide attempters had contact with their general practitioner or psychiatrist 4 weeks before the suicidal act and the point prevalence of depressive disorders in primary care is around 10% [22]. Education and training of primary care doctors might be successful in reducing suicide rates since they can play a priority role in suicide prevention [4, 22].

(b) The time spent in high-risk illness phases might be the most important determinant of risk for suicide attempts among patients with mood disorders [4, 6]. Psychiatric patients with MDD were followed during 5 years; the incidence of suicide attempts was 21-fold during the depressive episodes and 4-fold during partial remission, compared to the time in full remission [4]. In patients with bipolar disorder, the incidence of suicide attempts was 38-fold during mixed and depressive mixed phases and 18-fold during depressive episodes [4]. Effective management of these high-risk states in order to reduce time spent in a major depressive or mixed mood episode may be crucial for prevention [4]. In particular, agitated dysphoric states in a depressive episode have been associated the most with suicide in patients with both bipolar disorder and MDD [6]. Some recommend the integration of the concept of predominant polarity for the proper selection of available maintenance treatments for bipolar disorder as the predominantly depressive polarity has been associated with a higher risk of suicide than the predominantly manic polarity [37].

(c) Early diagnosis and intervention is paramount as it has been reported that a third of all suicidal acts occurred within the first few years from onset of MDD [6]. Suicide prevention efforts should start before the first suicide attempt happens, as between 50 and 60% of patients die on their first attempt [31].

(d) For patients who survive their first suicide attempt, the subsequent year has been found to be critical periods to use preventive strategies since most of the patients who eventually die by suicide after a first attempt do so in the first year after [31].

(e) Addressing modifiable risk factors:
  - Comorbid alcohol and drug abuse should be prevented, diagnosed, and treated early as its presence increases the risk for suicide [4, 7, 46]. Integrating health care for both conditions carries better outcomes than managing each one separately, but studies show that this rarely happens [46]. Primary care providers may play a role in improving care outcomes and reducing mortality in this population by screening and identifying this comorbidity [46].

- Anxiety disorder and borderline personality disorder should also be treated [4]. Anxiety symptoms should be considered an important warning sign of suicidal ideation even after resolution of depressive symptoms [41].
- Decreasing high impulsivity and aggressive traits [4].
- Comorbid cardiovascular diseases should be addressed as they increase the risk for suicide. This starts with promotion of a healthy lifestyle and referrals for medical screening and care [7]. Other medical conditions known to increase suicidal risk should be addressed as well.
- Assessing and addressing insomnia symptoms should be a prevention and treatment target in order to reduce suicide risk in patients with depression. A referral for cognitive behavioral therapy for insomnia is recommended with or without medication management [23].

(f) Strengthening protective risk factors such as meaningful and important relationships.

(g) Level of care:

- Rapid hospitalization is effective for short-term reduction of suicidal risk in acute suicidal crises, but is not known to have long-term preventive effects on suicide risk [6].

(h) Psychological treatments:

- There is evidence supporting the efficacy of cognitive behavioral therapy (CBT), combined with pharmacological treatment, for prevention of both relapse and new suicidal behavior in patients with bipolar disorder [7]. Cognitive therapy in a randomized clinical trial reduced repetitions of suicide attempts among patients with a recent suicide attempt or state, most of them with MDD [4].
- Other psychotherapeutic interventions as well as psychoeducation and training to improve social skills and active problem solving might reduce patient's suicidal ideation in patients with bipolar disorder, but there is no robust evidence to support this [7].
- Dialectic behavioral psychotherapy studies suggest that it is effective for suicide prevention among specific subgroups of patients with mental illness [15].
- Psychosocial and family interventions might play a role in the prevention of suicide by educating the individual support network about the damaging effects of reinforcing negative self-appraisals and feelings of burdensomeness [26].

(i) Biological treatments: Successful acute and long-term treatment of MDD and bipolar disorder markedly reduces suicide morbidity and mortality [22].

- MDD:

– Antidepressants:

Multiple studies support the suicide protective effect of acute and long-term use of antidepressants in patients with unipolar depressive episodes, for the reduction in risk of both suicide attempts and completed suicide in the majority of patients [22]. However, a meta-analysis on antidepressant monotherapy in unipolar major depression involving non-acutely suicidal and excluding the most severe cases showed a nonsignificant increase of suicidal behavior in patients receiving antidepressants compared to those taking placebo [22].

Another meta-analysis also found a significant increase in suicide attempts for patients taking selective serotonin reuptake inhibitors (SSRIs) compared with patients taking placebo, with no significant difference in the rate of completed suicides between both groups [22]. In 2004 the Food and Drug Administration (FDA) issued a warning about increased suicide risk among children and adolescent, mostly early in treatment. Other meta-analyses found that antidepressants lowered the risk of suicide and suicide behavior among treated patients compared to placebo [15].

Taken these results together, studies suggest that antidepressants prevent suicidal behavior in the most severe and acutely suicidal patients but can rarely induce these behaviors in the less severe and not acutely suicidal unipolar patients, particularly in the younger populations [22]. In addition, the initial activation [15, 22], agitation [6, 15], anger, dysphoria, restlessness, irritability [6], insomnia [6, 15], akathisia, mixed depression in latent bipolarity [15], behavioral disinhibition [6], and delayed onset of response [15] that can be seen with antidepressant medications might explain why patients become suicidal shortly after starting taking these medications [6, 22], especially when complicated by substance abuse, and in younger patients [6]. Therefore, providers must be especially vigilant during the first 10–14 days of treatment, when the risk of suicidal behavior is relatively more frequent. Practice guidelines continue to support the use of antidepressants for the treatment of depression with or without suicide risk in all age groups [15]. It is also important to understand that the risks associated with appropriate use of antidepressants are not high enough to outweigh the benefits in clinical practice and the protection that they provide against suicide [22].

Fluoxetine and sertraline appear to be associated with lower suicide risks when compared to other antidepressants such as paroxetine [22]. Fluoxetine has been reported to decrease anger, self-injurious behavior, and impulsive aggression [15]. In unipolar depression, tricyclic antidepressants may have a protective effect against suicide [15].

Subthreshold bipolarity and unrecognized bipolar depressive states might also explain a potential for nonresponse or worsening depression with antidepressant monotherapy [22].

Research on the effects of antidepressants on suicide risk carries a lot of difficulty methodologically. Some recommend avoiding antidepressants in the presence of depressive states accompanied by "mixed" symptoms such as agitation and anger and maybe using mood stabilizers or antipsychotic agents in order to reduce states associated with suicide [6].

Research is ongoing trying to find genetic markers that could identify patients at increased risk of suicide during antidepressant treatment [22].

- Lithium:

  The use of lithium in patients with MDD has shown to reduce the risk of suicides and suicide attempts [6, 22] with a similar risk reduction as in patients with bipolar disorder [22] but the effect sizes for prevention of suicide attempts seem to be largest in depression [15].

  Among patients with unipolar depression, a meta-analyses showed a reduction of the risk of death by suicide and by all causes, as well as a reduction of suicide risk 4–5-fold compared to placebo [15].

  The reduction of the risk of suicide doesn't only appear in patients with excellent response to medication but also in moderate responders and in poor responders. Therefore, the lack of clinical response in terms of symptomatology should not guide the clinician to discontinue lithium as it might still be having a protective effect in terms of suicide risk independent to its thymoregulatory properties [8, 22].

  The anti-suicidal effect of lithium might be related to a decrease in aggression and impulsiveness associated with depression or dysphoric agitated mixed high suicide risk states or it might be independent of its effect in mood since, as mentioned above, suicidal risk has been reduced even without a significant clinical response in mood stabilization [6].

  The combination of lithium and an antidepressant medication could reduce suicidal acts by decreasing suicidal ideation prior to the onset of the antidepressant effect [8].

- Bipolar disorder:

- Early diagnosis and intervention for bipolar disorder can decrease the lifetime prevalence of suicide attempts.
- Suicidal risk can be more effectively decreased by preventing rather than treating acute depressive episodes, which accounts for 40–50% of the time ill among patients with bipolar disorder [6].
- Medications: Maintenance treatment with mood stabilizers, including lithium and antiepileptic medications, has been the mainstay of treatment in patients with mood disorders. Lithium has shown in different studies to have a superior effect than antiepileptic medications against suicide attempts and completed suicide and also showed to increase the incidence ratio of attempt to suicides, which means lithium might lead to a reduced lethality in suicide attempts [7].
- Lithium:

  Not only has lithium been considered the first-line agent in the treatment of bipolar disorder based on its efficacy for both poles of the disease but it also has an effect in reducing suicide attempts and completed suicide among patients with a mood disorder [8].

  There is strong evidence showing a reduction in suicidal attempts and completions with the use of lithium in patients with bipolar disorder [6, 7]. The reduction in risk for attempted and completed suicides either in bipolar or in unipolar patients has been reported to be as high as 80% with long-term lithium treatment [8, 22], close to general population rates, and as high as 90% when completed suicides are excluded [22]. Long-term treatment with lithium reduces suicide attempts by about 10% and deaths by suicide by about 20% [8]. Also, the lethality of means used for suicide attempts was reduced with lithium treatment [8, 22]. The estimated number needed to treat with lithium to avoid one life-threatening or fatal act in one study was reported to be 23 (CI 21–25) [6].

In order to ensure the anti-suicidal efficacy of lithium it is recommended to maintain the lithium blood concentrations in efficient therapeutic range and to use it as a long-term maintenance treatment [8].

Even in the presence of a strong family history of suicidal behavior, treatment with lithium decreases suicide rates significantly [7].

Discontinuation of lithium maintenance treatment has led to an increase in the rate of suicidal acts [6, 8], with greater effect seen after abrupt and rapid versus gradual (over 2 weeks or longer) discontinuation. The suicidal behaviors later return to the levels present before the treatment was started [6].

The superior efficacy in reduction of suicide risk with lithium has been established in studies comparing it with placebo, anticonvulsant medications, and antidepressant medication [8].

Lithium might modulate impulsive and aggressive behavior, a phenotype associated with suicide in bipolar disorder. This effect might happen through the action of lithium on the serotoninergic system, specifically the 5-HT1B serotoninergic receptors, a specific molecular target for lithium [8]. The reduction in impulsive and aggressive behavior might also be mediated by an anti-inflammatory action of lithium [8].

– Anticonvulsants:

The evidence for a decrease in suicidal attempts and completed suicides with the use of anticonvulsant medications is weaker than that existing with lithium [6, 7, 22].

Despite evidence published about decrease in suicidal behavior with antiepileptic medications, in 2008 the Food and Drug Administration (FDA) issued an alert about increased risk of suicidal thoughts and behavior related to anticonvulsants. This alert came out based on the results of a meta-analysis of placebo-controlled trials involving 11 anticonvulsants. This study showed a higher rate of suicidal behavior or ideation with anticonvulsants than with placebo [6, 7] in patients with epilepsy but not in psychiatry patients [6]. This study was criticized and other studies in psychiatric populations have failed to reach the same conclusion [6, 7]. Therefore, research on the effect of anticonvulsants on suicidal risk remains inconsistent and inconclusive [6]. The evidence points towards an increase of depression in patients with epilepsy, that goes under-diagnosed and undertreated and progresses to suicidal ideation. The FDA black box warning generated increased discussion on the topic, in the metanaylisis that generated the FDA conclusion 199 clinical trials were examined, but only 33 of those studies were included, suicidal ideation and behavior was not one of the variables assessed prospectively sistematically, which makes it hard to make the conclusion that anticonvulsant medications increase suicidality, the effect of depression or mood disorders was also not taken into account. For further information on this topic please see chapter 6 in (Rudinzky and Meador 2011) [55].

– Antidepressants:

Studies suggest that the combination of antidepressants with mood stabilizers reduces but doesn't eliminate the elevated risk of suicide behaviors that has been associated with monotherapy with antidepressants. Therefore, if an antidepressant is needed to treat depressive episodes in patients with bipolar disorder, it is important to continue the patients on a mood stabilizer while they are taking an antidepressant. It is also recommended to use the antidepressant medication for as short time as possible [22].

However, results from an observational study suggest that prescribing antidepressant reduces suicidal behavior by 54% in bipolar disorder type 1 and by 35% in bipolar disorder type 2 [18].

– Antipsychotic medications:

Same as with antidepressants, studies suggest that the combination of antipsychotics, particularly first generation, with mood stabilizers reduces but doesn't eliminate the elevated risk of suicide that has been associated with the medications in patients on antipsychotic monotherapy. Therefore, if a typical antipsychotic is needed to treat breakthrough manic episodes, it is important to continue the patients on a mood stabilizer while they are taking the antipsychotic medication. It is also recommended to use the antipsychotic medication for as short time as possible and use mood stabilizer monotherapy as the main component of long-term pharmacotherapy [22].

The first FDA-approved treatment with an anti-suicide indication was clozapine for patients with schizophrenia or schizoaffective disorder [6, 15]. However, despite some evidence of effectiveness of this medication in bipolar disorder, including for patients who have not completely responded to other treatments and those with psychotic features, there is not enough evidence supporting that it carries an anti-suicidal effect in patients with bipolar disorder as it does in patients with schizophrenia [6].

(j) Anxiolytics and sedatives:
   - Although one would expect a beneficial effect of suicidal risk with the use of anxiolytics, the limited evidence available doesn't provide strong support for alteration of suicide risk, either short term or long term in patients with anxiety disorders or other psychiatric illnesses. On the other hand, behavioral disinhibition, especially when these medications are used in patients with substance-use disorders or personality disorders, may increase impulsivity and aggressive behaviors. Also, discontinuation of benzodiazepine treatment, especially abruptly, may increase suicidal risk [6].

(k) Ketamine:
   - Ketamine is an anesthetic medication that works as a noncompetitive N-methyl-D-aspartate (NMDA) glutamate receptor antagonist [15, 24]. It has shown to have a rapidly acting antidepressant effect and to acutely decrease suicidal ideation when used at sub-anesthetic dose of 0.5 mg/kg [24]. It has been studied in patients with treatment-resistant depression and bipolar disorder [15, 24]. The anti-suicidal effect occurs as early as 40 min after treatment [15, 24] and it has been reported to last for up to 5 days [24] for some, while others showed that the suicide scores returned to baseline range at 24–48 h post-infusions [15]. In a triple-blind randomized control study in 57 patients with treatment-resistant depression, 53% of ketamine-treated patients scored zero on all suicide measures compared with 24% of the midazolam group [15].

- The anti-suicidal effect of ketamine might not be solely due to its antidepressant or antianxiety effects, but also due to its impact on other factors associated with suicidal ideation such as hopelessness [24]. The efficacy of ketamine in treating conditions such as substance-use disorder, chronic pain, anxiety disorders, and PTSD, all strongly associated with suicidal behavior, might also have an impact in reduction of suicide risk in patients with coexisting mood disorders [24]. Also, a decrease in specific symptoms associated with suicide and commonly present in depression such as anhedonia, anxiety, hopelessness, rumination, hostility, and aggression might mediate the reduction of suicidal behavior [24]. A beneficial effect of ketamine on sleep might also be a reason for decreased suicidality with this medication [24]. Another potential mechanism for anti-suicidal effect with ketamine is the interruption of the kynurenine pathway and modulation of pro-inflammatory cytokine exacerbation [15].
- Ketamine is reported to be generally well tolerated and safe at the dose used for suicide risk reduction, with most commonly reported side effects being transiently increased blood pressure, pulse, and transient dissociative effects, drowsiness, blurred vision, poor coordination, and dizziness [24].
- While there are studies evidencing the anti-suicidal effect of ketamine in the acute setting, there is still not enough data showing effectiveness of ketamine for long-term prevention of suicidal behavior [24].

(l) Routine clinical testing of vitamin D levels could be beneficial in patients with suicidal symptoms, with subsequent supplementation in patients found to be deficient [11].

(m) Neurostimulation:

- Repetitive transcranial magnetic stimulation (rTMS):

– rTMS has shown to be effective in decreasing depression scores in patients with bipolar and unipolar depression and is considered an effective and well-tolerated treatment for patients who do not respond to, or cannot be treated with, antidepressant medications [56].

– Delivering high doses of left prefrontal rTMS has been feasible and safe, with few side effects and no worsening of suicidal thinking. Results from different studies suggested a rapid anti-suicidal effect but this effect was not different from the sham group [57, 58].

– rTMS has not been established as a treatment for suicidality but hypothesis on its effect on decreasing depression scores and modulating emotional and cognitive states associated with suicide risk suggests that more robust research is needed in this area [59].

- Electroconvulsive therapy (ECT):

– ECT is effective for short-term reduction of suicidal risk in patients with mood disorders but long-term preventive effects remain to be studied and there is no strong data evidencing maintenance of suicide risk reduction following discontinuation of ECT treatments [6, 15]. Progressive resolution of suicidal ideation is noted throughout the ECT course in patients at high acute suicide risk [15]. It remains the gold standard of treatment for suicidal depression [15]. Patients with mood disorders with acute suicide risk should be considered for ECT, unless suicide risk is related primarily to personality disorder or timely limited to substance abuse [60]. Early consideration should be warranted for patients with severe depressive mood accompanied by motor, vegetative, and cognitive dysfunction, as well as those with psychotic or melancholic depression, males older than 40 years with evidence of recurrent illness, and current alcohol abuse [60].

(n) Chronotherapy:

- Chronotherapy involves the therapeutic manipulation of sleep-wake cycles. The study of chronotherapeutic interventions in the adjunctive treatment of depression began in the 1970s when investigators noted a rapid, albeit transient, antidepressant response to sleep deprivation [61]. Another chronotherapeutic technique, bright-light therapy, has consistently shown benefit in the treatment of seasonal affective disorders [62]. Its use in the treatment of nonseasonal unipolar and bipolar depression has also shown promising results [63, 64].
- Triple chronotherapy (TCT):

– TCT is an approach that combines sleep deprivation, bright-light therapy, and sleep-phase advancement in the acute treatment of depression [3, 65, 66]. One of the first TCT studies in adults demonstrated a significant, acute antidepressant response in up to 70% of patients with bipolar depression, and a sustained response in up to 55% of patients at 1 month [65]. A more recent study employed an abbreviated protocol that included one night of sleep deprivation, followed by three nights of sleep-phase advancement and bright-light therapy in each of the four mornings of the intervention. This study demonstrated similar, accelerated antidepressant responses along with reduced suicidality and improved sleep quality [3].

Conclusions

Suicide is a leading cause of death in patients with mood disorder and the majority of the patients who commit suicide suffers from a mood disorder. The etiology for suicide in patients with mood disorders seems to be multifactorial involving several systems and neurological pathways interacting with genetic and environmental mechanisms. Assessing risk for suicide is an essential part of the overall assessment of patients with mood disorders. In addition to the known risk factors for suicide in the general population, disease-specific risk factors have been identified for patients suffering from mood disorders. High-risk states warrant especial monitoring and effective interventions. Strategies for prevention and treatment should be implemented in order to continue efforts to reduce suicide behaviors and deaths by suicide. Long-term use of lithium is associated with major reductions in the risk of suicide and suicide attempt in patients with bipolar disorder and major depression. More research is needed in order to reduce mortality and morbidity from suicide attempts and completed suicide.

References

1. Antypa N, Souery D, Tomasini M, Albani D, Fusco F, Mendlewicz J, Serretti A. Clinical and genetic factors associated with suicide in mood disorder patients. Eur Arch Psychiatry Clin Neurosci. 2016;266:181–93.
2. American Psychiatric Association (APA). Diagnosis and statistical manual of mental disorders. 5th ed. Arlington (VA): American Psychiatric Association; 2013.
3. Martiny K, Refsgaard E, Lund V, et al. Maintained superiority of chronotherapeutics vs. exercise in a 20-week randomized follow-up trial in major depression. Acta Psychiatr Scand. 2015;131(6):446–57.
4. Isometsa E. Suicidal behavior or mood disorders- who, when, and why? Can J Psychiatr. 2014;59(3):120–30.
5. Popovic D, Vieta E, Azorin J-M, Angst J, Bowden CL, Mosolov S, Young AH, Perugi G. Suicide attempts in major depressive episode: evidence from the BRIDGE-II-mix study. Bipolar Disord. 2015;17:795–803.
6. Tondo L, Baldessarini RJ. Suicidal behavior and mood disorders: response to pharmacological treatment. Curr Psychiatry Rep. 2016;18:88.
7. Latalova K, Kamaradova D, Prasko J. Suicide in bipolar disorder: a review. Psychiatr Danub. 2014;26(2):108–14.
8. Benard V, Vaiva D, Masson M, Geoffroy PA. Lithium and suicide prevention in bipolar disorder. L'Encephale. 2016;42:234–41.
9. Pavlova B, Perlis RH, Alda M, Uher R. Lifetime prevalence of anxiety disorders in people with bipolar disorder: a systematic review and meta-analysis. Lancet Psychiatry. 2015;2:710–7.
10. Schaffer A, Isometsa ET, Tondo L, et al. International society for bipolar disorders task force and suicide: meta-analyses and meta-regression of correlates of suicide attempts and suicide deaths in bipolar disorder. Bipolar Disord. 2014;17:1–16.
11. Grudet C, Malm J, Westrin A, Brundin L. Suicidal patients are deficient in vitamin D, associated with a pro-inflammatory status in the blood. Psychoneuroendocrinology. 2014;50:210–9.
12. O'Connor D, Ferguson E, Green JA, O'Carroll RE, O'Connor RC. Cortisol levels and suicidal behavior: a meta-analysis. Psychoneuroendocrinology. 2016;63:370–9.
13. O'Connor D, Green JA, Ferguson E, O'Carroll RE, O'Connor RC. Cortisol reactivity and suicidal behavior: investigating the role of hypothalamic-pituitary-adrenal axis responses to stress in suicide attempters and ideators. Psychoneuroendocrinology. 2017;75:183–91.
14. Kao WT, Yang MC, Lung FW. Association between HTR1B alleles and suicidal ideation in individuals with major depressive disorder. Neurosci Lett. 2017;638:204–10.
15. Al Jurdi RK, Swann A, Mathew SJ. Psychopharmacological agent and suicide risk reduction: ketamine and other approaches. Curr Psychiatry Rep. 2015;17:81.
16. Pawlak J, Dmitrzak-Weglarz M, Wilkosc M, Szczepankiewicz A, Leszczynska-Rodziewicz A, Zaremba D, Kapelski P, Rajewska-Rager A, Hauser J. Suicidal behavior as a quantitative trait and its genetic background. J Affect Disord. 2016;206:241–50.
17. Lopez-Castroman J, Courtent P, Baca-Garcia E, Oquendo MA. Identification of suicide risk in bipolar disorder. Bipolar Disord. 2015;17:22–3.
18. Saunders KEA, Hawton K. Suicidal behavior in bipolar disorder: understanding the role of affective states. Bipolar Disord. 2015;17:24–6.
19. Courtet P, Jaussent I, Genty C, Dupuy AM, Guillaume S, Ducasse D, Olie E. Increased CRP levels may be a trait marker of suicidal attempt. Eur Neuropsychopharmacol. 2015;25:1824–31.
20. Wilson S, Megan C, Fertuck E, Keilp J, Brodsky B, Mann JJ, Sonmez CC, Benjamin-Phillips C, Stanley B. Hear rate variability and suicidal behavior. Psychiatry Res. 2016;240:241–7.
21. Bernert RA, Luckenbaugh DA, Duncan WC, Iwata NG, Ballard ED, Zarate CA. Sleep architecture parameters as a putative biomarker of suicidal ideation in treatment-resistant depression. J Affect Disord. 2017;208:309–15.
22. Rihmer Z, Gonda X. Pharmacological prevention of suicide in patients with major mood disorders. Neurosci Biobehav Rev. 2013;37:2398–403.

23. Kay DB, Drombrovski AY, Buysse DJ, Reynolds CF III, Begley A, Szanto K. Insomnia is associated with suicide attempt in middle aged and older adults with depression. Int Psychogeriatr. 2016;28(4):613–9.
24. Mallick F, McCullumsmith CB. Ketamine for treatment of suicidal ideation and reduction of risk for suicidal behavior. Curr Psychiatry Rep. 2016;18:61.
25. Berutti M, Silva Dias R, Alver Pereira V, Lafer B. Association between history of suicide attempts and family functioning in bipolar disorder. J Affect Disord. 2016;192:28–33.
26. Owen R, Gooding P, Dempsey R, Jones S. A qualitative investigation into the relationships between social factors and suicidal thoughts and acts experienced by people with a bipolar disorder diagnosis. J Affect Disord. 2015;176:133–40.
27. Perez S, Marco JH, Garcia-Alandete J. Psychopathological differences between suicide ideators and suicide attempters in patients with mental disorders. Clin Psychol Psychother. 2017;24(4):1002–13.
28. Klonsky ED, Qiu T, Saffer BY. Recent advances in differentiating suicide attempters from suicide ideators. Curr Opin Psychiatry. 2017;30:15–20.
29. Aaltonen K, Naatanen P, Heikkinen M, Koivistro M, Baryshnikov I, Karpov B, Oksanen J, Melartin T, Suominen K, Joffe G, Paunio T, Isometsa E. Differences and similarities of risk factors for suicidal ideation and attempts among patients with depressive or bipolar disorders. J Affect Disord. 2016;193:318–30.
30. Zalpuri I, Rothschild AJ. Does psychosis increase her risk of suicide in patients with major depression? A systematic review. J Affect Disord. 2016;198:23–31.
31. Bostwick JM, Pabbati C, Geske J, McKean AJ. Suicide attempt as a risk factor for completed suicide: even more lethal than we knew. Am J Psychiatry. 2016;173:11.
32. Conejero I, Lopez-Castroman J, Giner L, Baca-Garcia E. Social demographic antecedent valley dangers of suicidal behavior: a review of recent literature. Curr Psychiatry Rep. 2016;13:94.
33. Schaffer A, Isometsa ET, Azorin JM, et al. A review of factors associated with greater likelihood of suicide attempts and suicide deaths in bipolar disorder: part II of her report of the International Society for Bipolar Disorders Task Force on suicide in bipolar disorder. Aust N Z J Psychiatry. 2015;49(11):1006–20.
34. Mertz DG, Kelleci M, Mizrak A, Semiz M, Demir MO. Factors associated with suicide attempts in patients with bipolar disorder type I. Psychiatr Danub. 2015;27(3):236–41.
35. Seo HJ, Wang HR, Jun TY, Woo YS, Bahk WM. Factors related to suicidal behavior in patients with bipolar disorder: the effect of mixed features on suicidality. Gen Hosp Psychiatry. 2016;38:91–6.
36. Cremaschi L, Dell'Osso B, Vismara M, Dobrea C, Buoli M, Ketter TA, Altamura C. Onset polarity in bipolar disorder: a strong association between first depressive episode and suicide attempts. J Affect Disord. 2017;209:182–7.
37. Carvalho AF, McIntyre RS, Dimelis D, Gonda X, Berk M, Nunes-Neto PR, Cha DS, Hyphantis TN, Angst J, Fountoulakis KN. Predominant polarity is of course specifier for bipolar disorder, and a systematic review. J Affect Disord. 2014;163:56–64.
38. Zimmerman M, Martinez J, Young D, Chelminski I, Morgan T, Dalrymple K. Comorbid bipolar disorder and borderline personality disorder and history of suicide attempts. J Personal Disord. 2014;28(3):358–64.
39. Werbeloff N, Markou M, Hayes JF, Pitman AL, Osborn DPJ. Individual and area-level risk factors for suicidal ideation and attempt in people with severe depression. J Affect Disord. 2016;205:387–92.
40. Wakefield JC, Schmitz MF. Feelings of worthlessness during a single complicated major depressive episode predict postremission suicide attempt. Acta Psychiatr Scand. 2016;133(4):257–65.
41. Baek JH, Heo JY, Fava M, Mischoulon D, Nierenberg A, Hong JP, Roh S, Jeon HJ. Anxiety symptoms are linked to new-onset suicidal ideation after 6 months of follow-up in outpatients with major depressive disorder. J Affect Disord. 2015;187:183–7.
42. Ramberg M, Stanley B, Ystgaard M, Mehlum L. Depressed suicide attempters with posttraumatic stress disorder. Arch Suicide Res. 2015;19:48–59.

43. Carter J, Arentsen TJ, Cordova J, Ruzek J, Reiser R, Suppes T, Ostacher MJ. Increased suicidal ideation in patients with co-Oecurring bipolar disorder and post-traumatic stress disorder. Arch Suicide Res. 2016;0:1–12.
44. Aas M, Henry C, Belliver F, Lajnef M, Gard S, Kahn JP, Lagerberg TV, Aminoff SR, Bjella T, Leboyer M, Andreassen OA, Melle I, Etain B. Affective lability mediates the association between childhood trauma and suicide attempts, mixed episodes and co-morbid anxiety disorders in bipolar disorders. Psychol Med. 2017;47(5):902–12.
45. Lan WH, Bai YM, Hsu JW, Huang KL, Su TP, Li CT, Yang AC, Lin WC, Chang WH, Chen TJ, Tsai SJ, Chen MH. Comorbidity of ADHD and suicide attempts among adolescents and young adults with bipolar disorder: a nationwide longitudinal study. J Affect Disord. 2015;176:171–5.
46. Carra G, Bartoli F, Crocamo C, Brady KT, Clerici M. Attempted suicide in people with co-occurring bipolar and substance use disorder: systematic review and meta-analysis. J Affect Disord. 2014;167:125–35.
47. Oquendo MA, Currier D, Liu SM, Hasin DS, Grant BF, Blanco C. Increased risk for suicidal behavior in comorbid bipolar disorder and alcohol use disorder: results from the National Epidemiologic Survey on alcohol and related conditions (NESARC). Clin Psychiatry. 2010;71:902–9.
48. Ballard ED, Vande Voort JL, Luckenbaugh DA, Machado-Vieira R, Tohen M, Zarate CA. Acute risk factors for suicide attempts and death: prospective findings from the STEP-BD study. Bipolar Disord. 2016;18:363–72.
49. Jylha P, Rosenstrom T, Mantere O, Suominen K, Melartin T, Vuorilehto M, Holma M, Riihimaki K, Oquendo MA, Keltikangas-Jarvinen L, Isometsa ET. Personality disorders and suicide attempts in unipolar and bipolar mood disorders. J Affect Disord. 2016;190:632–9.
50. Frias A, Baltasar I, Birmaher B. Comorbidity between bipolar disorder and borderline personality disorder: prevalence, explanatory theories, and clinical impact. J Affect Disord. 2016;202:210–9.
51. Hawkins M, Schaffer A, Reis C, Sinyor M, Herrmann N, Lanctot KL. Suicide in males and females with cardiovascular disease and comorbid depression. J Affect Disord. 2016;197:88–93.
52. Lam RW, McIntosh D, Wang JL, Enns MW, Kolivakis T, Michalak E, Sareen J, Song WY, Kennedy SH, MacQueen G, Milev RV, Parikh SV, Ravindran AV, the CANMAT Depression Work Group. Canadian network for mood and anxiety treatments (CANMAT) 2016 clinical guidelines for the Management of Adults with major depressive disorder: section I. Disease burden and principles of care. Can J Psychiatr. 2016;61(9):510–23.
53. Stange JP, Kleiman EM, Sylvia LG, Vieira-da Silva P, Berk M, Nierenberg AA, Deckersbach T. Specific mood symptoms confer risk for subsequent suicidal ideation in bipolar disorder with and without suicide attempt history: multi-wave data from STEP-BD. Depress Anxiety. 2016;33:464–72.
54. Calvacante Passos I, Mwangi B, Cao B, Hamilton J, Wu MJ, Zhang XY, Zunta-Soares GB, Quevedo J, Kauer-Sant-Anna M, Kapczinski F, Soares J. Identifying a clinical signature of suicidality among patients with mood disorders: a pilot study using a machine learning approach. J Affect Disord. 2016;193:109–16.
55. Rudzinksi LA, Meadork JJ. Epilepsy: 5 new things. Neurology. 2011;76(7 Suppl 2) S20–S25.
56. Carnell BL, Clarke P, Gill S, Galletly CA. How effective is repetitive transcranial magnetic stimulation for bipolar depression? J Affect Disord. 2017;209:270–2.
57. George MS, Raman R, Benedek DM, et al. A two-site pilot randomized 3 day trial of high dose left prefrontal repetitive transcranial magnetic stimulation (rTMS) for suicidal inpatients. Brain Stimul. 2014;7:421–31.
58. Desmyter S, Duprat R, Baeken C, Bijttebier S, van Heeringen K. The acute effects of accelerated repetitive transcranial magnetic stimulation on suicide risk in unipolar depression: preliminary results. Psychiatr Danub. 2014;26(Suppl 1):48–52.
59. Sher L, Mindes J, Novakovic V. Transcranial magnetic stimulation and the treatment of suicidality. Expert Rev Neurother. 2010;10(12):1781–4.
60. Fink M, Kellner CH, Vaughn McCall W. The role of ECT in suicide prevention. J ECT. 2014;30:5–9.

61. Pflug B, Tolle R. Disturbance of the 24-hour rhythm in endogenous depression and the treatment of endogenous depression by sleep deprivation. Int Pharmacopsychiatry. 1971;6(3):187–96.
62. Nussbaumer B, Kaminski-Hartenthaler A, Forneris CA, et al. Light therapy for preventing seasonal affective disorder. Cochrane Database Syst Rev. 2015;11:CD011269.
63. Tuunainen A, Kripke DF, Endo T. Light therapy for non-seasonal depression. Cochrane Database Syst Rev. 2004;2:CD004050.
64. Al-Karawi D, Jubair L. Bright light therapy for nonseasonal depression: meta-analysis of clinical trials. J Affect Disord. 2016;198:64–71.
65. Benedetti F, Riccaboni R, Locatelli C, Poletti S, Dallaspezia S, Colombo C. Rapid treatment response of suicidal symptoms to lithium, sleep deprivation, and light therapy (chronotherapeutics) in drug-resistant bipolar depression. J Clin Psychiatry. 2014;75(2):133–40.
66. Martiny K, Refsgaard E, Lund V, et al. A 9-week randomized trial comparing a chronotherapeutic intervention (wake and light therapy) to exercise in major depressive disorder patients treated with duloxetine. J Clin Psychiatry. 2012;73(9):1234–42.

Psychosis and Suicide

3

Tatiana Falcone, Migle Staniskyte,
and Jane Timmons-Mitchell

Overview

According to the World Health Organization (WHO), approximately 21 million people around the world are affected by schizophrenia, a severe and debilitating mental health disorder [1]. This illness is characterized by three forms of symptoms: positive, negative, and cognitive [2]. The positive symptoms include behaviors that are not present in healthy individuals, such as delusions, referring to false beliefs, and hallucinations, involving any of the five senses (most commonly, hearing voices and seeing objects and people that are not authentic). Negative symptoms include intrusive characteristics that affect one's emotions, such as decreased interest and satisfaction in everyday activities, flat affect, and inability to focus. The cognitive factors include decreased executive functions and working memory.

The median incidence of schizophrenia was described as 15.2 people per 100,000 by McGrath and colleagues [3]. A meta-analysis by Saha et al. identified a 0.3%–2.0% lifetime risk of developing schizophrenia with the median prevalence of 4.6 people per 1000 [4]. Perhaps the most common indicator of developing this disorder is family history. According to twin studies by Cardno and Gottesman, the lifetime risk increases from 1% in the general population to 10% in first-degree relatives of

T. Falcone, M.D., M.P.H. (✉)
Epilepsy Center/ Psychiatry Department,
Neurological Institute - Cleveland Clinic, Cleveland, OH, USA
e-mail: falcont1@ccf.org

M. Staniskyte, B.A.
Neurologic Institute, Cleveland Clinic, Cleveland, OH, USA
e-mail: stanism2@ccf.org

J. Timmons-Mitchell, Ph.D.
Begun Center for Violence Prevention Research and Education, Jack, Joseph, and Morton Mandel School of Applied Sciences, School of Medicine, Case Western Reserve University, Cleveland, OH, USA
e-mail: jct2@case.edu

T. Falcone, J. Timmons-Mitchell (eds.), *Suicide Prevention*,
https://doi.org/10.1007/978-3-319-74391-2_3

patients with schizophrenia [5]. This same study identified lifetime risk to be 40% in twins and 50% in patients whose parents suffer from this disorder. Schizophrenia is generally more dominant in males than females (1.4 men:1 woman) [4, 6], who exhibit symptoms at a significantly earlier age than females according to a study by Zhang and colleagues [7].

The emotional and financial hardship of this chronic neuropsychological disorder has long been overlooked and underestimated. The Global Burden of Disease study conducted by WHO in 2000 revealed that mental illness accounts for 15% of the total burden of disease in the world economy [8]. In this study, schizophrenia was estimated to be the seventh leading cause of years lived with disability (YLD) at a global level. Moreover, a personal impact study of schizophrenia (conducted by the European Psychiatric Services: Inputs Linked to Outcome Domains and Needs—EPSILON) found that out of 404 schizophrenic patients, 80% of them were unemployed and 65% were single [9]. Patients with this disorder have a lower quality of life, with intense social, psychological, and emotional impact on individuals' coping with the illness and their families and acquaintances.

Suicide and Schizophrenia

Individuals suffering from schizophrenia are at elevated risk for suicidal ideation, behavior, and attempt. According to a Danish study, the risk of patients with schizophrenia completing a suicide is approximately 20 times higher than that of the general population [10]. A study in the USA found that patients suffering from schizophrenia spectrum disorders are 12 times more likely to die by suicide than individuals without the disorder [11]. Approximately 1/3 of individuals with schizophrenia will attempt suicide [12], and an estimated 10% will complete [13]. Pompili et al. suggest that suicidal intent in patients with schizophrenia is stronger and more lethal than that of patients without schizophrenia who think about suicide [14]. Symptoms of depression appear to be one of most important risk factors in patients with schizophrenia experiencing suicidal ideation.

Suicide and First-Episode Psychosis

Joa et al. indicated that there is a critical connection between early onset psychosis and suicide [15]. Population studies analyzing the standardized mortality rates conclude that patients with schizophrenia are more likely to die by suicide in the first 5 years of the illness [16]. Other studies comparing early psychosis with chronic schizophrenia found rates of death by suicide 2.7 times higher in first-episode psychosis (FEP) [17]. Patients with schizophrenia are more likely to exhibit self-injurious behavior (SIB), and SIB increases the risk for suicide in this population [18].

Among patients with schizophrenia, studies have suggested that the most sensitive time period for death by suicide is in the first 10 years after the onset of symptoms, with about 50% in the first 2 years following diagnosis [19]. This high-sensitivity period is often referred to as first-episode psychosis (FEP), or the early phases of the schizophrenia spectrum disorders. According to Palmer et al., rates of suicide in first-admission cohorts are about three times as high as in the patients with chronic schizophrenia [11]. In a Norwegian study of 170 patients aged 18–65, over 1/3 of patients with FEP had experienced suicidal ideation (38.8%), and over ¼ had attempted suicide (25.9%) [20]. In the study, more than half of the patients who had attempted suicide did so in the duration of untreated psychosis (DUP). Barrett and colleagues suggested that there is a direct correlation between continued DUP and elevated risk of suicide attempts [20]. A Danish study also found suicide was highest during the first inpatient stay and after a recent discharge from the hospital [10]. In a meta-analysis by Melle and Barrett, 14–28% of individuals with first-episode psychosis attempted suicide before entering their first treatment [21].

A limited number of studies have assessed first-episode psychosis and suicide in the child and adolescent population. In a retrospective chart review of adolescent patients (12–18 years) with first-episode psychosis (FEP), 31% of patients attempted suicide. The rate of repeated attempts was higher than for adults with FEP [22].

Risk Factors

The identification of risk factors for suicidality in schizophrenia is of great interest to help decrease the risk of mortality by suicide. Some of the most common risk factors identified in patients with schizophrenia include early onset of schizophrenia, depressive symptoms, male gender, insight into the illness, high level of education, and positive symptoms.

Special risk factors were also identified in adolescents with psychosis like high IQ, and patients with more insight were more likely to feel depressed when they started feeling the impact of the psychosis in their life and their inability to perform previous roles to their full potential. Compared with the general population, adolescents who are diagnosed with schizophrenia are 70 times more likely to attempt suicide [23].

Other important risk factors include low self-esteem, hopelessness, agitation, and history of a previous suicide attempt. In patients with FEP, the presence of positive symptoms such as command hallucinations, depressive symptoms, and negative beliefs about psychosis including the fear of mental disintegration, isolation, impaired functioning, or inability of return to previous role impacted the ability of the patient to cope with the illness and increased the risk of suicide.

The duration of untreated psychosis, or poor adherence to treatment, is also an important risk factor for suicide in schizophrenia. The Opus trial [24] tracked suicidal ideation in a cohort of 547 adult patients aged 18–45; it helps us understand the trajectory of suicidal ideation in patients with schizophrenia. Researchers were able identify three groups. The first group was classified as Low Decreasing and included 61% of the cohort. Low Decreasing patients thought about suicide a couple of times before their recruitment to the study. During the next 2 years, this group reported no suicidal ideation. The second group was called Frequent Stable (33%). The Frequent Stable patients reported suicidal ideation many times in the year before the study recruitment. In the 2 years after recruitment, they continued to have suicidal ideation. The third group was designated as Frequent Increasing (6%). The Frequent Increasing patients had chronic suicidal ideation that increased over time. During the 2-year follow-up period, their suicidal ideation continued to increase from often to very often. Important characteristics identified in this group were more likely to be women, previous history of suicide attempt, and presence of hallucinations during the initial evaluation [24].

Protective Factors

The Centers for Disease Control and Prevention (CDC) lists the following protective factors which can mitigate the risks of suicide [25]:

Family and community support (connectedness)
Cultural and religious beliefs that discourage suicide and support instincts for self-preservation
Skills in problem solving and conflict resolution and nonviolent ways of handling disputes
Easy access to a variety of clinical interventions and support for help seeking
Effective clinical care for mental, physical, and substance abuse disorders and having a positive attitude toward treatment
Support from ongoing medical and mental health care relationship

Jill Harkavy-Friedman of the American Foundation for Suicide Foundation [26] adds additional factors, including having reasons for living, such as having someone/something to care for, like a child or a pet, and decreased access to lethal means.

Connectedness can include many categories. Of course interpersonal connectedness, with family and friends, is desirable. Studies have shown that people who are married or in long-term relationships have lower rates of suicide, especially among men. Among people with psychosis, social relationships are likely to suffer. Marriages and long-term relationships are frequently disrupted [27]. Families often remain involved. If families are accepting, inclusive, flexible, and calm, they can provide a buffer for the psychotic person as well as an atmosphere of unconditional support. For many families, the caregiver burden of having a family member with psychosis is so great that these bonds are strained. The National Alliance on Mental Illness (NAMI, www.nami.org) was formed to provide support for families struggling with the demands of caring for a psychotic relative.

Belonging to a faith community can provide structure for connectedness which is often lacking among psychotic people. Faith communities have many advantages for the mentally ill [28]. They are accessible in the communities where people live. They are welcoming, although there may be different levels of tolerance from one community to the next. Activities occur frequently and are generally free. Importantly, a person receives thanks from others for participation. Perhaps for these reasons, the World Health Organization (WHO) considers religion and spirituality as important contributors to quality of life overall [29]. Studies have shown that they are indeed important in promoting the quality of life for schizophrenic patients [30].

In the resilience literature, research has determined that children who are uniquely good at something (i.e., recognized by their peers and teachers) are less likely to succumb to a variety of stressors, including behavioral and emotional disorders [31]. Some children are recognized for being good athletes; others exhibit artistic or musical ability. Some children are good in math. Each of these strengths creates an avenue to pursue belonging that can buffer against adverse experiences. Those who are good in math are likely to finish school and to be employed. Employment is a protective factor since it helps structure the day, provides income, and allows for social interaction with co-workers. Earning a paycheck is a primary contributor to self-esteem, since it is a tangible recognition that one is a contributing member of society. Those who are good athletes can join teams where they develop positive peer relationships while learning structure and goal-directed problem solving. Cooperation is rewarded with better athletic performance, which enhances self-esteem. Those who have artistic or musical ability can contribute to creating beauty in the environment, enhancing worship, or performing as part of a group. Research shows that music lessons help to train the brain in focusing and improved impulse control, both of which could mitigate the effects of psychosis on the impulse of suicide [32].

Perhaps the single most important protective factor for suicide in psychotic people is restricting access to lethal means. Most suicides result from impulsive acts [33]; among psychotic people, this is even more strongly the case. If nothing is readily available, the likelihood that a person will complete suicide decreases dramatically [34].

Restricting access to guns is an important step in reducing suicides. Whereas most people who attempt suicide using a gun die from their injuries (Over 80%), most people attempting suicide using other means (at least in the USA) do not complete suicide. A 2013 study [35] shows that there is a significant difference in gun deaths, with states having strict gun laws having fewer suicides than those with lax gun laws. At one point, persons with severe mental illness were restricted from purchasing guns; however, that regulation has been overturned [36]. The combination of impulsivity, judgment that is strained by illness and possibly non-compliance with medication, and the presence of a gun is often lethal for persons with psychosis.

Assessment

Because the risk of suicide is great among patients with psychosis, it is important to screen and assess for suicide risk. Ideally, screening would occur at each encounter, to be followed by full assessment as needed, as is done in the protocol for the Veterans Administration (VA). In a comprehensive effort to prevent veteran suicides, the VA has established a rigorous protocol to identify and refer veterans at risk of suicide for further services: at every contact with the VA, veterans are given the PHQ-2 followed by the PHQ-9 if needed [37]. The Substance Abuse and Mental Health Services Administration (SAMHSA) has developed a pocket card outlining the steps in suicide assessment.

Screening Measures

In addition to the PHQ-2 and PHQ-9, which are described in the chapter on Primary Care Behavioral Health, and the ASQ and other measures described in the chapter on Youth Suicide, the SBQ-R (Suicidal Behaviors Questionnaire-Revised) is listed on the SAMHSA website as a good screening tool for suicide among patients with psychosis [38]. The SBQ-R has been validated on clinical and nonclinical samples of adolescents and adults, in both inpatient and outpatient settings. The four items of the SBQ-R assess different dimensions of suicide potential, including lifetime suicide ideation and/or attempt, frequency of suicidal ideation in the past 12 months, threat of suicide attempt, and self-reported likelihood of future suicidal behavior. Among psychiatric inpatients, 1/3 of whom had been diagnosed with schizophrenia, the sensitivity of the scale (true-positive rate) was 80% and the specificity was 91% (true-negative rate).

Two scales have been developed specifically to assess suicide among schizophrenic patients [39]. One of these, the SSRS (the Schizophrenia Suicide Risk Scale), was developed from knowledge about the use of other screening measures with schizophrenic patients [40]. Schizophrenic patients who completed suicide were paired with schizophrenic patients who had not completed suicide. Although the design of the study was good, the resulting sensitivity of the scale at 32% is low, meaning that only about 1/3 of schizophrenic patients who are at high risk for suicide are correctly identified by the scale.

Other standard scales are sometimes used to assess suicidality in schizophrenia, with mixed results. Kasckow et al. [41] report a number of studies that have employed scales including the HAM-D (Hamilton Rating Scale for Depression), the CDRS (Calgary Depression Rating Scale), and the PANSS (Positive and Negative Syndrome Scale), coupled with CGI (Clinical Global Impression), to assess change in depression with the addition of different psychotropic medications. In two double-blind placebo-controlled studies, citalopram was found to be superior in reducing depressive and suicidal symptoms [42, 43]. The dependent variable was HAM-D score greater than 7.

Assessment Measures

The C-SSRS (Columbia Suicide Severity Rating Scale) assessment process includes both a screener and a guided interview format if the results of screening are positive. Often referred to as the "gold standard" of suicide assessment, the Columbia has been used with thousands of patients in a wide variety of settings [44]. The initial Columbia administration establishes lifetime prevalence, while subsequent administrations ask about incidents since the last time the measure was administered.

The Columbia has been integrated into clinics treating psychotic patients. Administration helps staff feel more confident and delivers good care to patients. In California, since 2010, the Columbia has been used to guide care for first-episode psychosis (FEP) patients in four countywide clinics [45]. As part of usual care, all clinicians are trained in the C-SSRS, so that they can document findings in the medical chart and review outcomes as part of ongoing evaluation. Niendam reports that, while clinicians are at first apprehensive and observe that including the C-SSRS adds time to the assessment, after conducting it, they are excited and confident and notice additional ways which including the Columbia can benefit their patients.

The Columbia has been included in research with subclinical samples of young adults, in which both psychosis and suicide were assessed to be salient "trans diagnostic clinical causes... that do not cause one another."

The second scale, the InterSePT Suicide Scale (ISST) [46], was developed as part of the multisite InterSePT study group on schizophrenia. The ISST scale with the previously developed Scale for Suicidal Ideation [47], a 19-item interview screener, adapted as a self-report measure and called the Beck Scale for Suicide Ideation (BSI). Pinninti et al. [48] used the BSI to determine suicide risk in patients, over 2/3 of whom were diagnosed as having schizophrenic or schizoaffective disorders. Higher scores on the measure were strongly related to having been admitted for and/or having made a previous suicide attempt.

The ISST was developed while studying which medications would more successfully prevent suicidal behavior in high-risk schizophrenic and schizoaffective patients [49]. In constructing the ISST, the BSI was used as a point of departure, deleting redundant items and those that did not correlate strongly with predicting suicidality. The resulting 12 items are administered in a semi-structured interview lasting between 20 and 30 min, which is why this is categorized as an assessment measure. Following the establishment of good interrater reliability ($\kappa = 0.90$), convergent validity was established with a number of other measures. The Calgary Depression Scale, the Positive and Negative Symptom Scale, the Scale of Functioning, and the Extrapyramidal Symptom Rating Scale were administered, and an adaptation of Clinical Global Impression for Severity of Suicidality (CGI-SS) was conducted. A factor analysis was conducted that explained over half of the variance using a three factor solution; of interest, the three factors are similar to those found in the original BSS. Additional convergent validity was established in the Ayer et al. [50] study; the ISST and the Calgary Depression Scale showed similarly high levels of specificity. Using an intricate design, the ISST was able to demonstrate discriminant validity for patients who either made a suicide attempt or were hospitalized to prevent an attempt relative to those who did not throughout the 2-year duration of the study.

Treatment

The aim for the psychiatrist treating a patient with schizophrenia should be to manage the psychotic symptoms as early as possible. Frequently assess for the ability of the patient to control the positive symptoms; at every visit assess for suicide, and if the patient is reporting any suicidal thoughts, refer to the appropriate level of care. If the patient is going to be managed in the community, intensive case management and close follow-up are required. The aim of the treatment should be to increase social support; teach the patient and family about positive coping skills [19].

If the patient is admitted to the hospital for acute suicidal thoughts, certain measures can be put into place to prevent suicide during the hospitalization. Optimizing pharmacotherapy is primary. The patient might need to be in direct 1:1 supervision until they are able to contract for safety. If the patient is clearly psychotic and internally stimulated, group participation is unlikely until symptoms are more in control. There are important comorbidities to take into account when treating patients with schizophrenia. Substance abuse is one: reviewing the results of urine toxicology to assess the need for further substance abuse treatment is key. It is also important to take extra measures to ensure that the patient is cooperating with the medication plan. Patients may question the importance of medication and choose not to take their medication. Since medication adherence is of primary importance, psychoeducation with the patient and family can improve medication adherence [51, 52].

Early Intervention

There is evidence that early intervention and early detection of psychotic symptoms will reduce the suicidal risk; we will review some of the early intervention programs [53]. In the last 20 years, research in the field of schizophrenia has provided evidence to understand the pathophysiology of this illness. The earlier patients with psychosis are identified and treated, the better the prognosis. Strategies in early intervention programs focus on identifying patients early and implementing treatment early, which will improve symptom treatment and decrease worsening of the disease. Strategies evaluated by the early intervention programs include medication management using antipsychotic medications, family interventions, psychoeducation for the patient and family, and programs to help decrease the stigma of schizophrenia among the general population. Some authors describe early intervention as the key to prevent chronic disability in schizophrenia. Some programs target duration of untreated psychosis as a measure of the effectiveness of an intervention program.

Early intervention programs have progressively grown around the world in the last 20 years. The first programs were established in Australia and in the UK and then expanded to Germany, the USA, Canada, Scandinavia, and Switzerland. The goal of some programs is to improve the capacity of local existing community mental health. Other programs use the "hub and spoke" model, where the hub is the core central specialist service that supports all the resources and services needed in each individual car. Case management and psychoeducation play a key role in managing patients with schizophrenia. The more the patient knows about the prognosis, importance of treatment, and signs of relapse, the more likely it will be that the patient will actively participate in treatment.

One of the pioneer programs on early intervention was Orygen Youth Health in Melbourne, Australia. This program started in the 1980s and later became the Early Psychosis Prevention and Intervention Center (EPPIC). It was attached to a psychiatric hospital but was focused on helping patients with first-episode psychosis. In 1992, the treatment was transported to the community, and several outpatient clinics were established to provide community-focused service, home-based treatment, and intensive case management. Another important goal of the program was to increase community awareness and decrease stigma about psychosis. The principles of this program include focusing on early intervention and providing early assessment and treatment. Interventions are clinically staged to the illness. The program is youth-friendly, stigma-free, and patient centered. The main goal is to help the patient and the family feel empowered and to be an active part of their treatment team. Studies demonstrating the effectiveness of the approach contributed to its becoming an evidence-based practice; it has spread around the world. Despite all the efforts, the suicide rate for patients with schizophrenia has not decreased, and the Orygen group also is setting up new strategies for suicide prevention.

In 2008, NIMH funded the North American Prodromal Longitudinal study, which includes several centers investigating the role of early detection and early intervention in North America. The project RAISE (Recovery After an Initial Schizophrenia Episode) is a large-scale program evaluating the role of coordinated care for the treatment of early psychosis [54]. To date, the results are similar to the Orygen program: it is very important to focus efforts on early detection and intervention in psychosis. RAISE has also demonstrated that coordinated specialty care can be delivered in the community and can be very effective. The goals of RAISE are to decrease relapse, prevent future psychotic episodes, reduce long-term disability, and help patients with schizophrenia get their lives back so they can effectively fulfill their goals.

Cognitive Behavioral Therapy

Cognitive behavioral therapy (CBT) is a therapeutic approach that has been widely used for the past several decades in order to effectively treat various psychiatric disorders. This therapeutic method is based on the concept that negative cognitions influence emotional stability and behaviors [55]. CBT has been employed with schizophrenia patients, especially those with first-episode psychosis, and has shown promise. Bateman et al. looked at whether CBT changes the level of suicidal ideation in patients with schizophrenia [56]. Using the Comprehensive Psychopathological Rating Scale (CPRS) as a tracking measure, their study showed a significant decrease in suicidal ideation at 9 months follow-up.

A meta-analysis by Zimmerman et al. suggested that CBT substantially lowers the positive signs of schizophrenia (i.e., hallucinations and delusions) and has also been shown to help individuals suffering from a brief psychotic episode [57]. In a study by Startup et al., TAU (treatment as usual) was compared with TAU plus CBT in patients with acute psychotic episodes [58]. Ratings of symptoms and social functioning at baseline and at 6 and 12 months revealed more improvement for the condition that included CBT.

In a randomized controlled trial comparing a cognitive behavioral treatment protocol for patients with psychosis (CBSPp) and treatment as usual (TAU), patients randomized into the CBSPp group showed significantly greater improvement on measures of suicidal ideation and suicide probability [59]; however, in another multicenter study when CBT was compared to TAU, positive advantages in symptoms and recovery time were shown, but no differences for hospitalization or relapse rates were seen [60].

Multisystemic Therapy-Psychiatric

Multisystemic Therapy-Psychiatric (MST-P) is a variant of Multisystemic Therapy. MST-P has been listed as a promising practice by the Suicide Prevention Resource Center (SPRC) and as an evidence-based practice on NREPP (SAMHSA's National Registry of Evidence Based Programs and Practices). In studies of MST-P which included youth with thought disorders, decreases in suicide attempts have been reported. MST-P is one of the few evidence-based treatments for youth with psychosis.

MST is a family- and community-based intervention that uses intense contact with families to understand the functional basis of behavioral problems. Strengths of the youth and family are used to address challenges. A goal of treatment is to teach parents the skills needed to supervise and monitor youth so that additional services are not usually needed. MST provides service delivery at home and in the community 24 h a day, 7 days a week according to the needs of the family. Length of treatment usually ranges between 3 and 5 months; however, unlike other home-based models, there is no prescribed length of service. MST therapists focus on empowering parents to develop natural support systems and remove barriers to improve their effectiveness as parents. By working with parents, teachers, coaches, leaders of faith communities, and others, MST aims to restructure a youth's ecology to support prosocial development and decrease delinquent behavior. Intervention development is guided by an analytic process that reflects the nine principles that serve to operationalize MST. The nine principles that guide MST intervention development are detailed in previous publications (e.g., see [61]).

MST-P was developed because of the prevalence of severe mental health needs in the adolescent population referred. Some of the strategies used to reduce the risk of self-harm include in-home safety assessment and safety planning to eliminate risks for self-harm, increased eyes on supervision of youth by family members, decreased contact with peers and activities that may be triggers for self-harm, and increased empowerment of adults to structure youth activities. Strategies used by MST-P to address serious psychiatric illness include integrating psychiatrists into the treatment team, integrating evidence-based psychiatric interventions, and training therapists to assess for psychiatric problems and coordinate with psychiatrists.

Staffing of an MST-P team includes a full-time crisis case worker and a part-time child psychiatrist. Therapists receive additional training in how to effectively address safety with suicidal and psychotic behavior, how to recognize and treat psychiatric issues, and how to recognize and treat substance use problems.

MST-P was first evaluated in a study funded by the National Institute of Mental Health (NIMH) published in 1999 [62]. A second randomized clinical trial was published in 2004 [63]. In randomized clinical trials, MST-P assessed both mental health needs, including thought disorders, using the Global Severity Index of the Brief Symptom Index (GSI-BSI). Suicide attempts were assessed using a single item taken from the Youth Risk Behavior Survey (YRBS) which asks how many times the youth attempted suicide in the past 12 months ("How many times did you actually attempt suicide?"). Responses range from 0 (0 times) to 4 (6 or more times). One study found that MST-P was more effective in reducing self-reported suicide attempts ($p < 0.001$) than the comparison group of youth who were hospitalized briefly to address suicide attempts [62]. Youth in the MST Psychiatric condition were much also less likely ($p < 0.001$) to be rehospitalized (57%) and, if they were hospitalized, had fewer days of hospitalization (72%) compared with youth who were hospitalized and released 1–2 weeks later. MST-P also reduced the number of days in out of home placement by 49%. According to the SPRC, "The treatment provided greater and more rapid reductions in suicide attempts than hospitalization. There were no significant differences for suicidal ideation."

Medications

In the management of acute psychosis, hospitalization may be needed, particularly at the initial stage. Patients are often agitated and unable to take care of themselves. The treatment of acute psychotic symptoms is antipsychotic medication. Managing patients in acute psychosis can be very challenging; if the agitation is severe, the patient may have to be physically restrained to protect against themselves and for the safety of others. Antipsychotic medications (either first or second generation) are the gold standard treatment for the management of psychosis. It is important to gather all medical history from previous treatments so that allergic reaction to previous treatment (acute dystonic reaction) is identified. In the initial stages of the treatment, the combination of the antipsychotic with anticholinergic medications (benztropine) and/or benzodiazepines (such as lorazepam or clonazepam) may be indicated for acute management of the psychotic episode.

The primary goal in the first psychotic episode is the remission of the psychotic symptoms; medication should always be titrated slowly to decrease the risk of adverse side effects [64]. After the initial symptoms are controlled, some studies report that low doses of the same medication can be effective in preventing relapse [65, 66]. Psychoeducation is key to explain to the patient and family the role of medication, the nature and course of the illness, and the risk of relapse if the medication is stopped. Studies about discontinuation of the medication after the resolution of the psychotic symptoms in patients with schizophrenia is very controversial, because of the high risk of relapse [67]. The relapse rate reported in the first year after medication discontinuation can be up to 78% and by the end of the second year increased up to 98% [65].

The Clinical Antipsychotic Trial of Intervention Effectiveness (CATIE) is one of the landmark studies on the treatment of schizophrenia in the real world. CATIE helped us understand that effectiveness for first-generation and second-generation antipsychotics is very similar. Many patients on the first-generation antipsychotics discontinued treatment secondary to side effects: metabolic side effects for patients on olanzapine was an important reason for discontinuation [68]. In the follow-up study when patients failed to improve with the atypical antipsychotic, those who tried clozapine reported better control of symptoms compared to other antipsychotics [69]. A similar study was performed in the UK, the Cost Utility of the Latest Antipsychotic Drugs in Schizophrenia Study (CUtLASS). Conclusions were similar to those of CATIE: no substantial difference between first- or second-generation antipsychotics in the quality of life of patients with schizophrenia was found [70].

After the symptoms are controlled, maintaining good engagement with the patient and the family, including ongoing psychoeducation about the need for ongoing treatment, is key [71]. Psychopharmacologic treatment is the cornerstone to preventing suicide in schizophrenia, since decreasing the psychotic symptoms gives the patient more control over delusions and suicidal thoughts and behavior. In a study evaluating patients with schizophrenia who died by suicide, more than half were either under-medicated or noncompliant with their medication; interestingly, 23% of the sample were treatment-resistant schizophrenia [72]. Treatment-resistant schizophrenia is defined as patients who failed to respond to at least two adequate trials of antipsychotics for at least 6 weeks and have poor social and occupational functioning.

Meltzer and collaborators studied 1000 patients with schizophrenia and schizoaffective disorder who reported suicidal thoughts and concluded that clozapine was more effective in decreasing suicidality in this population than olanzapine [49]. Clozapine continues to be underutilized, perhaps due to side effects of agranulocytosis, seizures, and myocarditis for some patients [73]. In a recent meta-analysis of 21 randomized controlled studies (2364 patients) using clozapine for treatment-resistant schizophrenia, the authors concluded that clozapine was superior for treatment-refractory schizophrenia. However, if no signs of clinical response were evident by 6 months, other medications should be considered [74].

Despite advances in psychopharmacology and the proven effectiveness of antipsychotic medications, most patients will have residual symptoms (some of them negative symptoms, some of them positive symptoms, some cognitive deficits). Many patients are unable to return to previous levels of functioning after the first psychotic episode. Psychosocial interventions are key to helping the patient regain as much social and occupational functioning as possible. Even those who achieve good remission of the psychotic symptoms are at increased risk of attempting suicide: the realization that the illness will have a lasting impact on their life stresses already strained coping mechanisms. Programs that focus on helping the patient to access all their basic needs, such as care coordination, are important. If the patient is unable to return to the previous level of functioning, training in vocational skills can be beneficial [75].

Family communication, and how the family copes and interacts with the patient, should be a focus of treatment. Adverse family environment (expressed emotion) is one of the bigger predictors of relapse in schizophrenia. The major characteristics of communication patterns in families with EE include highly critical, hostile, and emotionally overinvolved; intense, with multiple negative exchanges; and oppositionality. In the 1950s, after the first studies using chlorpromazine to treat schizophrenia were published, George Brown and collaborators examined the reasons for readmission to the hospital following discharge [76]. Brown's group concluded that the type of family communication in the home to which the patient was discharged had a strong effect on relapse as cause of readmission; families exhibiting patterns of EE had higher readmission rates than other families.

Researchers evaluating critical comments during the interview with patient and family reported that the interaction observed in the office is normally reflective of the interaction at home. High EE caregivers tend to react more negatively toward the negative symptoms of schizophrenia, exhibiting more frustration and anger about patients who are isolated, not engaging with the family or in their own personal care, and not participating in chores in the house.

Some interventions have focused on psychosocial strategies to reduce EE by educating the caregiver to reduce high EE. Interventions are based on teaching the patient and the family about schizophrenia, how to manage crisis, problem solving skills, debunking myths, decreasing stigma, and how to provide appropriate emotional support. In a crucial study by Goldstein et al., a 6-week therapy focused on teaching families effective communication skills and problem solving skills. Families who improved on these skills had patients who displayed reduced relapse rates for up to 6 months [77]. Others were able to replicate similar findings.

Conclusion

Among the 21 million people in the world with schizophrenia, the risk of suicide is high. Some studies indicate that about ¼ of schizophrenics will attempt suicide, while others place the estimate higher. There is agreement that the time between diagnosis and engagement with evidence-based treatment for FEP is a time of high risk for suicide. Risk factors for suicide among people with psychosis include very-early-onset schizophrenia, depressive symptoms, male gender, insight into the illness, high level of education, positive symptoms, and duration of illness. Protective factors include problem solving skills, having a positive attitude and connection to treatment, being connected to others, participating in a faith community, and having responsibility, like taking care of a pet.

Several evidence-based intervention strategies provide hope for the best possible outcome. Connecting with treatment providers early after the discovery of psychosis is key, as is working with a psychiatrist to find the most helpful medication regimen. Evidence-based treatments are comprehensive in scope. Three are discussed in the chapter: Early Psychosis Prevention and Intervention Center (EPPIC) which began in Australia, cognitive behavioral therapy (CBT) for suicide in psychosis, and Multisystemic Therapy-Psychiatric. These interventions target aspects of psychotic symptoms that place patients at greater risk of suicide, including sequencing behavior and interrupting the sequence of action that flows from a cognitive reaction to a behavior. Despite the risks, many patients with schizophrenia can learn to manage symptoms associated with suicidality.

References

1. World Health Organization. Schizophrenia: fact sheet. 2016. http://www.who.int/mediacentre/factsheets/fs397/en/.
2. National Institute of Mental Health. Schizophrenia. 2017. https://www.nimh.nih.gov/health/publications/schizophrenia-booklet/index.shtml.
3. McGrath J, Saha S, Chant D, Welham J. Schizophrenia: a concise overview of incidence, prevalence, and mortality. Epidemiol Rev. 2008;30(1):67–76.
4. Saha S, Chant D, Welham J, McGrath J. A systematic review of the prevalence of schizophrenia. PLoS Med. 2005;2(5):e141.
5. Cardno AG, Gottesman II. Twin studies of schizophrenia: from bow-and-arrow concordances to star wars Mx and functional genomics. Am J Med Genet. 2000;97(1):12–7.
6. McGrath J, Saha S, Welham J, El Saadi O, MacCauley C, Chant D. A systematic review of the incidence of schizophrenia: the distribution of rates and the influence of sex, urbanicity, migrant status and methodology. BMC Med. 2004;2(1):13.
7. Zhang XY, Chen DC, Xiu MH, Yang FD, Haile CN, Kosten TA, et al. Gender differences in never-medicated first-episode schizophrenia and medicated chronic schizophrenia patients. J Clin Psychiatry. 2012;73(7):1025–33.
8. Mathers CD, Stein C, Ma Fat D, Rao C, Inoue M, Tomijima N, et al. Global Burden of Disease 2000: version 2 methods and results. Geneva: World Health Organization; 2002. http://www.who.int/healthinfo/paper50.pdf
9. Wijngaarden van B, Schene AH, Koeter M, Vazquez-Barquero JL, Knudsen HC, Lasalvia A, et al. Caregiving in schizophrenia: development, internal consistency and reliability of the Involvement Evaluation Questionnaire-European Version. Br J Psychiatry. 2000;77(39):s21–7.
10. Nordentoft M, Laursen TM, Agerbo E, Qin P, Høyer EH, Mortensen PB. Change in suicide rates for patients with schizophrenia in Denmark, 1981–97: nested case-control study. BMJ. 2004;329(7460):261.
11. Palmer BA, Pankratz VS, Bostwick JM. The lifetime risk of suicide in schizophrenia: a reexamination. Arch Gen Psychiatry. 2005;62(3):247–53.
12. Andreasen NC, Black DW, editors. Introductory textbook of psychiatry. 4th ed. Arlington: American Psychiatric Publishing; 2006.
13. Siris SG. Suicide and schizophrenia. J Psychopharmacol. 2001;15(2):127–35.
14. Pompili M, Mancinelli I, Tatarelli R. Suicide and schizophrenia. Psych Serv. 2003;54(5):747–8.
15. Joa I, Johannessen JO, Langeveld J, Friis S, Melle I, Opjordsmoen S, et al. Baseline profiles of adolescent vs. adult-onset first-episode psychosis in an early detection program. Acta Psychiatr Scand. 2009;119(6):494–500.
16. Munk-Jørgensen P, Mortensen PB. Social outcome in schizophrenia: a 13-year follow-up. Soc Psychiatry Psychiatr Epidemiol. 1992;27(3):129–34.
17. Brown S. Excess mortality of schizophrenia: a meta-analysis. Br J Psychiatry. 1997;171(6):502–8.
18. Haw C, Hawton K, Sutton L, Sinclair J, Deeks J. Schizophrenia and deliberate self-harm: a systematic review of risk factors. Suicide Life Threat Behav. 2005;35(1):50–62.
19. Montross LP, Zisook S, Kasckow J. Suicide among patients with schizophrenia: a consideration of risk and protective factors. Ann Clin Psychiatry. 2005;17(3):173–82.

20. Barrett EA, Sundet K, Faerden A, Nesvåg R, Agartz I, Fosse R, et al. Suicidality before and in the early phases of first episode psychosis. Schizophr Res. 2010;119(1):11–7.
21. Melle I, Ann Barrett E. Insight and suicidal behavior in first-episode schizophrenia. Expert Rev Neurother. 2012;12(3):353–9.
22. Falcone T, Mishra L, Carlton E, Lee C, Butler R, Janigro D, et al. Suicidal behavior in adolescents with first-episode psychosis. Clin Schizophr Relat Psychoses. 2010;4(1):34–40.
23. Kelleher I, Corcoran P, Keeley H, Wigman JT, Devlin N, Ramsay H, et al. Psychotic symptoms and population risk for suicide attempt: a prospective cohort study. JAMA Psychiat. 2013;70(9):940–8.
24. Madsen T, Karstoft KI, Secher RG, Austin SF, Nordentoft M. Trajectories of suicidal ideation in patients with first-episode psychosis: secondary analysis of data from the OPUS trial. Lancet Psychiatry. 2016;3(5):443–50.
25. US Public Health Service. The Surgeon General's call to action to prevent suicide. Washington, DC: US Department of Health and Human Services; 1999. http://www.surgeongeneral.gov/library/calltoaction/default.htm
26. Harkavy-Friedman J. Suicide risk among people with psychosis: focus on first episode. SAMHSA sponsored webinar; June 28, 2016. https://www.nasmhpd.org/content/part-i-recognizing-suicidal-ideation-and-behavior-individuals-first-episode-psychosis.
27. Bilsker D, White J. The silent epidemic of male suicide. B C Med J. 2011;53(10):529–34.
28. Grover S, Davuluri T, Chakrabarti S. Religion, spirituality, and schizophrenia: a review. Indian J Psychol Med. 2014;36(2):119–24.
29. Culliford L. Spirituality and clinical care: spiritual values and skills are increasingly recognised as necessary aspects of clinical care. BMJ. 2002;325(7378):1434–6.
30. Shah R, Kulhara P, Grover S, Kumar S, Malhotra R, Tyagi S. Contribution of spirituality to quality of life in patients with residual schizophrenia. Psychiatry Res. 2011;190(2):200–5.
31. Cowen EL, Wyman PA, Work WC. Resilience in highly stressed urban children: concepts and findings. Bull N Y Acad Med. 1996;73(2):267–84.
32. Kraus N, Chandrasekaran B. Music training for the development of auditory skills. Nat Rev Neurosci. 2010;11(8):599–605.
33. Simon TR, Swann AC, Powell KE, Potter LB, Kresnow MJ, O'Carroll PW. Characteristics of impulsive suicide attempts and attempters. Suicide Life Threat Behav. 2001;32:49–59.
34. Nock MK, Borges G, Bromet EJ, Cha CB, Kessler RC, Lee S. Suicide and suicidal behavior. Epidemiol Rev. 2008;30(1):133–54.
35. Fleegler EW, Lee LK, Monuteaux MC, Hemenway D, Mannix R. Firearm legislation and firearm-related fatalities in the United States. JAMA Intern Med. 2013;173(9):732–40.
36. Barrett T. House rolls back Obama gun background check rule. CNN Politics. 3 Feb 2017. http://www.cnn.com/2017/02/02/politics/house-vote-guns-mental-illnesses/.
37. Sundararaman R, Panangala SV, Lister SA. Suicide prevention among veterans: congressional research service report to Congress. Congressional Research Service: Washington, DC; 2008.
38. Osman A, Bagge CL, Gutierrez PM, Konick LC, Kopper BA, Barrios FX. The Suicidal Behaviors Questionnaire-Revised (SBQ-R): validation with clinical and nonclinical samples. Assessment. 2001;8(4):443–54.
39. Preston E, Hansen L. A systematic review of suicide rating scales in schizophrenia. Crisis. 2005;26(4):170–80.
40. Taiminen T, Huttunen J, Heilä H, Henriksson M, Isometsä E, Kähkönen J, et al. The Schizophrenia Suicide Risk Scale (SSRS): development and initial validation. Schizophr Res. 2001;47(2):199–213.
41. Kasckow J, Felmet K, Zisook S. Managing suicide risk in patients with schizophrenia. CNS Drugs. 2011;25(2):129–43.
42. Zisook S, Kasckow JW, Lanouette NM, Golshan S, Fellows I, Vahia I, et al. Augmentation with citalopram for suicidal ideation in middle-aged and older outpatients with schizophrenia and schizoaffective disorder who have subthreshold depressive symptoms: a randomized controlled trial. J Clin Psychiatry. 2010;71(7):915–22.

43. Zisook S, Kasckow JW, Golshan S, Fellows I, Solorzano E, Lehman D, et al. Citalopram augmentation for subsyndromal symptoms of depression in middle-aged and older outpatients with schizophrenia and schizoaffective disorder: a randomized controlled trial. J Clin Psychiatry. 2009;70(4):562–71.
44. Posner K, Brown GK, Stanley B, Brent DA, Yershova KV, Oquendo MA, et al. The Columbia–Suicide Severity Rating Scale: initial validity and internal consistency findings from three multisite studies with adolescents and adults. Am J Psychiatry. 2011;168(12):1266–77.
45. Niendam T. Integrating the C-SSRS into FEP clinical practice. SAMHSA sponsored webinar; June 28, 2016. https://www.nasmhpd.org/content/part-i-recognizing-suicidal-ideation-and-behavior-individuals-first-episode-psychosis.
46. Lindenmayer JP, Czobor P, Alphs L, Nathan AM, Anand R, Islam Z, et al. The InterSePT scale for suicidal thinking reliability and validity. Schizophr Res. 2003;63(1):161–70.
47. Beck AT, Steer RA, Ranieri WF. Scale for suicide ideation: psychometric properties of a self-report version. J Clin Psychol. 1988;44(4):499–505.
48. Pinninti N, Steer RA, Rissmiller DJ, Nelson S, Beck AT. Use of the Beck Scale for suicide ideation with psychiatric inpatients diagnosed with schizophrenia, schizoaffective, or bipolar disorders. Behav Res Ther. 2002;40(9):1071–9.
49. Meltzer HY, Alphs L, Green AI, Altamura AC, Anand R, Bertoldi A, et al. Clozapine treatment for suicidality in schizophrenia: international suicide prevention trial (InterSePT). Arch Gen Psychiatry. 2003;60(1):82–91.
50. Ayer DW, Jayathilake K, Meltzer HY. The InterSePT suicide scale for prediction of imminent suicidal behaviors. Psychiatry Res. 2008;161(1):87–96.
51. Hawton K, Sutton L, Haw C, Sinclair J, Deeks JJ. Schizophrenia and suicide: systematic review of risk factors. Br J Psychiatry. 2005;187(1):9–20.
52. Hunt IM, Kapur N, Robinson J, Shaw J, Flynn S, Bailey H, et al. Suicide within 12 months of mental health service contact in different age and diagnostic groups. Br J Psychiatry. 2006;188(2):135–42.
53. Melle I, Johannesen JO, Friis S, Haahr U, Joa I, Larsen TK, et al. Early detection of the first episode of schizophrenia and suicidal behavior. Am J Psychiatry. 2006;163(5):800–4.
54. Kreyenbuhl JA, Medoff DR, McEvoy JP, Smith TE, Hackman AL, Nossel IR, et al. The RAISE connection program: psychopharmacological treatment of people with a first episode of schizophrenia. Psychiatr Serv. 2016;67(12):1300–6.
55. Beck AT. Cognitive therapy: nature and relation to behavior therapy. Behav Ther. 1970;1(2):184–200.
56. Bateman K, Hansen L, Turkington D, Kingdon D. Cognitive behavioral therapy reduces suicidal ideation in schizophrenia: results from a randomized controlled trial. Suicide Life Threat Behav. 2007;37(3):284–90.
57. Zimmermann G, Favrod J, Trieu VH, Pomini V. The effect of cognitive behavioral treatment on the positive symptoms of schizophrenia spectrum disorders: a meta-analysis. Schizophr Res. 2005;77(1):1–9.
58. Startup M, Jackson MC, Bendix S. North Wales randomized controlled trial of cognitive behaviour therapy for acute schizophrenia spectrum disorders: outcomes at 6 and 12 months. Psychol Med. 2004;34(03):413–22.
59. Tarrier N, Kelly J, Maqsood S, Snelson N, Maxwell J, Law H, et al. The cognitive behavioural prevention of suicide in psychosis: a clinical trial. Schizophr Res. 2014;156(2):204–10.
60. Tarrier N, Lewis S, Haddock G, Bentall R, Drake R, Kinderman P, et al. Cognitive-behavioural therapy in first-episode and early schizophrenia. Br J Psychiatry. 2004;184(3):231–9.
61. Henggeler SW, Schoenwald SK, Borduin CM, Rowland MD, Cunningham PB. Multisystemic treatment of antisocial behavior in children and adolescents. New York: Guilford; 1998.
62. Henggeler SW, Rowland MD, Randall J, Ward DM, Pickrel SG, Cunningham PB, et al. Home-based multisystemic therapy as an alternative to the hospitalization of youths in psychiatric crisis: clinical outcomes. J Am Acad Child Adolesc Psychiatry. 1999;38(11):1331–9.

63. Huey SJ, Henggeler SW, Rowland MD, Halliday-Boykins CA, Cunningham PB, Pickrel SG, et al. Multisystemic therapy effects on attempted suicide by youths presenting psychiatric emergencies. J Am Acad Child Adolesc Psychiatry. 2004;43(2):183–90.
64. Remington G, Kapur S, Zipursky R. APA practice guideline for schizophrenia: risperidone equivalents. Am J Psychiatry. 1998;155(9):1301–2.
65. Robinson DG, Woerner MG, Alvir JM, Geisler S, Koreen A, Sheitman B, et al. Predictors of treatment response from a first episode of schizophrenia or schizoaffective disorder. Am J Psychiatry. 1999;156(4):544–9.
66. Schooler N, Rabinowitz J, Davidson M, Emsley R, Harvey PD, Kopala L, et al. Risperidone and haloperidol in first-episode psychosis: a long-term randomized trial. Am J Psychiatry. 2005;162(5):947–53.
67. Crow TJ, MacMillan JF, Johnson AL, Johnstone EC. A randomised controlled trial of prophylactic neuroleptic treatment. Br J Psychiatry. 1986;148(2):120–7.
68. Lieberman JA, Stroup TS, McEvoy JP, Swartz MS, Rosenheck RA, Perkins DO, et al. Effectiveness of antipsychotic drugs in patients with chronic schizophrenia. N Engl J Med. 2005;353(12):1209–23.
69. McEvoy JP, Lieberman JA, Stroup TS, Davis SM, Meltzer HY, Rosenheck RA, et al. Effectiveness of clozapine versus olanzapine, quetiapine, and risperidone in patients with chronic schizophrenia who did not respond to prior atypical antipsychotic treatment. Am J Psychiatry. 2006;163(4):600–10.
70. Schooler NR. Relapse and rehospitalization: comparing oral and depot antipsychotics. J Clin Psychiatry. 2003;64:14–7.
71. Essock SM, Covell NH, Davis SM, Stroup TS, Rosenheck RA, Lieberman JA. Effectiveness of switching antipsychotic medications. Am J Psychiatry. 2006;163(12):2090–5.
72. Heilä H, Isometsä ET, Henriksson MM, Heikkinen ME, Marttunen MJ, Lönnqvist JK. Suicide victims with schizophrenia in different treatment phases and adequacy of antipsychotic medication. J Clin Psychiatry. 1999;60(3):200–8.
73. Forrester T, Siskind D, Winckel K, Wheeler A, Hollingworth S. Increasing clozapine dispensing trends in Queensland, Australia 2004–2013. Pharmacopsychiatry. 2015;48:164–9.
74. Pankowski D, Kowalski J, Gawęda Ł. Skuteczność treningu metapoznawczego u osób chorujących na schizofrenię: narracyjny przegląd systematyczny badań opublikowanych w latach 2009–2015. Psychiatr Pol. 2016;50(4):787–803.
75. Rapp CA, Goscha RJ. The principles of effective case management of mental health services. Psychiatr Rehabil J. 2004;27(4):319.
76. Brown GW. Experiences of discharged chronic schizophrenic mental hospital patients in various types of living groups. Milbank Mem Fund Q. 1959;37:105–31.
77. Goldstein MJ, Rodnick EH, Evans JR, May PR, Steinberg MR. Drug and family therapy in the aftercare of acute schizophrenics. Arch Gen Psychiatry. 1978;35(10):1169–77.

Part II

Special Populations

Suicide in Children

4

Elizabeth C. Lanzillo, Lisa M. Horowitz, and Maryland Pao

Introduction

One of the most challenging mental health presentations for mental health clinicians to assess and manage is the patient with suicidal thoughts and/or behaviors. This is especially challenging with children and adolescents. Suicide risk changes at each developmental stage of a young person's life, increasing with age throughout adolescence and early adulthood [1, 2]. Risk of suicide increases in the late teen years, coinciding with increased risk of mood disorder onset [2]. As with many types of mental health concerns, a one-size-fits-all approach covering all youth will not be effective.

Given that nearly half of all mental illness onset begins in childhood [2, 3], intervening as early as possible is critical. Developmental trajectories are important factors to consider in youth suicide prevention and are the main characteristics that set children apart from adults (Fig. 4.1). These developmental considerations include factors such as variable physical growth; differences in cognition or the ability to think abstractly; language proficiency, including the ability to communicate one's needs and wants; and social competence, which plays an influential role in a young person's ability to make and keep friends and to feel accepted or isolated. These streams of development all occur at different times and at varying paces in children and adolescents [2].

Converging upon these developmental pathways are critical risk factors such as onset of mental illness, a family history of mental illness, and, the most potent risk factor, a history of suicidal ideation or behavior. In addition, other comorbid psychiatric conditions, such as substance or alcohol use disorders, may help promote the transition from suicidal ideation to suicidal behavior. Some psychological traits

E. C. Lanzillo, B.A. (✉) · L. M. Horowitz, Ph.D., M.P.H. · M. Pao, M.D.
Intramural Research Program, National Institute of Mental Health,
National Institutes of Health, Bethesda, MD, USA
e-mail: elizabeth.lanzillo@nih.gov; horowitzl@mail.nih.gov; paom@mail.nih.gov

T. Falcone, J. Timmons-Mitchell (eds.), *Suicide Prevention*,
https://doi.org/10.1007/978-3-319-74391-2_4

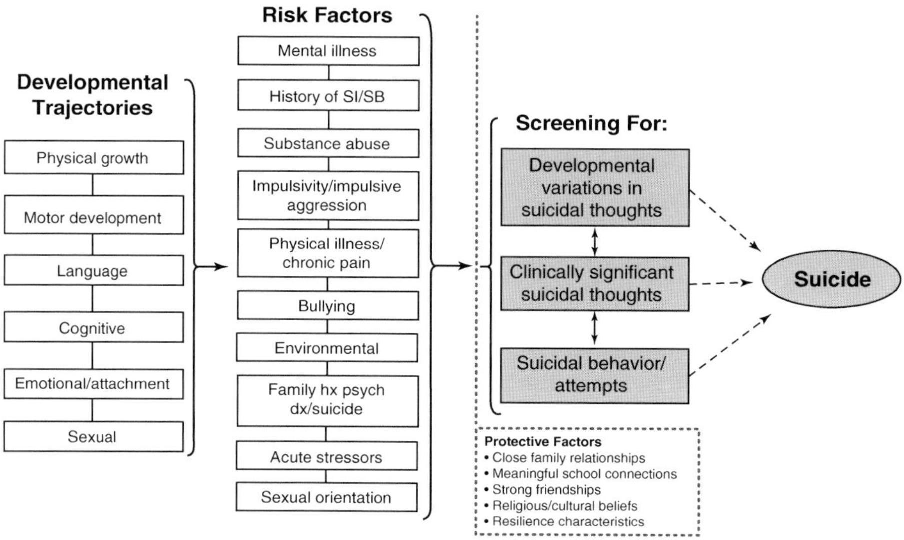

Fig. 4.1 Developmental considerations in youth suicide [2]. *SI* suicidal ideation, *SB* suicidal behavior, *hx* history of, *dx* diagnosis

manifested in youth can increase risk, such as impulsive aggression in which a child may have a tendency to react aggressively to frustrating situations or have other maladaptive coping strategies. Environmental factors such as psychosocial stressors, poverty, and "non-intact" families may contribute to feelings of hopelessness or helplessness. Moreover, many youth have acute stressors that include interpersonal conflict, loss, and academic or social challenges in school. These factors can all increase a young person's risk for suicide. Ideally, protective factors such as strong relationships with trusted adults, academic success, or religious beliefs can modify these risk factors and reduce risk for suicidal behaviors; however, these are not always sufficiently protective and cannot be relied upon [2].

The following chapter will discuss the language around suicide, the epidemiology of youth suicide, risk and protective factors, and assessment and treatment of suicidal ideations and behaviors.

Terminology

The provided definitions for suicidal thoughts and behaviors were obtained from consensus papers on the topic of terminology [4–7].

Suicide: the act of intentionally ending one's own life; in research, it implies a completed act. The language of suicide has evolved over the decades. The use of "committing suicide" or a "successful suicide" is discouraged when referring to a death by suicide as such terminology often carries negative connotations. Stating that an individual "*committed* suicide" suggests that people who kill themselves carried out a criminal act or another act of wrongdoing. Relatedly, the phrase "successful suicide" implies that causing one's own death could actually be viewed as a success or that a suicide attempt not resulting in death is a "failure." This language implicitly either subtly endorses the act of killing oneself or denies the possibility of recovery from suicidal behavior. For these reasons, current accepted terminology includes the terms completed suicide, death or die by suicide, or killing oneself.

Nonfatal suicidal thoughts and behaviors

- *Suicide ideation*: thoughts of engaging in behavior to end one's own life
- *Suicide plan*: the formulation of a specific method through which one intends to die
- *Suicide attempt*: engagement in potentially self-injurious behavior in which there is at least some intent to die

Suicidality: refers to the continuum of suicidal ideation, thoughts and behaviors, plans and attempts. All points along the continuum, from passive thoughts of wanting to be dead to suicide attempt with intent to die are all important and noteworthy, because each manifestation has been linked to completed suicide. Therefore, all suicidality should be taken seriously. Moreover, any youth who is frequently having thoughts of suicide, even in the absence of imminent danger, is most likely experiencing significant emotional distress that warrants further evaluation.

Non-suicidal self-injury[1]: self-injury in which a person has no intent to die (e.g., cutting).

Epidemiology

Suicide is an international public health threat and the second leading cause of death for young people ages 10–24 worldwide. This is also true in the United States, where more than 5900 youths killed themselves in 2015, a youth death rate greater than that of HIV, septicemia, diabetes, influenza/pneumonia, stroke, heart disease, and cancer combined [8]. While pediatric mortality from major medical conditions such as childhood leukemia has decreased in recent years [9], the youth suicide rate has increased significantly from 1999 to 2014 [10]. The suicide rate has increased over the past 70 years, with a 24% increase between 1999 and 2014 [10].

Youth Ages 5–11 Years

Suicide among young children is a rare occurrence, yet in 2014 suicide ranked as the 10th leading cause of death for children ages 5–11 in the United States [11]. The majority of epidemiologic studies of suicide have excluded children younger than

[1] Will not be discussed in this chapter.

10 years, examining trends within specific age groups generally starting with children only as young as 10. One of the few studies focusing on younger children examined data from the Web-based Injury Statistics Query and Reporting System of the Centers for Disease Control and Prevention and identified 657 deaths by suicide among children aged 5–11 years between 1993 and 2012. Overall, the suicide rate remained stable during this time period. However, when the data were stratified by race, a significant increase in the suicide rate among black children (from 1.36 to 2.54 per 1 million) and a significant decrease for white children (from 1.14 to 0.77) was noted [12]. Further research is warranted to investigate in more detail this potential racial disparity, which was seen mostly in black boys under age 12. Suffocation is the most common method of suicide in this age group, accounting for 71.4% of deaths by suicide in 2014, followed by firearms (26.5%) [8]. A follow-up study analyzed data from the National Violent Death Reporting System to compare characteristics and precipitating circumstances of suicide between elementary school-aged children (5–11 years) and early adolescent (12–14 years) decedents between 2003 and 2012. The findings revealed that children who died by suicide were more commonly male and black and died by hanging/strangulation/suffocation, compared to the early adolescents who completed suicide. Among the suicide decedents who had previously diagnosed mental health problems, children had a higher incidence of attention-deficit disorder with or without hyperactivity and less often experienced depression or dysthymia than the early adolescents who died by suicide. Authors postulated that impulsivity might be more prominent in younger children who die by suicide than depression [13]. Another striking finding was that 29% of these young decedents disclosed their suicide intent prior to killing themselves [13]. This presents an important opportunity for rescue and lends more evidence that healthcare providers and adults in trusted positions (e.g., parents, teachers, coaches, etc.) should be educated on how to identify warning signs of suicide and ask children about suicidal thoughts. The findings from this recent study highlight the need for both common and developmentally specific suicide prevention strategies during the elementary school-aged and early adolescent years [13].

Youth Ages 10–14 Years

While younger preteens and teens have a lower rate of suicide than the older adolescents, there has been a significant rise in the suicide rate among youth ages 10–14. In 2014, suicide ranked as the second leading cause of death for this age group, accounting for 425 deaths and surpassing the death rate for the most common killer of young people, traffic accidents [8, 11]. While the death rate from car accidents has been halved over the past 15 years, the suicide rate has nearly doubled, increasing from 0.9 in 2007 to 2.1 in 2014 per 100,000 population. Although more boys than girls killed themselves in 2014 (a rate of 2.6 per 100,000 for boys compared to 1.5 for girls), the suicide rate among girls increased drastically from 1999 to 2014, with a 200% percent increase during this time period (tripling from 0.5 per 100,000 in 1999 to 1.5 in 2014) [14]. The most common means of suicide is suffocation, which comprises approximately 53% of deaths by suicide for youth ages 10–14, followed by firearms (40.9%) and poisoning (4.2%) [11].

Youth Ages 15–19 Years

Suicide also ranks as the second leading cause of death among young people ages 15–19 years [11]. In this age group, 1384 teenagers died by suicide in 2014 [8]. Consistent with younger adolescents, suffocation is the most common method of suicide for people ages 15–19, accounting for nearly 50% of suicide deaths in 2014, followed by firearms (42.2%) [8].

While the youth suicide rates in this country and around the world are tragically high, youth suicide is a relatively rare event. More common than completed suicide are suicidal thoughts and behaviors. The United States measures these behaviors in the form of the Youth Risk Behavior Surveillance System (YRBSS). The YRBSS is a survey conducted every 2 years to monitor health-risk behaviors that contribute to the leading causes of death and disability among youth and adults. For the purpose of this chapter, results published from a 2015 report were reviewed and included prevalence rates of suicidal behaviors among high school students (grades 9–12) [15]. The survey is given to high school students at public and private schools in the 50 states and the District of Columbia. Students are asked to anonymously self-report many behaviors including tobacco use, alcohol and other drug use, sexual behaviors, physical inactivity, and suicidal thoughts, plans, and behaviors. The results indicate that suicidal thoughts are highly prevalent in high schools around the country; nearly 18% of high school students report having seriously considered attempting suicide in the 12 months prior to the survey. More concerning is that 8.6% of high school students nationwide attempted suicide one or more times during the 12 months before the survey. While more male than female adolescents die by suicide each year, female adolescents seriously consider attempting suicide at a higher rate than male adolescents (24.4% of females vs. 12.2% of males) [15, 16]. Notably, as the YRBSS only reaches youth in school, these are likely to be underestimates of the true prevalence in youth who are truant, medically ill, or otherwise out of school.

Youth Ages 19–24 Years

Suicide continues to be the second leading cause of death for young adults ages 19–24 [11]. In 2014, 3245 people ages 19–24 died by suicide [8]. In contrast to the other age groups, firearms are the most common method of suicide for people aged 19–24 (46.7% of deaths), followed by suffocation (36.5%) [8].

Risk Factors

Psychopathology

The presence of psychiatric disorders is a well-known risk factor for suicidal thoughts and behaviors. Among adolescent suicide attempters and completers, 80–90% has a diagnosed psychiatric disorder [17]. The most prevalent disorders among suicidal youth are mood, anxiety, conduct, and substance use disorders [17]. Youth with comorbid psychiatric disorders, particularly mood, disruptive, and substance abuse disorders, are at an elevated risk for suicidal thoughts and behaviors. Nevertheless, a common misconception is that only youth with mental illness are at risk for suicide. A recent study examining mortality data to collect information about antecedents of death by suicide among youth in England revealed that 61% of youth who died by suicide had no reported mental health diagnoses [18].

Depression

Depression is highly prevalent among youth who think about, attempt, and die by suicide. Results from psychological autopsy studies indicate that up to 60% of adolescent suicide completers had a depressive disorder at the time of death [19–21]. A prospective study examining the relationship between suicide risk and contemporaneous psychiatric disorders among 180 adolescents recently hospitalized on psychiatric inpatient units found that major depressive disorder was associated with a more than fivefold increase in rate of suicide attempts [22]. Findings from the study also demonstrate that the relationship between suicide attempts and major depression strengthens with age [22]. Of note, depression and dysthymic disorder were identified to be more common among repeat than first-time attempters [22].

Previous Suicidal Behavior

A previous suicide attempt is one of the strongest risk factors for suicide completion and future suicide attempts [20, 23]. Hawton and colleagues found that female and male adolescents and young adults ages 10–24 who presented to the hospital after deliberate self-harm were at 35 and 75 times, respectively, higher risk of suicide over the course of the following year than the general population [24]. While there is a dearth of research on the time period post-suicide attempt during which an individual is at risk for reattempt, Suokas and colleagues found that the highest risk of death by suicide occurs during the 6 months following the suicide attempt [25]. However, long-term follow-up studies indicate that the risk of suicide continues to be elevated for many years after the initial suicide attempt [25, 26]. Much of the existing data on suicide attempt to suicide completion is from adult studies. In a 14-year follow-up study of 1018 adults who attempted suicide by self-poisoning and were treated in the emergency department (ED), 6.7% of the sample died by suicide over the course of the follow-up period [25]. Among those who completed suicide, 50% died during the 2 years following the index attempt. However, deaths by suicide occurred more than a decade after the index attempt [25]. Importantly, it is unclear if these adult studies are generalizable to youth. More research is needed, particularly among youth, to examine the time period after a suicide attempt during which the individual is at highest risk.

Despite the potential for individuals who previously attempted suicide to make a future attempt, the majority of individuals who die by suicide do so on their first attempt [27]. A recent study found that nearly 60% of people who killed themselves did so as a result of their first attempt to die by suicide [28]. These data underscore the need and critical importance of identifying individuals at risk prior to the onset of suicidal behavior. Limiting suicide risk screening and assessment to high-risk individuals who have a suicide attempt history will fail to capture the majority of people who die the first time they try to kill themselves [28]. Even more disconcerting are studies about the characteristics of youth suicide attempters. A study that examined pediatric patients in the ED after a suicide attempt found that 85% of the patients did not discuss their suicidal thoughts with anyone and 30–60% had not told anyone about their previous attempt(s). Moreover, 90% of the attempts went unknown to their parents. Perhaps the most disquieting finding from this study was that nearly 70% of these suicide attempters reported a time interval less than 30 min between thinking about killing themselves and attempting [29]. Once again, this highlights the need to be proactive in probing youth about suicidal thoughts and helping them to develop effective coping strategies to manage difficult stressors in the future. Accordingly, more research to better understand possible differences between people who die on their first attempt and those who do not is critical for suicide prevention.

Substance Abuse

Substance use disorders are highly associated with increased risk for suicide, particularly among older adolescent males with comorbid mood or disruptive disorders [17, 19, 30]. Alcohol has detrimental and substantial psychopharmacological impacts on the brain. As such, it may be a proximal risk of suicidal behavior among young people. Drinking alcohol to excess can cause stress or increase co-occurring psychopathology and therefore may potentially be a distal risk factor for youth suicidal behavior [30]. Findings from a psychological autopsy study comparing adolescents who died by suicide to a community control sample of adolescents, matched on demographic characteristics, found that 35% of suicide completers met criteria for a substance abuse disorder, 22% for alcohol abuse, and 25% for illicit drug abuse. Of note, the presence of any substance abuse disorder was six times greater among male adolescent suicide completers, compared to the community control sample [20]. A study by Aseltine and colleagues found that youth ages 13 years and younger who engaged in heavy episodic drinking (HED) in the past year were approximately 2.6 times more likely to report a suicide attempt compared to youth who did not report recent HED [31]. Among youth 18 years and older, those who reported past year HED were 1.2 times more likely to report a suicide attempt as compared to youth of the same age who did not participate in HED [31].

Family Factors

Cash and Bridge identified several family factors that are associated with increased risk of suicide and suicidal behavior among youth. Such factors include family discord, loss of a parent, poor relationship between the parent and child, and maltreatment [17]. However, more research is warranted to better understand how related variables, such as adolescent or parental psychopathology, may impact these family factors and youth suicidal behavior [17, 32, 33]. In addition, it is important to consider how family factors may influence suicidal behavior differently throughout development. A study examining characteristics and precipitating circumstances of suicide in elementary school-aged children relative to early adolescent decedents found that children who died by suicide were more likely than adolescents to experience problems with family members [13].

Familial Transmission of Suicidal Behaviors

There has been extensive research demonstrating that suicidal behavior is transmitted from parent to child [32, 33]. A study of 181 people who attempted suicide found that 35% reported a family history of suicide or suicide attempt [34]. Findings from adoption, twin, and family studies indicate that the familial transmission of suicidal behavior is genetic and is transmitted independent of parental psychopathology [17, 33]. The genetic transmission appears to be mediated by intermediate phenotypes such as impulsive aggression, neuroticism, or neurocognitive deficits [32, 33]. A prospective study examining early-onset suicidal behavior among offspring of parents with mood disorders identified a higher rate of incident suicide attempts among offspring of probands who had made suicide attempts (4.1%), compared with offspring of parents with mood disorders who had not made attempts (0.6%) [35].

At present, the most convincing explanatory model of this transmission is Brent and Mann's stress-diathesis model [36]. According to the model, parents may pass suicidal tendencies to their children due to the convergence of the following elements: "child and parent psychopathology, suboptimal family environment, childhood abuse, the presence of impulsive aggression or neurocognitive deficits and life stress" [33, 36]. However, the researchers emphasize that significant individual variation exists in the risk factors and processes that lead to suicide [33, 36]. More research is needed to enhance our understanding of the sequence and relation of salient factors associated with the familial transmission of suicidality [33].

Childhood Trauma

Childhood exposure to physical abuse or violent sexual abuse places an individual at significantly higher risk for suicidal ideation, suicide attempts, and suicide completion [34, 37, 38]. A study examining the effect of preadolescent physical abuse on adolescent suicidal behavior found a significant association between preadolescent abuse and increased risk of both suicidal ideation and suicide attempt. The findings indicated that 27% of physically abused adolescents, compared to 8% of control group adolescents with no history of abuse, reported suicidal ideation. Furthermore, 21% of abused adolescents reported a suicide attempt, compared to only 4% of control adolescents [39]. The researchers also tested several mediation models and concluded that the relationship between childhood physical abuse and suicidal behavior was not mediated by attachment to friends or family, internalizing or externalizing pathology, or life events [39], highlighting the strength of the relationship between physical abuse and adolescent suicidal behavior. Another study examining suicide risk following childhood sexual abuse found that the suicide rate among young people who had experienced sexual abuse was 10.7–13.0 times greater than the national suicide rate. Moreover, while there were no suicides in the control group during the follow-up period, 32% of the sexually abused children had attempted suicide, and 43% had thought about suicide since they were sexually abused [40].

Sexual Orientation and Gender Identity

Sexual and gender minority (SGM) youth are at greater risk for suicidal behavior relative to heterosexual and/or non-transgender adolescents [41]. While 8% of the general youth population report past year suicide attempts [42], rates of past year suicide attempts among SGM youth are estimated to be between 27 and 37% [43, 44].

Sexual Orientation

Data from the YRBSS indicate that rates of past year suicide attempts among lesbian, gay, and bisexual high school students are nearly five times higher than heterosexual students [42, 45]. Findings of the YRBSS also reveal that rates of suicidal behavior are higher among bisexual youth than lesbian and gay-identified youth, with bisexual females reporting the highest prevalence of suicidal ideation (42.1%), suicide planning (34.8%), and suicide attempts (30.1%) [46]. Research demonstrates that identifying as lesbian, gay, or bisexual coupled with additional risk factors including parental psychological abuse during childhood, increased parental efforts to discourage childhood gender atypical behavior, and early openness about sexual orientation are associated with an elevated likelihood of having attempted suicide [47].

A potential additional risk factor for suicidal behavior in LGBTQ youth is the political milieu of the region in which they live. This factor was examined in a recent study on the association between same-sex marriage policies and adolescent suicide attempts. Through an analysis of YRBSS data from 1999 to 2015, the authors found that same-sex marriage policies were associated with a 0.6% point reduction in suicide attempts. This represents a 7% relative reduction in the proportion of high school students attempting suicide owing to same-sex marriage policies [45].

Gender Identity

According to the National Transgender Discrimination Survey, 45% of transgender youth ages 18–24 reported a history of attempted suicide [48]. Similar to sexual minority youth, there are specific risk factors that increase the likelihood of suicidal behavior among transgender individuals such as disclosure of gender identity, family rejection, prior verbal or physical harassment or bullying at school, treatment refusal by a doctor or healthcare provider, and homelessness [48]; but overall, there is a lack of research specifically examining risk of suicide among transgender youth. The only known study to date specifically of male-to-female and female-to-male transgender youth found a significant association between a history of a suicide attempt and experiences of past parental verbal and physical abuse and lower body esteem [49].

Bullying

Numerous studies have identified bullying as a risk factor for suicidal behavior among youth. A study by Klomek and colleagues examined associations between childhood bullying behaviors at 8 years of age and subsequent suicidal behavior in a large sample of Finnish children [50]. The findings indicated that boys who were both bullies and victims of bullying had a higher likelihood of suicidal behavior as compared to boys who had no history of bullying behaviors or who were only victims of bullying. Among girls, those who were victims of bullying were more likely to exhibit suicidal behaviors, compared to girls who were neither perpetrators nor victims of bullying [50]. Another study examining suicide risk in pediatric patients presenting to the ED found that among the 11.5% of patients who reported recent bullying victimization, 55% screened positive for suicide risk [51]. In addition to traditional forms of bullying, cyberbullying has increasingly become a problem among adolescents [52]. A large study of middle school-aged adolescents found that youth who were offenders or victims of either traditional bullying or cyberbullying were more likely to report suicidal ideation and suicide attempts, compared to students who had not experienced peer bullying [53]. The findings also revealed a stronger association with suicidal behavior for victimization than offending [53]. More research specifically on cyberbullying as it relates to suicidal behavior among youth is warranted. In addition, future research should seek to detect factors potentially mediating the relationship between bullying and suicidal behavior.

Academic Pressure

A recent study investigating child-specific and young person-specific antecedents of suicide in England identified 145 suicides in people under the age of 20 between

January 2014 and April 2015. Among the youth who had died by suicide during the study period, 51% had experienced academic pressures prior to their death. Furthermore, four youth completed suicide on the day of an exam or the following day [18].

Recent "suicide clusters" at high schools known for their academic rigor in the United States highlight the potential for highly competitive academic contexts to have negative, even devastating consequences for youth mental health. Suicide clusters occur when multiple deaths by suicide take place in close succession and proximity. In 2009, five teens in the Palo Alto region of California killed themselves in a span of 9 months. Only 5 years later, the region was hit by another suicide cluster when another four teens died by suicide [54]. In response to such suicide clusters, Joshi and colleagues suggest that when faced with significant stress, suicidal youth may be more attracted to death and less able to develop alternatives to suicide [55]. The researchers highlight the need for prevention efforts focusing on school-based mental health education and promotion. Such interventions may include awareness and education curricula, suicide screening, gatekeeper training, skills training, and peer leadership [55]. Detailed information about these interventions can be found in their 2015 study "School Based Suicide Prevention: Content, Process, and the Role of Trusted Adults and Peers."

The majority of research addressing the relationship between academic stress and suicidal behavior has focused on East Asian populations. As cultural factors may influence the way academic pressure manifests among youth, comparative research specific to other groups is warranted.

Autism Spectrum Disorder (ASD) and/or Intellectual Disabilities (ID)

There is a dearth of research on suicide risk among adolescents with ASD/ID, but recent studies suggest that youth with ASD and/or ID are at elevated risk for suicide [56, 57]. Clinicians do not fully understand how suicidal thoughts are expressed in ASD/ID and how they may vary from that of typically developing youth, making it difficult to accurately detect suicide risk in this population [58]. Communication difficulties inherent in ASD, such as identifying and communicating self-states, expressing abstract concepts of death and dying, the use of idiosyncratic or stereotyped language, and circumscribed interests, affect attempts to measure suicide risk [59]. More research is warranted to better capture the prevalence of suicidal thoughts and behaviors in this population.

Medical Illness

Several studies have identified physical illness as a risk factor for suicide [18, 60–64]. Historically, suicide risk associated with medical illness has focused on adult and elderly populations and adult survivors of childhood cancer [65–67], but an increasing number of studies have shown that physical illness also increases risk for suicide among youth. Youth with medical illnesses such as epilepsy, asthma, and endocrine disorders appear to be at higher risk than those without these medical conditions [68, 69]. A recent study examining mental health and substance abuse (MHSA) hospitalization patterns in children with comorbid epilepsy found that children with epilepsy who were hospitalized for MHSA conditions were over three times as likely to have suicide ideation or a suicide attempt as the reason for admission, compared to children without epilepsy [69]. Another study that investigated the incidence of suicide deaths among youth with current asthma found the rate of suicide mortality to be more than twice as high at the study baseline compared to youth with no history of asthma [68]. In addition, a study examining the antecedents of youth suicide in England found that over one-third of the youth who killed themselves during the time period of interest had a medical illness [18]. More research is necessary to establish the specific medical conditions, or combinations of conditions, that confer the greatest risk of suicidal thoughts and behavior among youth. Awareness of the increased risk for suicidal tendencies among youth with physical illnesses is critical for healthcare professionals, who need to become more aware of youths' concomitant psychological symptoms.

Implication of Assessment and Management by Risk Factor

- Diagnose and treat depression and other comorbid psychiatric conditions (pharmacotherapy, psychotherapy, hospitalization).
- Diagnose and treat youth substance abuse (substance programs).
- *Be alert to previous suicide attempts.*
- Diagnose and treat parent psychopathology (refer parent for treatment).
- Assess for family discord and poor relationship between the parent and child (family therapy).
- Assess for child abuse and report appropriately (CPS/parent anger management therapy).
  - Assess for the presence of impulsive aggression or neurocognitive deficits and ability to manage life stress (neuropsychological testing, coping skills).
  - Assess for bullying—physical and cyber (limit social media).
  - Assess sexual orientation/gender identity/gender attraction/natal sex (seek appropriate guidance).
  - Assess school/academic pressures/self-imposed expectations (psychotherapy/family therapy/school guidance).
  - Assess for comorbid medical illness (appropriate medical treatment/psychological screening/psychotherapy/coping skills).

Protective Factors

While there is extensive literature examining risk factors for youth suicide, significantly less is known about the factors that may protect youth from suicidal thoughts and behavior. Protective factors are defined as factors that decrease the probability of a negative outcome among those at risk [70, 71]. As highlighted by Cha and Nock, a protective factor is not defined by the absence of a risk factor, but, instead, it is a third variable that modifies the strength or direction of the relation between a risk factor and outcome [70].

Social Connectedness

Social connectedness has been identified as a potential protective factor for suicidal behavior and associated risk factors of suicide [72, 73]. A study that examined associations of age, gender, and psychosocial factors during adolescence with risk of suicide between the ages of 19 and 23 found that low levels of family support were associated with suicide attempts in early adulthood for females and low levels of support from friends were predictive of suicide attempts for males [74]. Another study that investigated risk and protective factors for medically serious suicide attempts among a sample of 18–24-year-olds who presented to the ED following a suicide attempt found a direct relationship between social connectedness and lower risk of suicidal behavior. According to their findings, social connectedness is a stronger protective factor among youth with high levels of depressive symptomatology, compared to those with lower levels of depressive symptoms [75].

Internal Locus of Control

An individual's locus of control refers to the extent to which they perceive reinforcement to be contingent upon their own actions or attributes [76]. Findings from the previously discussed study of 18–24-year-olds presenting to the ED after attempting suicide found that an internal locus of control protects against medically serious suicide attempts [75]. In addition, a qualitative study seeking to understand how adolescents overcome suicidality from the perspective of previously suicidal female adolescents identified recognition of choice and personal control as instrumental to overcoming suicidality [77].

Effective Coping Strategies

A study comparing the coping responses of hospitalized adolescent suicide attempters to hospitalized non-attempters matched on diagnosis and demographic characteristics found that suicide attempters made fewer effortful approach and more automatic-approach coping responses and were judged by trained raters to have coped less effectively to stressful episodes, relative to the comparison group of hospitalized adolescents who did not attempt suicide. The findings also indicated that higher coping effectiveness at baseline assessment was predictive of a greater decline in suicidal behavior across a 2-year follow-up period [78].

Religiosity

Many studies have identified religion as a protective factor against suicide. There are various aspects of religiousness that may protect an individual from suicidal behavior, such as religious prohibitions against killing oneself that may act as a strong deterrent [79], or the social network it provides [80].

The majority of research to date on the potential for religiosity to be a protective factor against suicide has been retrospective in design, with the use of psychological autopsy studies relying on proxy informants. A 2014 study was the first longitudinal study to prospectively examine protective factors against death by suicide [80]. The researchers sought to determine whether individuals who frequently attend religious services were less likely to die by suicide than individuals who did not attend regularly. Data was collected on a sample of 20,014 people between 1988 and 1994, and follow-up mortality data was collected from baseline until the end of 2006. The findings indicated that people who frequently attended religious services were less likely to die by suicide. More specifically, individuals who attended religious services at least 24 times per year were less than half as likely to die by suicide as individuals who attended less frequently. This protective effect predicted suicide up to 16 years later and remained after accounting for other predictors of suicide. Importantly, this was a small sample which may limit the generalizability of these data.

Few studies have examined how religiosity is protective against suicidal behavior specifically among adolescents. One of the studies identified focused on a youth sample consisted of 1615 adolescents aged 15–19 at three high schools in Canada [81]. The researchers found that religious attendance was protective against suicidal ideation in females; however, depression accounted for this relationship. In addition, religious importance was a weak protective factor for suicidal thoughts among females, but this relationship became insignificant after including measures of social trust and substance use. Associations between suicidal ideation and religious importance or religious attendance were not identified in males [81].

Importance of Screening as Means of Prevention

As a result of the striking number of adolescents who die by such each year, along with the even greater and ever growing number of youth experiencing suicidal thoughts and behaviors, there has been a nationwide push to screen for suicide risk in various settings. In 2004, the Garrett Lee Smith Memorial Act was signed into Congress, highlighting the need for early intervention services, including suicide risk screening, to be incorporated into school systems, educational institutions, juvenile justice systems, mental health and substance use programs, and foster care systems, among other organizations [82]. As recently as February 2016, The Joint Commission, the accrediting organization for healthcare programs in hospitals throughout the United States, issued a Sentinel Event Alert recommending that all medical patients in all medical settings (inpatient hospital units, outpatient practices, EDs) be screened for suicide risk [83]. To accurately identify youth who may be at risk for suicide, it is critical that the screening instruments utilized are psychometrically sound and validated in both the setting and population being screened.

Risk for suicide changes at different developmental stages. Specifically, suicide risk increases with age throughout adolescence and early adulthood, levels off, and then rises again later in life. While suicide is a rare event among children under the age of 12, it does occur [12, 13]. In fact, as discussed in the epidemiology section of this chapter, a recent report by the Centers for Disease Control and Prevention indicates that the suicide death rate for children ages 10–14 has surpassed the death rate due to motor vehicle accidents for this age group [14]. Furthermore, as half of all mental illness onset occurs in childhood [3], this is a critical time to intervene. In addition to identifying youth who are at risk, screening for suicide among adolescents may thwart the progression of suicidal ideation to suicidal behavior [2].

Currently, the majority of suicide risk screening in medical settings occurs in a non-standardized manner, typically only with patients who appear at high risk or present with suicidal ideation. Moreover, suicide risk screening items and practices vary across and within hospitals and medical practices, depending on the knowledge and training of staff which is often limited [2]. To accurately and consistently identify distressed youth, a paradigm shift in which validated screening tools are implemented throughout hospitals and other medical settings is critical. Staff must be appropriately trained to use clinical practice guidelines developed for safely managing adolescents who screen positive. It is also essential to screen universally, as opposed to only screening patients who present with psychiatric concerns or are deemed to be at risk.

In order for universal screening in medical settings to be feasible and nondisruptive to workflow, the initial screening tool needs to be brief, highly sensitive and specific, and validated on the targeted population [2, 82]. A screening tool that is highly *sensitive* will correctly identify almost all of the adolescents who are at elevated risk for suicide. Therefore, the more sensitive the tool, the less likely that it will fail to capture an individual who is at risk [72]. It is also critical that the screening tool utilized be highly *specific*, meaning the tool does not identify as suicidal an individual who is not at heightened risk [72]. There are several measures available to screen youth for suicide risk in medical settings (see Table 4.1). Before implementing a suicide risk screening tool, it is imperative that a plan for managing patients who screen positive be established. This will be discussed in greater detail in the following section on assessment.

Opposition to suicide risk screening often stems from the concern that asking youth about suicide will lead to iatrogenic effects of subsequent suicidal ideation; in other words, the concern that asking youth questions about suicide will "put the idea into their head" is commonly raised. In 2005, Gould et al. measured distress before and after screening high school students for suicide risk. This landmark article established that asking youth about suicide was not harmful and did not lead to increased distress or suicidal thoughts in the post-screening assessments [88]. More recently, Mathias and colleagues addressed this concern through an examination of

Table 4.1 Suicide risk screening tools

Tool	Setting used	Format	Reference
Ask Suicide-Screening Questions (ASQ)	Pediatric emergency department, inpatient hospital units, outpatient clinics, and primary care	Brief questionnaire consisting of 4 "yes/no" questions; a "yes" response to any question is considered a positive screen, and an additional acuity question is asked to determine imminent risk	Horowitz et al. [59]
Beck Scale for Suicide Ideation	Inpatient hospital units; outpatient clinics and primary care	Semi-structured interview consisting of 19 items to assess [1] active suicidal desire, [2] specific plans for suicide, and [3] passive suicidal desire	Beck et al. [84]
Behavioral health screen (BHS)	Pediatric outpatient clinics and primary care	Internet-based tool that addresses a range of mental health problems and behaviors including suicide	Diamond [85]
Columbia Suicide Severity Scale (C-SSRS)	Pediatric emergency department, inpatient hospital units, outpatient clinics, and primary care	Semi-structured clinical interview that assesses the types and severity of suicidal ideation and behavior	Posner et al. [86]
Patient Health Questionnaire for Adolescents (PHQ-A)	Pediatric outpatient clinics and primary care	Self-administered questionnaire consisting of 9 questions that assess anxiety, eating, mood, and substance use disorders; question #9 addresses suicidal thoughts	Johnson et al. [87]

adolescents who had previously been treated in an inpatient psychiatric setting. The researchers repeatedly tested suicidal ideation at 6-month intervals over the course of 2 years. The findings demonstrated a significant decline in suicidal ideation in the context of repeated assessment, indicating that asking youth about suicidal thoughts is not associated with an increase in thoughts about suicide [89]. This concern has been examined by other researchers who have also concluded that asking about suicidal thoughts and behavior does not induce or increase such thoughts and experiences [88, 90].

Cultural Considerations

Pena and Caine highlight the potential for screening instruments to be less reliable, and consequently, less effective with communities that include greater ethnic and language diversity than the population upon which the tool was initially developed [82]. Importantly, populations may differ in their understanding of suicide and the terminology used to discuss suicide. As such, it is imperative to verify the meaning of items if screening tools are translated into other languages, and pilot testing of tools is advised prior to full-scale implementation [82]. It is also important to explain to parents/guardians and the patients themselves why they are being screened for suicide risk. While it is critical to be culturally sensitive, the reason for screening should be explained in the context of the culture of safety or mission of the healthcare setting where screening is taking place.

Assessment

Three components are necessary for implementing suicide risk screening:

1. Suicide risk screening
   If patient screens negative, and clinician judgment is in agreement, no further action is necessary. If patient screens positive for suicide risk, refuses to answer the screening questions, or the clinician is uncomfortable with the manner in which the patient answered the questions, then the following two steps are necessary.
2. Brief suicide safety assessment
3. Full mental health evaluation/full safety assessment (if deemed necessary after conducting brief suicide safety assessment)

The first step is screening for suicide risk. It is essential to distinguish between a suicide risk *screen* and a suicide risk *assessment*. A suicide risk screen seeks to cast a wide net to identify youth who may be at heightened risk for suicidal thoughts and behavior [72]. Screening tools should be brief, easy to use and interpret, and evidenced-based with strong psychometric properties and may be administered by nonmental health clinicians. If an individual screens positive for suicide risk, or is suspected of having suicidal ideation or behavior, they warrant a brief yet thorough suicide safety assessment (step 2). This brief suicide safety assessment should be conducted by a mental health clinician to gather more comprehensive information about risk, protective factors, and the nature and severity of elevated risk. The brief assessment will enable the medical team to better understand the individual's level of risk and make a determination for next steps.

Guidelines are available to utilize when conducting a brief suicide safety assessment. One commonly used instrument for such an assessment is the Columbia Suicide Severity Scale (CSSRS) [86]. The CSSRS helps the clinician determine whether the patient is at low, moderate, or high risk. Another instrument to guide clinicians in this assessment is the ASQ brief suicide safety assessment (BSSA), which was specifically developed for use with the Ask Suicide-Screening Questions (ASQ) tool [59] (see Figs. 4.2, 4.3, 4.4, and 4.5 for the ASQ and the BSSA for the ED, outpatient, and inpatient pediatric settings). The BSSA provides language for clinicians to ask about frequency of suicidal thoughts, a suicide plan, past suicidal behavior, various psychiatric symptoms, and support and safety. The BSSA also includes questions to be addressed to parents/guardians of youth under the age of 18. Importantly, the guide reminds the clinician to discuss means restriction and safety planning, two critical intervention strategies that have been proven effective [91]. By the end of the brief safety assessment, the mental health clinician should have the necessary information to better understand the patient's level of risk and

asQ
Ask Suicide-Screening Questions

NIMH TOOLKIT

Suicide Risk Screening Tool

Ask the patient:

1. **In the past few weeks, have you wished you were dead?** ❍ Yes ❍ No

2. **In the past few weeks, have you felt that you or your family would be better off if you were dead?** ❍ Yes ❍ No

3. **In the past week, have you been having thoughts about killing yourself?** ❍ Yes ❍ No

4. **Have you ever tried to kill yourself?** ❍ Yes ❍ No

   If yes, how? ______________________________

   ____

   ____

   When? ______________________________

   ____

If the patient answers **Yes** *to any of the above, ask the following acuity question:*

5. **Are you having thoughts of killing yourself right now?** ❍ Yes ❍ No

   If yes, please describe: ______________________________

Next steps:

- If patient answers "No" to all questions 1 through 4, screening is complete (not necessary to ask question #5). No intervention is necessary (**Note: Clinical judgment can always override a negative screen*).
- **If patient answers "Yes" to any of questions 1 through 4, or refuses to answer, they are considered a positive screen. Ask question #5 to assess acuity:**
  - ☐ "Yes" to question #5 = **acute positive screen** (imminent risk identified)
    - **Patient requires a STAT safety/full mental health evaluation. Patient cannot leave until evaluated for safety.**
    - Keep patient in sight. Remove all dangerous objects from room. Alert physician or clinician responsible for patient's care.
  - ☐ **"No"** to question #5 = **non-acute positive screen** (potential risk identified)
    - **Patient requires a brief suicide safety assessment to determine if a full mental health evaluation is needed. Patient cannot leave until evaluated for safety.**
    - Alert physician or clinician responsible for patient's care.

Provide resources to all patients

- 24/7 National Suicide Prevention Lifeline 1-800-273-TALK (8255) En Español: 1-888-628-9454
- 24/7 Crisis Text Line: Text "HOME" to 741-741

asQ Suicide Risk Screening Toolkit NATIONAL INSTITUTE OF MENTAL HEALTH (NIMH) NIH 6/13/2017

Fig. 4.2 Ask Suicide-Screening Questions tool

determine if a full mental health evaluation is necessary (see Treatment section for description of safety planning). If deemed necessary after conducting the brief suicide safety assessment, a comprehensive mental health evaluation should be conducted by a mental health clinician (step 3).

NIMH TOOLKIT: EMERGENCY DEPARTMENT

asQ Ask Suicide-Screening Questions

Brief Suicide Safety Assessment

What to do when a pediatric patient screens positive for suicide risk:

- Use after a patient **(10 - 24 years)** screens positive for suicide risk on the asQ
- Assessment guide for mental health clinicians, MDs, NPs, or PAs
- Prompts help determine disposition

1 Praise patient *for discussing their thoughts*

"I'm here to follow up on your responses to the suicide risk screening questions. These are hard things to talk about. Thank you for telling us. I need to ask you a few more questions."

2 Assess the patient

If possible, assess patient alone *(depending on developmental considerations and parent willingness)*

Review patient's responses from the asQ

Frequency of suicidal thoughts

Determine if and how often the patient is having suicidal thoughts. Ask the patient: "In the past few weeks, have you been thinking about killing yourself?" **If yes, ask:** "How often?" (once or twice a day, several times a day, a couple times a week, etc.)

"Are you having thoughts of killing yourself right now?" **(If "yes," patient requires an urgent/STAT mental health evaluation and cannot be left alone. A positive response indicates imminent risk.)**

Suicide plan

Assess if the patient has a suicide plan, regardless of how they responded to any other questions (ask about method and access to means). Ask the patient: "Do you have a plan to kill yourself? Please describe." **If no plan, ask:** "If you were going to kill yourself, how would you do it?"

Note: If the patient has a very detailed plan, this is more concerning than if they haven't thought it through in great detail. If the plan is feasible (e.g., if they are planning to use pills and have access to pills), this is a reason for greater concern and removing or securing dangerous items (medications, guns, ropes, etc.).

Past behavior *(Strongest predictor of future attempts)*

Evaluate past self-injury and history of suicide attempts (method, estimated date, intent). Ask the patient: "Have you ever tried to hurt yourself?" "Have you ever tried to kill yourself?" **If yes, ask:** "How? When? Why?" and assess intent: "Did you think [method] would kill you?" "Did you want to die?" (for youth, intent is as important as lethality of method) **Ask:** "Did you receive medical/psychiatric treatment?"

Symptoms

Depression: "In the past few weeks, have you felt so sad or depressed that it makes it hard to do the things you would like to do?"

Anxiety: "In the past few weeks, have you felt so worried that it makes it hard to do the things you would like to do or that you feel constantly agitated/on-edge?"

Impulsivity/Recklessness: "Do you often act without thinking?"

Hopelessness: "In the past few weeks, have you felt hopeless, like things would never get better?"

Irritability: "In the past few weeks, have you been feeling more irritable or grouchier than usual?"

Substance and alcohol use: "In the past few weeks, have you used drugs or alcohol?" **If yes, ask:** "What? How much?"

Other concerns: "Recently, have there been any concerning changes in how you are thinking or feeling?"

Support & Safety

Support network: "Is there a trusted adult you can talk to? Who? Have you ever seen a therapist/counselor?" **If yes, ask:** "When?"

Safety question: "Do you think you need help to keep yourself safe?" (A "no" response does not indicate that the patient is safe, but a "yes" is a reason to act immediately to ensure safety.)

Reasons for living: "What are some of the reasons you would NOT kill yourself?"

3 Interview patient and parent/guardian together

***If patient is ≥ 18, ask patient's permission for parent to join.**

Say to the parent: "After speaking with your child, I have some concerns about his/her safety. We are glad your child spoke up as this can be a difficult topic to talk about. We would now like to get your perspective."

- "Your child said (reference positive responses on the asQ). Is this something he/she shared with you?"
- "Does your child have a history of suicidal thoughts or behaviors that you're aware of?" **If yes, say:** "Please explain."
- "Does your child seem sad or depressed? Withdrawn? Anxious? Impulsive? Hopeless? Irritable? Reckless?"
- "Are you comfortable keeping your child safe at home?"
- "How will you secure or remove potentially dangerous items (guns, medications, ropes, etc.)?"
- "Is there anything you would like to tell me in private?"

4 Determine disposition

After completing the assessment, choose the appropriate disposition.

- ❑ Emergency psychiatric evaluation: **Patient is at imminent risk for suicide (current suicidal thoughts).** Urgent/STAT page psychiatry; keep patient safe in ED
- ❑ Further evaluation of risk is necessary: Request full mental health/safety evaluation in the ED
- ❑ No further evaluation in the ED: Create safety plan for managing potential future suicidal thoughts and discuss securing or removing potentially dangerous items (medications, guns, ropes, etc.)
  - ❍ Send home with mental health referrals

  or
  - ❍ No further intervention is necessary at this time

5 Provide resources to all patients

- 24/7 National Suicide Prevention Lifeline: 1-800-273-TALK (8255), En Español: 1-888-628-9454
- 24/7 Crisis Text Line: Text "HOME" to 741-741

asQ Suicide Risk Screening Toolkit NATIONAL INSTITUTE OF MENTAL HEALTH (NIMH) NIH 7/14/2017

Fig. 4.3 Brief suicide safety assessment (BSSA) for youth in the emergency department

This evaluation should include detailed information about:

- An understanding of the person's current situation and any stressors or risk factors described above
- Psychiatric review of symptoms (sleep, appetite, energy, somatic symptoms, mood including signs of irritability, depression or mania, anxiety including

NIMH TOOLKIT: OUTPATIENT

asQ — Ask Suicide-Screening Questions

Brief Suicide Safety Assessment

What to do when a pediatric patient screens positive for suicide risk:

- Use after a patient **(10 - 24 years)** screens positive for suicide risk on the asQ
- Assessment guide for mental health clinicians, MDs, NPs, or PAs
- Prompts help determine disposition

1 Praise patient *for discussing their thoughts*

"I'm here to follow up on your responses to the suicide risk screening questions. These are hard things to talk about. Thank you for telling us. I need to ask you a few more questions."

2 Assess the patient *(If possible, assess patient alone depending on developmental considerations and parent willingness.)*

Review patient's responses from the asQ

Frequency of suicidal thoughts

Determine if and how often the patient is having suicidal thoughts.

Ask the patient: "In the past few weeks, have you been thinking about killing yourself?" **If yes, ask:** "How often?" (once or twice a day, several times a day, a couple times a week, etc.) "When was the last time you had these thoughts?"

"Are you having thoughts of killing yourself right now?" **(If "yes," patient requires an urgent/ STAT mental health evaluation and cannot be left alone. A positive response indicates imminent risk.)**

Suicide plan

Assess if the patient has a suicide plan, regardless of how they responded to any other questions (ask about method and access to means).

Ask the patient: "Do you have a plan to kill yourself?" **If yes, ask:** "What is your plan?" **If no plan, ask:** "If you were going to kill yourself, how would you do it?"

Note: If the patient has a very detailed plan, this is more concerning than if they haven't thought it through in great detail. If the plan is feasible (e.g., if they are planning to use pills and have access to pills), this is a reason for greater concern and removing or securing dangerous items (medications, guns, ropes, etc.).

Past behavior

Evaluate past self-injury and history of suicide attempts (method, estimated date, intent).

Ask the patient: "Have you ever tried to hurt yourself?" "Have you ever tried to kill yourself?"

If yes, ask: "How? When? Why?" and assess intent: "Did you think [method] would kill you?" "Did you want to die?" (for youth, intent is as important as lethality of method) **Ask:** "Did you receive medical/psychiatric treatment?"

Note: Past suicidal behavior is the strongest risk factor for future attempts.

Symptoms — Ask the patient about:

Depression: "In the past few weeks, have you felt so sad or depressed that it makes it hard to do the things you would like to do?"

Anxiety: "In the past few weeks, have you felt so worried that it makes it hard to do the things you would like to do or that you feel constantly agitated/on-edge?"

Impulsivity/Recklessness: "Do you often act without thinking?"

Hopelessness: "In the past few weeks, have you felt hopeless, like things would never get better?"

Anhedonia: "In the past few weeks, have you felt like you couldn't enjoy the things that usually make you happy?"

Isolation: "Have you been keeping to yourself more than usual?"

Irritability: "In the past few weeks, have you been feeling more irritable or grouchier than usual?"

Substance and alcohol use: "In the past few weeks, have you used drugs or alcohol?" **If yes, ask:** "What? How much?"

Sleep pattern: "In the past few weeks, have you had trouble falling asleep or found yourself waking up in the middle of the night or earlier than usual in the morning?"

Appetite: "In the past few weeks, have you noticed changes in your appetite? Have you been less hungry or more hungry than usual?"

Other concerns: "Recently, have there been any concerning changes in how you are thinking or feeling?"

Social Support & Stressors

(For all questions below, if patient answers yes, ask them to describe.)

Support network: "Is there a trusted adult you can talk to? Who? Have you ever seen a therapist/counselor?" **If yes, ask:** "When?"

Family situation: "Are there any conflicts at home that are hard to handle?"

School functioning: "Do you ever feel so much pressure at school (academic or social) that you can't take it anymore?"

Bullying: "Are you being bullied or picked on?"

Suicide contagion: "Do you know anyone who has killed themselves or tried to kill themselves?"

Reasons for living: "What are some of the reasons you would NOT kill yourself?"

asQ Suicide Risk Screening Toolkit NATIONAL INSTITUTE OF MENTAL HEALTH (NIMH) 7/14/2017

Fig. 4.4 Brief Suicide Safety Assessment (BSSA) for Youth in the Outpatient Setting—(**a**) Front, (**b**) Back

panic, PTSD, OCD symptoms, hallucinations, delusions, reality testing, level of alertness, impulsivity)

- Developmental history including any physical or cognitive disabilities or impairments and remediation

NIMH TOOLKIT: OUTPATIENT

asQ Ask Suicide-Screening Questions

Brief Suicide Safety Assessment

3 Interview patient & parent/guardian together

If patient is ≥ 18 years, ask patient's permission for parent/guardian to join.

Say to the parent: "After speaking with your child, I have some concerns about his/her safety. We are glad your child spoke up as this can be a difficult topic to talk about. We would now like to get your perspective."

- "Your child said… (reference positive responses on the asQ). Is this something he/she shared with you?"
- "Does your child have a history of suicidal thoughts or behavior that you're aware of?" **If yes, say:** "Please explain."
- "Does your child seem:
  - o Sad or depressed?"
  - o Anxious?"
  - o Impulsive? Reckless?"
  - o Hopeless?"
  - o Irritable?"
  - o Unable to enjoy the things that usually bring him/her pleasure?"
  - o Withdrawn from friends or to be keeping to him/herself?"
- "Have you noticed changes in your child's:
  - o Sleeping pattern?"
  - o Appetite?"
- "Does your child use drugs or alcohol?"
- "Has anyone in your family/close friend network ever tried to kill themselves?"
- "How are potentially dangerous items stored in your home?" (e.g. guns, medications, poisons, etc.)
- "Does your child have a trusted adult they can talk to?" (Normalize that youth are often more comfortable talking to adults who are not their parents)
- "Are you comfortable keeping your child safe at home?"

At the end of the interview, ask the parent/guardian: "Is there anything you would like to tell me in private?"

4 Make a safety plan with the patient

Include the parent/guardian, if possible.

Create a safety plan for managing potential future suicidal thoughts. A safety plan is different than making a "safety contract"; asking the patient to contract for safety is NOT effective and may be dangerous or give a false sense of security.

Say to patient: "Our first priority is keeping you safe. Let's work together to develop a safety plan for when you are having thoughts of suicide."

Examples: "I will tell my mom/coach/teacher." "I will call the hotline." "I will call ________."

Discuss coping strategies to manage stress (such as journal writing, distraction, exercise, self-soothing techniques).

Discuss means restriction (securing or removing lethal means): "Research has shown that limiting access to dangerous objects saves lives. How will you secure or remove these potentially dangerous items (guns, medications, ropes, etc.)?"

Ask safety question: "Do you think you need help to keep yourself safe?" (A "no" response does not indicate that the patient is safe; but a "yes" is a reason to act immediately to ensure safety.)

5 Determine disposition

After completing the assessment, choose the appropriate disposition plan. *If possible, nurse should follow-up with a check-in phone call (within 48 hours) with all patients who screened positive.*

- ❑ **Emergency psychiatric evaluation:** **Patient is at imminent risk for suicide (current suicidal thoughts).** Send to emergency department for extensive mental health evaluation (unless contact with a patient's current mental health provider is possible and alternative safety plan for imminent risk is established).
- ❑ **Further evaluation of risk is necessary:** Review the safety plan and send home with a mental health referral as soon as patient can get an appointment (preferably within 72 hours).
- ❑ **Patient might benefit from non-urgent mental health follow-up:** Review the safety plan and send home with a mental health referral.
- ❑ **No further intervention is necessary at this time.**

For all positive screens, follow up with patient at next appointment.

6 Provide resources to all patients

- **24/7 National Suicide Prevention Lifeline 1-800-273-TALK (8255) En Español: 1-888-628-9454**
- **24/7 Crisis Text Line: Text "HOME" to 741-741**

asQ Suicide Risk Screening Toolkit NATIONAL INSTITUTE OF MENTAL HEALTH (NIMH) NIH 7/14/2017

Fig. 4.4 (continued)

- Past psychiatric history including any type of treatment, hospitalizations, or previous suicide attempts
- Family history especially family psychiatric history
- History of physical or sexual abuse or any previous child protection involvement
- Past medical history

asQ Ask Suicide-Screening Questions

NIMH TOOLKIT: INPATIENT

Brief Suicide Safety Assessment

What to do when a pediatric patient screens positive for suicide risk:

- Use after a patient **(10 - 24 years)** screens positive for suicide risk on the asQ
- Assessment guide for mental health clinicians, MDs, NPs, or PAs
- Prompts help determine disposition

1 Praise patient *for discussing their thoughts*

"I'm here to follow up on your responses to the suicide risk screening questions. These are hard things to talk about. Thank you for telling us. I need to ask you a few more questions."

2 Assess the patient *(If possible, assess patient alone depending on developmental considerations and parent willingness.)*

Review patient's responses from the asQ

Frequency of suicidal thoughts

Determine if and how often the patient is having suicidal thoughts.

Ask the patient: "In the past few weeks, have you been thinking about killing yourself?" **If yes, ask:** "How often?" (once or twice a day, several times a day, a couple times a week, etc.) "When was the last time you had these thoughts?"

"Are you having thoughts of killing yourself right now?" **(If "yes," patient is at imminent risk and requires an urgent/STAT mental health evaluation and cannot be left alone. Notify patient's medical team.)**

Suicide plan

Assess if the patient has a suicide plan, regardless of how they responded to any other questions (ask about method and access to means).

Ask the patient: "Do you have a plan to kill yourself?" **If yes, ask:** "What is your plan?" **If no plan, ask:** "If you were going to kill yourself, how would you do it?"

Note: If the patient has a very detailed plan, this is more concerning than if they haven't thought it through in great detail. If the plan is feasible (e.g., if they are planning to use pills and have access to pills), this is a reason for greater concern and removing or securing dangerous items (medications, guns, ropes, etc.).

Past behavior

Evaluate past self-injury and history of suicide attempts (method, estimated date, intent).

Ask the patient: "Have you ever tried to hurt yourself?" "Have you ever tried to kill yourself?"

If yes, ask: "How? When? Why?" and assess intent: "Did you think [method] would kill you?" "Did you want to die?" (for youth, intent is as important as lethality of method) **Ask:** "Did you receive medical/psychiatric treatment?"

Note: Past suicidal behavior is the strongest risk factor for future attempts.

Symptoms Ask the patient about:

Depression: "In the past few weeks, have you felt so sad or depressed that it makes it hard to do the things you would like to do?"

Anxiety: "In the past few weeks, have you felt so worried that it makes it hard to do the things you would like to do or that you feel constantly agitated/on-edge?"

Impulsivity/Recklessness: "Do you often act without thinking?"

Hopelessness: "In the past few weeks, have you felt hopeless, like things would never get better?"

Anhedonia: "In the past few weeks, have you felt like you couldn't enjoy the things that usually make you happy?"

Isolation: "Have you been keeping to yourself more than usual?"

Irritability: "In the past few weeks, have you been feeling more irritable or grouchier than usual?"

Substance and alcohol use: "In the past few weeks, have you used drugs or alcohol?" **If yes, ask:** "What? How much?"

Sleep pattern: "In the past few weeks, have you had trouble falling asleep or found yourself waking up in the middle of the night or earlier than usual in the morning?"

Appetite: "In the past few weeks, have you noticed changes in your appetite? Have you been less hungry or more hungry than usual?"

Other concerns: "Recently, have there been any concerning changes in how you are thinking or feeling?"

Social Support & Stressors

(For all questions below, if patient answers yes, ask them to describe.)

Support network: "Is there a trusted adult you can talk to? Who? Have you ever seen a therapist/counselor?" **If yes, ask:** "When?"

Family situation: "Are there any conflicts at home that are hard to handle?"

School functioning: "Do you ever feel so much pressure at school (academic or social) that you can't take it anymore?"

Bullying: "Are you being bullied or picked on?"

Suicide contagion: "Do you know anyone who has killed themselves or tried to kill themselves?"

Reasons for living: "What are some of the reasons you would NOT kill yourself?"

asQ Suicide Risk Screening Toolkit NATIONAL INSTITUTE OF MENTAL HEALTH (NIMH) NIH 7/14/2017

Fig. 4.5 Brief Suicide Safety Assessment (BSSA) for Youth in the Inpatient Medical Setting—(**a**) Front, (**b**) Back

asQ Ask Suicide-Screening Questions

NIMH TOOLKIT: INPATIENT

Brief Suicide Safety Assessment

3 Interview patient & parent/guardian together

If patient is ≥ 18 years, ask patient's permission for parent/guardian to join.

Say to the parent: "After speaking with your child, I have some concerns about his/her safety. We are glad your child spoke up as this can be a difficult topic to talk about. We would now like to get your perspective."

- "Your child said… (reference positive responses on the asQ). Is this something he/she shared with you?"
- "Does your child have a history of suicidal thoughts or behavior that you're aware of?" **If yes, say:** "Please explain."
- "Does your child seem:
  - o Sad or depressed?"
  - o Anxious?"
  - o Impulsive? Reckless?"
  - o Hopeless?"
  - o Irritable?"
  - o Unable to enjoy the things that usually bring him/her pleasure?"
  - o Withdrawn from friends or to be keeping to him/herself?
- "Have you noticed changes in your child's:
  - o Sleeping pattern?"
  - o Appetite?"
- "Does your child use drugs or alcohol?"
- "Has anyone in your family/close friend network ever tried to kill themselves?"
- "How are potentially dangerous items stored in your home?" (e.g. guns, medications, poisons, etc.)
- "Does your child have a trusted adult they can talk to?" (Normalize that youth are often more comfortable talking to adults who are not their parents)
- "Are you comfortable keeping your child safe at home?"

At the end of the interview, ask the parent/guardian: "Is there anything you would like to tell me in private?"

4 Make a safety plan with the patient

Include the parent/guardian, if possible.

Create a safety plan for managing potential future suicidal thoughts. A safety plan is different than making a "safety contract"; asking the patient to contract for safety is NOT effective and may be dangerous or give a false sense of security.

Say to patient: "Our first priority is keeping you safe. Let's work together to develop a safety plan for when you are having thoughts of suicide."

Examples: "I will tell my mom/coach/teacher." "I will call the hotline." "I will call ________."

Discuss coping strategies to manage stress (such as journal writing, distraction, exercise, self-soothing techniques).

Discuss means restriction (securing or removing lethal means): "Research has shown that limiting access to dangerous objects saves lives. How will you secure or remove these potentially dangerous items (guns, medications, ropes, etc.)?"

Ask safety question: "Do you think you need help to keep yourself safe?" (A "no" response does not indicate that the patient is safe; but a "yes" is a reason to act immediately to ensure safety.)

5 Determine disposition

After completing the assessment, choose the appropriate disposition plan.

- ❑ **Emergency psychiatric evaluation:** **Patient is at imminent risk for suicide (current suicidal thoughts).** Keep patient safe on the unit. Follow the standard of care for a suicidal patient (e.g. remove dangerous objects, 1:1 observer). Request a STAT, emergency psychiatric evaluation.
- ❑ **Further evaluation of risk is necessary:** Request a comprehensive mental health/safety evaluation prior to discharge.
- ❑ **Patient might benefit from non-urgent mental health follow-up post-discharge:** No further mental health evaluation in the hospital is needed at this time. Review safety plan for potential future suicidal thoughts and refer patient for a follow-up mental health evaluation in the community, post-discharge.
- ❑ **No further intervention is necessary at this time.**

6 Provide resources to all patients

- **24/7 National Suicide Prevention Lifeline 1-800-273-TALK (8255) En Español: 1-888-628-9454**
- **24/7 Crisis Text Line: Text "HOME" to 741-741**

asQ Suicide Risk Screening Toolkit NATIONAL INSTITUTE OF MENTAL HEALTH (NIMH) NIH 7/14/2017

Fig. 4.5 (continued)

- Medications (prescribed and over-the-counter)
- Substance use (legal and illegal)
- Social and school history
- Mental status exam (see ASQ BSSA for Outpatients, Fig. 4.4)

The following case examples help clarify when a full mental health evaluation is necessary.

Case example #1: A pediatric patient admitted to an ED for abdominal pain or an asthmatic episode screens positive on a suicide risk screening tool because they attempted suicide in the past; upon conducting a brief suicide safety assessment, it is discovered that the patient's parent is aware of the past attempt and the patient is currently receiving regular mental health treatment. Since this individual is determined not to be in imminent danger and is already connected with mental healthcare, it would not be necessary to conduct a full mental health evaluation in the ED.

Case example #2: A pediatric patient presents to the ED with the same medical chief complaint as the patient in example #1 (i.e., abdominal pain or an asthmatic episode). The patient screens positive for suicide risk. During the brief suicide safety assessment, the patient reveals that he is having frequent thoughts of suicide, has developed a feasible and worrisome suicide plan, has little hope for the future, and has never revealed these thoughts to anyone. In this case, an additional full mental health evaluation is warranted and necessary to guide next steps of how to safely connect this patient with much-needed mental health care.

Developmental considerations are important when assessing suicide risk. Assessments should be tailored so that the patient clearly understands what is being asked. It is important to avoid leading questions and to be direct (i.e., "Are you having thoughts about killing yourself" rather than, "You are not having any thoughts about killing yourself, are you?"). While clinicians may feel anxious and more comfortable asking the latter question, doing so will almost certainly lead the patient to respond dishonestly. It is also important to praise the patient for his or her willingness to speak up about a topic that is difficult for many to discuss. Clinicians should make an effort to recognize that many people have these thoughts but should stress the importance of developing effective coping mechanisms to refrain from acting on suicidal thoughts. For youth in particular, it is critical to address the frequency of thoughts. Someone who is thinking of suicide often cannot focus on other important things in life, such as schoolwork, social situations, family relationships, extracurricular activities, hobbies, and most importantly, joy. Developmental considerations may also affect what a child or adolescent believes to be a lethal method. When assessing level of risk, it is essential to understand a child's *intent* to die. The following case example highlights the importance of considering intent when discussing method.

Case example #3: A 10-year-old patient presents to his primary care physician for an annual checkup. During intake, the patient is screened for suicide risk and screens positive because he attempted suicide in the past. During the follow-up brief suicide safety assessment, the patient is asked to describe his attempt and reveals that he took four Tylenol. Although this amount of medication is not lethal, the patient fully intended to die and believed that this dose would result in death. As such, this suicide attempt should be treated with significance equivalent to an attempt involving a highly lethal method.

Patient Physical Examination

There is no specific medical test that indicates if someone is suicidal or how suicidal someone is outside of querying the person directly. In a general medical practice, if a person presents as suicidal as a sudden change in mental status, a basic medical evaluation may be warranted that includes a physical exam and tests for a general medical condition. Testing will include complete blood count, electrolytes, and urine and blood toxicology screening.

Physical Exam

- Examination assessing for any evidence of hematologic, neurologic, endocrine, gastrointestinal, autoimmune, or infectious diseases
- Evidence of previous suicide attempts or self-injury cuts and scars
- Evidence of physical or sexual abuse
- Vital signs for any significant fever, heart rate, or blood pressure changes
- Height and weight (and percentile) that may be suggestive of failure to thrive, eating disorder, short stature, or gigantism that may lead to teasing/bullying
- Possible medication side effects (e.g., dilated pupils, tachycardia, high blood pressure, nausea)

Laboratory Evaluation

- Toxicology screen/blood alcohol and drug screen (know what your laboratory screen does and does not test for—most screens will not pick up synthetic cannabinoids or other illicit drugs)
- Complete blood count and chemistry panel (electrolytes with liver function tests) to rule out medical etiologies
- Pregnancy test (if indicated)

Management

For the acutely suicidal patient, the main goal is keeping the patient safe. This will vary depending where treatment is taking place. For outpatient treatment, patients in imminent risk may need to be sent to the ED for closer monitoring and determination whether or not psychiatric hospitalization is warranted. In the ED or the inpatient setting, keeping the patient safe usually entails 24-h closed observation in the acute situation. Depending on the age, size, and determination of the person, the reliability of the family, and the patient's relationship with the clinician, this is managed in a variety of settings ranging from home to day hospital to full hospitalization with 1:1 constant observation. Clinicians try to put the person in the least restrictive environment that still maintains personal safety. The frequency of assessment will be largely related to how reliable the clinician believes the person to be with regard to behavior since there is no blood or imaging test for suicidality and clinicians must rely heavily on self-report. It is generally believed that past behavior predicts future behavior, so youth who have made previous attempts should be monitored more closely and for a longer duration.

Once a patient is deemed to have suicidal thoughts or behaviors, they should be continually monitored at future visits and check-ins. Even if the patient feels the issue has resolved, sensitive inquiry is still warranted at future visits, such as, "I know you are feeling better, but I wanted to ask if you have been having any thoughts about killing yourself lately."

Treatments

Treatment of a suicidal child or adolescent is focused on the short-term goals of keeping the youth safe while addressing the precipitating events (immediate stressors), helping the youth find alternative coping skills and problem solving. This generally requires that the parent of the child partner with a mental health clinician to help the youth stay safe. This also means reducing or buffering the stressor such as bullying, academic pressure, or family conflicts. It may require removing the child from the home if there is ongoing physical or sexual abuse. If the child is hopeless and severely depressed, inpatient psychiatric hospitalization may be necessary. Longer-term perpetuating or predisposing factors may require ongoing interventions with school officials or mental health clinicians including a psychiatrist to address psychiatric disorders or treatment programs to address ongoing substance use disorders. Thus, treatments may include outpatient psychotherapies including psychodynamic and interpersonal therapy, cognitive behavioral therapy, dialectical behavior therapy, family therapy, or social skills group to psychopharmacologic interventions for underlying psychiatric disorders such as ADHD, depression, anxiety, psychosis, or schizophrenia.

Treating youth with medications should be done cautiously and monitored closely. Antidepressants such as SSRIs or tricyclic antidepressants are often a first-line treatment. Lithium has been shown to have anti-suicidal properties and may be considered under some circumstances in adolescents. Ketamine, a rapidly acting antidepressant in adults, has also been shown to have rapid onset of anti-suicidal properties, but has not yet been fully studied in adolescents; trials are underway. Methods such as non-invasive neuromodulation including transcranial magnetic stimulation and electroconvulsive therapy are also being studied.

There is no single effective gold standard treatment modality for suicidal youth. Often a combination of cognitive behavior therapy (CBT) and pharmacological treatment is recommended. Many treatments have reduced suicidal ideation but are less effective in achieving the goal of treatment—preventing future suicide attempts [92]. There are also a number of interventions that are currently being studied in clinical trials, like Cognitive Behavior Therapy for Suicide Prevention (CBT-SP) [93]. Treatments such as the Collaborative Assessment and Management of Suicidality (CAMS) [94], have been shown to be effective in adults and are being adapted and tested for use with adolescent patients. Another treatment that has shown some reduction in suicide attempts post- treatment is Integrated Cognitive Behavior Therapy (ICBT) [95]. Some promising family-based interventions like the SAFETY Program [96] and the Family-based Crisis Intervention [97] are currently being examined for effectiveness in emergency departments and outpatient clinics.

Selective Serotonin Reuptake Inhibitors (SSRIs) and Suicidality

Antidepressant trials and SSRI prescriptions in children and adolescents increased rapidly from the late 1990s until 2003 when British regulators raised concerns about paroxetine and suicidality in children. In 2004, the US Food and Drug Administration (FDA), based on a meta-analysis that found children randomly assigned to antidepressants had twice the rate of suicidal ideation and behavior as compared to children randomly assigned to placebo (but no actual deaths), added a black box warning to all antidepressants [98, 99]. At that time, the FDA highlighted recommendations for close patient monitoring upon antidepressant initiation [100]. In May 2007, the black box warning was expanded to specifically include 18–24-year-olds [101].

Following the black box warning, overall use of antidepressants in children and adolescents decreased, and the pattern of drug use changed; decreased use of paroxetine and increased use of fluoxetine, the only FDA-approved SSRI for depressed youth as young as 6 years, has been described [102–104]. Practice patterns have shifted with more patients being referred to psychiatric specialists and lower doses at initiation though the frequency of visits does not appear to have been impacted [105, 106].

Since 2005, several studies have suggested that the increased rates of suicide in youth in the United States might be related to the decreased rates of antidepressant prescription [107–109]. Furthermore, Bridge et al. concluded that antidepressants, relative to placebo, are modestly efficacious for the treatment of pediatric major depressive disorder and that the benefits of antidepressants appear to be greater than the risks of suicidal ideation or suicide attempts [110]. In summary, there is modest evidence that antidepressants may be helpful in moderate to severe depression in young children with fluoxetine as the only FDA-approved SSRI for depression in young children. The black box warning remains in place for 18–24-year-olds with careful monitoring guidelines for suicidality suggested.

As is true of all pediatric medical treatments, especially involving mental healthcare, engaging parents is of paramount importance in the treatment of suicidal youth. It is critical to cultivate a positive and effective working alliance with parents/guardians. Parents may feel guilty or blamed for having a child with suicidal thoughts and/or behaviors. Sometimes, parents are at the core of their children's suicidal problems, so their involvement can be challenging; their participation may be therapeutic, or it could be troublesome. Nevertheless, it is important to actively engage parents in the treatment while at the same time respecting your patient's need for privacy and independence. Assure parents that while it is important to keep much of what your patient tells you confidential, you will always inform them should you have any safety concerns. Make sure to obtain the parent's perspective on the situation, as they will have insights and information that no one else can give you. It is not uncommon for parents to minimize or deny their child's suicidal thoughts. Be sure to speak pointedly about the high risks of suicidal thinking and the great need for treating all talk of suicide seriously. Make sure to partner with parents around designing the treatment plan, as they can be an aide in ensuring adherence to the plan. Educate the parents about how to recognize and respond to risk factors and warning signs of suicide. Keep parents updated with treatment progress and challenges [72, 111].

Make a Safety Plan with the Patient

Create a safety plan for managing potential future suicidal thoughts. A safety plan is different than making a "safety contract"; asking the patient to contract for safety is an antiquated method that mental health clinicians utilized in which they asked the patient to sign a contract stating that they would not kill themselves. This is not effective and may be dangerous, as it can give the clinician a false sense of security. In actuality, the only value in a safety contract is if a patient cannot agree. Regardless, this method is no longer considered valid. Instead, developing safety plans with patients and their families is advised. Tell the patient that your first priority is to keep them safe, and partner with them to create strategies to utilize if suicidal thoughts should arise in the future. Which trusted adult will they tell? Do they have the phone number for this adult? Do they have the suicide hotline or crisis text line available on their phone? Discuss means of restriction with the parents, and educate how to safely store or remove any lethal means in the home.

Ability to Consent/Legal/Confidentiality

Legally, adults at age 18 years have the ability to consent to treatment. This may vary by state to as young as 12 years of age, with regard to consent for substance abuse or mental health treatment without parental permission, so it is important to know one's state laws [112]. It is important to establish at the beginning of mental health treatment, particularly with adolescents and young adults, the boundaries of confidentiality which may not exclude parents when information concerning self-harm, suicidal thoughts and behaviors, or harm to others is revealed. As there is increasing evidence that, although incredibly rare, children as young as 3 or 4 years can make suicidal comments, it is important to alert parents or caregivers to any suicidal statements made in order to seek early treatment that includes family participation.

Often youth will not want you to disclose suicidal ideation to their parents. Remind them that by law you must do so. Also, tell them that you take these thoughts very seriously and the most important thing is to make sure they are safe, and that is why you must alert their parent/guardian about their suicidal thoughts.

Documentation

Accurate documentation is critical. As with all medical interactions, if the evaluation is not documented in a timely manner, it can be viewed as if it did not happen. The evaluator should document the absence or presence of known risk factors described above as well as any protective factors identified. Attempt to elicit any current stressors. Documentation should specifically address absence or presence of suicidal thoughts (if present: content, severity, frequency, controllability, impulsivity), history of previous attempts (if present: number, precipitants, method, and results), and access to lethal means. Documentation should be as objective as possible without overreporting or underreporting the suicidality. Document mental status exam including mood, anxiety, cognitive status, presence of psychosis, and suicidal or homicidal intent.

When working with children, adolescents, and young adults, in addition to speaking with them, it is important to gather collateral information from parents, school, or other relevant sources. This additional information may play a role in the formulation and plan. This too should be documented.

Documentation should include the clinician's judgment of the level of risk of suicide resulting in a documented action plan, e.g., outpatient therapy, partial hospitalization, or hospitalization. If a clinician deviates from the standard of care, she/he should indicate the reasons and may consider referring the patient for a second opinion [72].

Resources

All patients suspected to be at risk for suicide should be given, at minimum, the following two resources:

1. National Suicide Prevention Lifeline 1-800-273-TALK (8255)
2. Crisis Text Line: Text "START" to 741-741

The patient should be told that both of these resources can be contacted 24 hours a day, 7 days a week, and that there is always a trained person available to speak to them. Encourage youth to put these contact numbers in their cell phones and to share the contacts with their friends. In addition, any local resources, such as community mental health clinics, should also be provided.

Conclusion

There is nothing simple about assessing a child or adolescent for suicide risk. It is a humbling experience even for the most seasoned clinician. Once a patient expresses suicidal thoughts, unease in the clinician should be expected. We do not yet have crystal balls (or biomarkers) that can determine who will be safe and who will attempt suicide. While more research on suicidal thoughts and behaviors may develop better models of prediction, we will never be able to know exactly who will harm themselves and who will not. For these reasons, it is important to err on the side of caution every time. Put the patient's safety first, as best as you can, and know that there are limits to our ability to protect. Detecting suicide risk and managing those that screen positive is one of the most difficult endeavors in the field of mental healthcare. Yet, with appropriate training, ongoing learning experiences, and thoughtful interventions, every healthcare provider can have the chance to make a difference and hopefully save precious lives.

Acknowledgments The authors wish to thank Jarrod Smith for his thoughtful proofreading and careful attention to detail.

References

1. Gould MS, Greenberg TE, Velting DM, Shaffer D. Youth suicide risk and preventive interventions: a review of the past 10 years. J Am Acad Child Adolesc Psychiatry. 2003;42(4):386–405.
2. Horowitz LM, Bridge JA, Boudreaux ED. Screening youth for suicide risk in medical settings: time to ask questions. Am J Prev Med. 2014;47(3):S170–5.
3. Kessler RC, Berglund P, Demler O, Jin R, Merikangas KR, Walters EE. Lifetime prevalence and age-of-onset distributions of DSM-IV disorders in the National Comorbidity Survey Replication. Arch Gen Psychiatry. 2005;62(6):593–602.
4. Nock MK, Borges G, Bromet EJ, Cha CB, Kessler RC, Lee S. Suicide and suicidal behavior. Epidemiol Rev. 2008;30(1):133–54.
5. O'Carroll PW, Berman AL, Maris RW, Moscicki EK, Tanney BL, Silverman MM. Beyond the Tower of Babel: a nomenclature for suicidology. Suicide Life Threat Behav. 1996;26(3):237–52.
6. Posner K, Oquendo MA, Gould M, Stanley B, Davies M. Columbia Classification Algorithm of Suicide Assessment (C-CASA): classification of suicidal events in the FDA's pediatric suicidal risk analysis of antidepressants. Am J Psychiatry. 2007;164(7):1035–43.
7. Silverman MM, Berman AL, Sanddal ND, O'Carroll PW, Joiner TE. Rebuilding the tower of babel: a revised nomenclature for the study of suicide and suicidal behaviors part 1: background, rationale, and methodology. Suicide Life Threat Behav. 2007;37(3):248–63.
8. Centers for Disease Control and Prevention. Web-based Injury Statistics Query and Reporting System (WISQARS): fatal injury reports, national and regional, 1999–2015. https://webappa.cdc.gov/sasweb/ncipc/mortrate10_us.html.
9. US Cancer Statistics Working Group. United States cancer statistics: 1999–2013 incidence and mortality web-based report. Atlanta: US Department of Health and Human Services, Centers for Disease Control and Prevention and National Cancer Institute. https://nccd.cdc.gov/uscs/.
10. Curtin SC, Warner M, Hedegaard H. Increase in suicide in the United States, 1999–2014. NCHS Data Brief. 2016;241:1–8.

11. Centers for Disease Control and Prevention. WISQARS leading causes of death reports, national and regional. 2014. https://www.cdc.gov/injury/wisqars/leading_causes_death.html.
12. Bridge JA, Asti L, Horowitz LM, Greenhouse JB, Fontanella CA, Sheftall AH, et al. Suicide trends among elementary school–aged children in the United States from 1993 to 2012. JAMA Pediatr. 2015;169(7):673–7.
13. Sheftall AH, Asti L, Horowitz LM, Felts A, Fontanella CA, Campo JV, et al. Suicide in elementary school-aged children and early adolescents. Pediatrics. 2016;138(4):e20160436.
14. Centers for Disease Control and Prevention. Morbidity and Mortality Weekly Report (MMWR). https://www.cdc.gov/mmwr/volumes/65/wr/mm6543a8.htm?s_cid=mm6543a8_w.
15. Centers for Disease Control and Prevention. Youth Risk Behavior Surveillance System (YRBSS). https://www.cdc.gov/healthyyouth/data/yrbs/.
16. Grunbaum JA, Kann L, Kinchen S, Ross J, Hawkins J, Lowry R, et al. Youth risk behavior surveillance—United States, 2003. MMWR Surveill Summ. 2004 May;53(2):1–96.
17. Cash SJ, Bridge JA. Epidemiology of youth suicide and suicidal behavior. Curr Opin Pediatr. 2009;21(5):613.
18. Rodway C, Tham SG, Ibrahim S, Turnbull P, Windfuhr K, Shaw J, et al. Suicide in children and young people in England: a consecutive case series. Lancet Psychiatry. 2016;3(8):751–9.
19. Brent DA, Baugher M, Bridge J, Chen T, Chiappetta L. Age- and sex-related risk factors for adolescent suicide. J Am Acad Child Adolesc Psychiatry. 1999;38(12):1497–505.
20. Shaffer D, Gould MS, Fisher P, Trautman P, Moreau D, Kleinman M, Flory M. Psychiatric diagnosis in child and adolescent suicide. Arch Gen Psychiatry. 1996;53(4):339–48.
21. Shafii M, Steltz-Lenarsky J, Derrick AM, Beckner C, Whittinghill JR. Comorbidity of mental disorders in the post-mortem diagnosis of completed suicide in children and adolescents. J Affect Disord. 1988;15(3):227–33.
22. Goldston DB, Daniel SS, Erkanli A, Reboussin BA, Mayfield A, Frazier PH, et al. Psychiatric diagnoses as contemporaneous risk factors for suicide attempts among adolescents and young adults: developmental changes. J Consult Clin Psychol. 2009;77(2):281.
23. Borges G, Angst J, Nock MK, Ruscio AM, Walters EE, Kessler RC. A risk index for 12-month suicide attempts in the National Comorbidity Survey Replication (NCS-R). Psychol Med. 2006;36(12):1747–57.
24. Hawton K, Zahl D, Weatherall R. Suicide following deliberate self-harm: long-term follow-up of patients who presented to a general hospital. Br J Psychiatry. 2003;182(6):537–42.
25. Suokas J, Suominen K, Isometsä E, Ostamo A, Lönnqvist J. Long-term risk factors for suicide mortality after attempted suicide: findings of a 14-year follow-up study. Acta Psychiatr Scand. 2001;104(2):117–21.
26. Hall DJ, O'Brien F, Stark C, Pelosi A, Smith H. Thirteen-year follow-up of deliberate self-harm, using linked data. Br J Psychiatry. 1998;172(3):239–42.
27. Busch KA, Fawcett J, Jacobs DG. Clinical correlates of inpatient suicide. J Clin Psychiatry. 2003;64(1):14–9.
28. Bostwick JM, Pabbati C, Geske JR, McKean AJ. Suicide attempt as a risk factor for completed suicide: even more lethal than we knew. Am J Psychiatry. 2016;173(11):1094–100.
29. Negron R, Piacentini J, Graae F, Davies M, Shaffer D. Microanalysis of adolescent suicide attempters and ideators during the acute suicidal episode. J Am Acad Child Adolesc Psychiatry. 1997;36(11):1512–9.
30. Esposito-Smythers C, Spirito A. Adolescent substance use and suicidal behavior: a review with implications for treatment research. Alcohol Clin Exp Res. 2004;28(5 Suppl):77s–88s.
31. Aseltine RH, Schilling EA, James A, Glanovsky JL, Jacobs D. Age variability in the association between heavy episodic drinking and adolescent suicide attempts: findings from a large-scale, school-based screening program. J Am Acad Child Adolesc Psychiatry. 2009;48(3):262–70.
32. Brent DA, Melhem N. Familial transmission of suicidal behavior. Psychiatr Clin North Am. 2008;31(2):157–77.

33. Nock MK, editor. The Oxford handbook of suicide and self-injury. New York: Oxford University Press; 2014.
34. Rajalin M, Hirvikoski T, Jokinen J. Family history of suicide and exposure to interpersonal violence in childhood predict suicide in male suicide attempters. J Affect Disord. 2013;148(1):92–7.
35. Melhem NM, Brent DA, Ziegler M, Iyengar S, Kolko D, Oquendo M, et al. Familial pathways to early-onset suicidal behavior: familial and individual antecedents of suicidal behavior. Am J Psychiatry. 2007;164(9):1364–70.
36. Brent DA, Mann JJ. Familial pathways to suicidal behavior—understanding and preventing suicide among adolescents. N Engl J Med. 2006;355(26):2719–21.
37. Joiner TE, Sachs-Ericsson NJ, Wingate LR, Brown JS, Anestis MD, Selby EA. Childhood physical and sexual abuse and lifetime number of suicide attempts: a persistent and theoretically important relationship. Behav Res Ther. 2007;45(3):539–47.
38. Jokinen J, Forslund K, Ahnemark E, Gustavsson JP, Nordström P, Asberg M. Karolinska Interpersonal Violence Scale predicts suicide in suicide attempters. J Clin Psychiatry. 2010;71(8):1025–32.
39. Salzinger S, Rosario M, Feldman RS, Ng-Mak DS. Adolescent suicidal behavior: associations with preadolescent physical abuse and selected risk and protective factors. J Am Acad Child Adolesc Psychiatry. 2007;46(7):859–66.
40. Plunkett A, O'Toole B, Swanston H, Oates RK, Shrimpton S, Parkinson P. Suicide risk following child sexual abuse. Ambul Pediatr. 2001;1(5):262–6.
41. O'Brien KH, Putney JM, Hebert NW, Falk AM, Aguinaldo LD. Sexual and gender minority youth suicide: understanding subgroup differences to inform interventions. LGBT Health. 2016;3(4):248–51.
42. Youth KL. Risk behavior surveillance—United States, 2015. MMWR Surveill Summ. 2016;65(6):1–174.
43. Eisenberg ME, Resnick MD. Suicidality among gay, lesbian and bisexual youth: the role of protective factors. J Adolesc Health. 2006;39(5):662–8.
44. Veale J, Saewyc E, Frohard-Dourlent H, Dobson S, Clark B. Being safe, being me: results of the Canadian Trans Youth Health survey, vol. 79. Vancouver, BC: Stigma and Resilience; 2015.
45. Raifman J, Moscoe E, Austin SB, McConnell M. Difference-in-differences analysis of the association between state same-sex marriage policies and adolescent suicide attempts. JAMA Pediatr. 2017;171(4):350–6. https://doi.org/10.1001/jamapediatrics.2016.4529.
46. Stone DM, Luo F, Ouyang L, Lippy C, Hertz MF, Crosby AE. Sexual orientation and suicide ideation, plans, attempts, and medically serious attempts: evidence from local youth risk behavior surveys, 2001–2009. Am J Public Health. 2014;104(2):262–71.
47. D'Augelli AR, Grossman AH, Salter NP, Vasey JJ, Starks MT, Sinclair KO. Predicting the suicide attempts of lesbian, gay, and bisexual youth. Suicide Life Threat Behav. 2005;35(6):646–60.
48. Haas AP, Rodgers PL, Herman JL. Suicide attempts among transgender and gender nonconforming adults. 2014. http://escholarship.org/uc/item/8xg8061f.
49. Grossman AH, D'Augelli AR. Transgender youth and life-threatening behaviors. Suicide Life Threat Behav. 2007;37(5):527–37.
50. Klomek AB, Sourander A, Niemelä S, Kumpulainen K, Piha J, Tamminen T, et al. Childhood bullying behaviors as a risk for suicide attempts and completed suicides: a population-based birth cohort study. J Am Acad Child Adolesc Psychiatry. 2009;48(3):254–61. https://doi.org/10.1097/CHI.0b013e318196b91f.
51. Stanley IH, Horowitz LM, Bridge JA, Wharff EA, Teach SJ. Bullying and suicide risk among pediatric emergency department patients. Pediatr Emerg Care. 2016;32(6):347–51.
52. Hinduja S, Patchin JW. Bullying beyond the schoolyard: preventing and responding to cyberbullying. Thousand Oaks: Corwin Press; 2014.
53. Hinduja S, Patchin JW. Bullying, cyberbullying, and suicide. Arch Suicide Res. 2010;14(3):206–21. https://doi.org/10.1080/13811118.2010.494133.

54. Rosin H. The Silicon Valley suicides: why are so many kids with bright prospects killing themselves in Palo Alto? Washington, DC: The Atlantic; 2015.
55. Joshi SV, Hartley SN, Kessler M, Barstead M. School-based suicide prevention: content, process, and the role of trusted adults and peers. Child Adolesc Psychiatr Clin N Am. 2015;24(2):353–70.
56. Bennett M. The importance of interviewing adults on the autism spectrum about their depression and suicidal ideation experiences. J Autism Dev Disord. 2016;46(4):1492–3. https://doi.org/10.1007/s10803-015-2674-4.
57. Mayes SD, Gorman AA, Hillwig-Garcia J, Syed E. Suicide ideation and attempts in children with autism. Res Autism Spectr Disord. 2013;7(1):109–19.
58. Hannon G, Taylor EP. Suicidal behaviour in adolescents and young adults with ASD: findings from a systematic review. Clin Psychol Rev. 2013;33(8):1197–204.
59. Horowitz LM, Bridge JA, Teach SJ, Ballard E, Klima J, Rosenstein DL, et al. Ask Suicide-Screening Questions (ASQ): a brief instrument for the pediatric emergency department. Arch Pediatr Adolesc Med. 2012;166(12):1170–6.
60. Karmakar C, Luo W, Tran T, Berk M, Venkatesh S. Predicting risk of suicide attempt using history of physical illnesses from electronic medical records. JMIR Mental Health. 2016;3(3):e19. https://doi.org/10.2196/mental.5475.
61. Misono S, Weiss NS, Fann JR, Redman M, Yueh B. Incidence of suicide in persons with cancer. J Clin Oncol. 2008;26(29):4731–8.
62. Qin P, Webb R, Kapur N, Sørensen HT. Hospitalization for physical illness and risk of subsequent suicide: a population study. J Intern Med. 2013;273(1):48–58.
63. Webb RT, Kontopantelis E, Doran T, Qin P, Creed F, Kapur N. Suicide risk in primary care patients with major physical diseases: a case-control study. Arch Gen Psychiatry. 2012;69(3):256–64.
64. Zhou ES, Hu JC, Kantoff PW, Recklitis CJ. Identifying suicidal symptoms in prostate cancer survivors using brief self-report. J Cancer Surviv. 2015;9(1):59–67.
65. Brinkman TM, Zhang N, Recklitis CJ, Kimberg C, Zeltzer LK, Muriel AC, et al. Suicide ideation and associated mortality in adult survivors of childhood cancer. Cancer. 2014;120(2):271–7.
66. Recklitis CJ, Diller LR, Li X, Najita J, Robison LL, Zeltzer L. Suicide ideation in adult survivors of childhood cancer: a report from the Childhood Cancer Survivor Study. J Clin Oncol. 2009;28(4):655–61.
67. Shah SS, Dellarole A, Peterson EC, Bregy A, Komotar R, Harvey PD, et al. Long-term psychiatric outcomes in pediatric brain tumor survivors. Childs Nerv Syst. 2015;31(5):653–63.
68. Kuo CJ, Chen VC, Lee WC, Chen WJ, Ferri CP, Stewart R, et al. Asthma and suicide mortality in young people: a 12-year follow-up study. Am J Psychiatry. 2010;167(9):1092–9.
69. Thibault DP, Mendizabal A, Abend NS, Davis KA, Crispo J, Willis AW. Hospital care for mental health and substance abuse in children with epilepsy. Epilepsy Behav. 2016;57:161–6. https://doi.org/10.1016/j.yebeh.2016.01.031.
70. Cha CB, Nock MK. Emotional intelligence is a protective factor for suicidal behavior. J Am Acad Child Adolesc Psychiatry. 2009;48(4):422–30.
71. Kazdin AE. Research design in clinical psychology. 4th ed. Boston: Pearson; 2003.
72. King CA, Foster CE, Rogalski KM. Teen suicide risk: a practitioner guide to screening, assessment, and management. New York: Guilford Press; 2013.
73. King CA, Merchant CR. Social and interpersonal factors relating to adolescent suicidality: a review of the literature. Arch Suicide Res. 2008;12(3):181–96.
74. Lewinsohn PM, Rohde P, Seeley JR, Baldwin CL. Gender differences in suicide attempts from adolescence to young adulthood. J Am Acad Child Adolesc Psychiatry. 2001;40(4):427–34.
75. Donald M, Dower J, Correa-Velez I, Jones M. Risk and protective factors for medically serious suicide attempts: a comparison of hospital-based with population-based samples of young adults. Aust N Z J Psychiatry. 2006;40(1):87–96.
76. Pearce CM, Martin G. Locus of control as an indicator of risk for suicidal behaviour among adolescents. Acta Psychiatr Scand. 1993;88(6):409–14.

77. Everall RD, Altrows KJ, Paulson BL. Creating a future: a study of resilience in suicidal female adolescents. J Couns Dev. 2006;84(4):461.
78. Piquet ML, Wagner BM. Coping responses of adolescent suicide attempters and their relation to suicidal ideation across a 2-year follow-up: a preliminary study. Suicide Life Threat Behav. 2003;33(3):288–301.
79. Dervic K, Oquendo MA, Grunebaum MF, Ellis S, Burke AK, Mann JJ. Religious affiliation and suicide attempt. Am J Psychiatry. 2004;161(12):2303–8.
80. Kleiman EM, Liu RT. Prospective prediction of suicide in a nationally representative sample: religious service attendance as a protective factor. Br J Psychiatry. 2014;204(4):262–6.
81. Rasic D, Kisely S, Langille DB. Protective associations of importance of religion and frequency of service attendance with depression risk, suicidal behaviours and substance use in adolescents in Nova Scotia, Canada. J Affect Disord. 2011;132(3):389–95.
82. Pena JB, Caine ED. Screening as an approach for adolescent suicide prevention. Suicide Life Threat Behav. 2006;36(6):614–37.
83. The Joint Commission. Detecting and treating suicide ideation in all settings. 2016. https://www.jointcommission.org/assets/1/18/SEA_56_Suicide.pdf.
84. Beck AT, Kovacs M, Weissman A. Assessment of suicidal intention: the scale for suicide ideation. J Consult Clin Psychol. 1979;47(2):343.
85. Diamond G, Levy S, Bevans KB, Fein JA, Wintersteen MB, Tien A, et al. Development, validation, and utility of internet-based, behavioral health screen for adolescents. Pediatrics. 2010;126(1):e163–70.
86. Posner K, Brown GK, Stanley B, Brent DA, Yershova KV, Oquendo MA, et al. The Columbia–Suicide Severity Rating Scale: initial validity and internal consistency findings from three multisite studies with adolescents and adults. Am J Psychiatry. 2011;168(12):1266–77.
87. Johnson JG, Harris ES, Spitzer RL, Williams JB. The patient health questionnaire for adolescents: validation of an instrument for the assessment of mental disorders among adolescent primary care patients. J Adolesc Health. 2002;30(3):196–204.
88. Gould MS, Marrocco FA, Kleinman M, Thomas JG, Mostkoff K, Cote J, et al. Evaluating iatrogenic risk of youth suicide screening programs: a randomized controlled trial. JAMA. 2005;293(13):1635–43.
89. Mathias CW, Michael Furr R, Sheftall AH, Hill-Kapturczak N, Crum P, et al. What's the harm in asking about suicidal ideation? Suicide Life Threat Behav. 2012;42(3):341–51.
90. Crawford MJ, Thana L, Methuen C, Ghosh P, Stanley SV, Ross J, et al. Impact of screening for risk of suicide: randomised controlled trial. Br J Psychiatry. 2011;198(5):379–84.
91. Barber CW, Miller MJ. Reducing a suicidal person's access to lethal means of suicide: a research agenda. Am J Prev Med. 2014;47(3):S264–72.
92. Koslow SH, Ruiz P, Nemeroff CB, editors. A concise guide to understanding suicide: epidemiology, pathophysiology and prevention. Cambridge: Cambridge University Press; 2014.
93. Stanley B, Brown G, Brent DA, Wells K, Poling K, Curry J, et al. Cognitive-behavioral therapy for suicide prevention (CBT-SP): treatment model, feasibility, and acceptability. J Am Acad Child Adolesc Psychiatry. 2009;48(10):1005–13.
94. Jobes DA. The Collaborative Assessment and Management of Suicidality (CAMS): an evolving evidence-based clinical approach to suicidal risk. Suicide Life Threat Behav. 2012;42(6):640–53.
95. Esposito-Smythers C, Spirito A, Kahler CW, Hunt J, Monti P. Treatment of co-occurring substance abuse and suicidality among adolescents: a randomized trial. J Consult Clin Psychol. 2011;79(6):728.
96. Asarnow JR, Berk M, Hughes JL, Anderson NL. The SAFETY program: a treatment-development trial of a cognitive-behavioral family treatment for adolescent suicide attempters. J Clin Child Adolesc Psychol. 2015;44(1):194–203.
97. Wharff EA, Ginnis KB, Ross AM, White EM, White MT, Forbes PW. Family-based crisis intervention with suicidal adolescents: a randomized clinical trial. Pediatr Emerg Care. 2017. https://doi.org/10.1097/PEC.0000000000001076.

98. Hammad TA, Laughren T, Racoosin J. Suicidality in pediatric patients treated with antidepressant drugs. Arch Gen Psychiatry. 2006;63(3):332–9.
99. Leslie LK, Newman TB, Chesney PJ, Perrin JM, Greenhouse JB, Kelleher KJ, et al. The food and drug Administration's deliberations on antidepressant use in pediatric patients. Pediatrics. 2005;116(1):233–5.
100. US Food and Drug Administration. FDA launches a multi-pronged strategy to strengthen safeguards for children treated with antidepressant medications. FDA News-For Immediate Release. 15 Oct 2014.
101. Stone M, Laughren T, Jones ML, Levenson M, Holland PC, Hughes A, et al. Risk of suicidality in clinical trials of antidepressants in adults: analysis of proprietary data submitted to US Food and Drug Administration. BMJ. 2009;339:b2880.
102. Bhatia SK, Rezac AJ, Vitiello B, Sitorius MA, Buehler BA, Kratochvil CJ. Antidepressant prescribing practices for the treatment of children and adolescents. J Child Adolesc Psychopharmacol. 2008;18(1):70–80.
103. Kurian BT, Ray WA, Arbogast PG, Fuchs DC, Dudley JA, Cooper WO. Effect of regulatory warnings on antidepressant prescribing for children and adolescents. Arch Pediatr Adolesc Med. 2007;161(7):690–6.
104. Nemeroff CB, Kalali A, Keller MB, Charney DS, Lenderts SE, Cascade EF, et al. Impact of publicity concerning pediatric suicidality data on physician practice patterns in the United States. Arch Gen Psychiatry. 2007;64(4):466–72.
105. Busch SH, Frank RG, Leslie DL, Martin A, Rosenheck RA, Martin EG, et al. Antidepressants and suicide risk: how did specific information in FDA safety warnings affect treatment patterns? Psychiatr Serv. 2010;61(1):11–6.
106. Morrato EH, Libby AM, Orton HD, deGruy III, MD FV, Brent DA, Allen R, et al. Frequency of provider contact after FDA advisory on risk of pediatric suicidality with SSRIs. Am J Psychiatry. 2008;165(1):42–50.
107. Gibbons RD, Brown CH, Hur K, Marcus SM, Bhaumik DK, Erkens JA, et al. Early evidence on the effects of regulators' suicidality warnings on SSRI prescriptions and suicide in children and adolescents. Am J Psychiatry. 2007;164(9):1356–63.
108. Gibbons RD, Hur K, Bhaumik DK, Mann JJ. The relationship between antidepressant prescription rates and rate of early adolescent suicide. Am J Psychiatry. 2006;163(11):1898–904.
109. Katz LY, Kozyrskyj AL, Prior HJ, Enns MW, Cox BJ, Sareen J. Effect of regulatory warnings on antidepressant prescription rates, use of health services and outcomes among children, adolescents and young adults. Can Med Assoc J. 2008;178(8):1005–11.
110. Bridge JA, Iyengar S, Salary CB, Barbe RP, Birmaher B, Pincus HA, et al. Clinical response and risk for reported suicidal ideation and suicide attempts in pediatric antidepressant treatment: a meta-analysis of randomized controlled trials. JAMA. 2007;297(15):1683–96.
111. Jobes DA. Managing suicidal risk: a collaborative approach. 2nd ed. New York: Guilford; 2016.
112. Kerwin ME, Kirby KC, Speziali D, Duggan M, Mellitz C, Versek B, et al. What can parents do? A review of state laws regarding decision making for adolescent drug abuse and mental health treatment. J Child Adolesc Subst Abuse. 2015;24(3):166–76.

5 Substance Abuse and Suicide

Youssef Mahfoud and Michael Ignatowski

Introduction

Substance use disorders (SUD) involve the recurrent use of alcohol and/or drugs leading to consuming larger amounts than intended, being unable to quit when attempting, cravings, and using in hazardous situations. They also include other clinical and functional impairment, such as health problems, disability, or social deficiency such as failure to meet major responsibilities at work, school, and home. Tolerance and withdrawal symptoms can often develop with continued use. The substance use disorders can be defined as mild, moderate, and severe depending on the degree of impairment and the number of diagnostic criteria met [1].

The 2015 National Survey on drug use in the United States revealed that over 175 million persons (65.7% of the population ages 12 and up) reported alcohol use in the past year, with over 66 million (24.9%) reporting binge drinking in the previous month. Another 12.5 million reported misusing prescription pain relievers, and over 300,000 reported using heroin in the past year. Overall, 7.8% of the population (20.8 million people) met diagnostic criteria for a substance use disorder for alcohol or illicit drugs, and another 1% met diagnostic criteria for both an alcohol and illicit drug use disorder. Only 2.2 million individuals (10.4%) received any type of treatment. Of those treated, only 63.7% received treatment in specialty substance use disorder treatment programs [2].

Y. Mahfoud, M.D., F.A.P.A., F.A.S.A.M. (✉)
Opioid Treatment Program, CWRU School of Medicine, Cleveland Louis Stokes VA Medical Center, Cleveland, OH, USA
e-mail: Youssef.Mahfoud@va.gov

M. Ignatowski, D.O.
CWRU School of Medicine, Cleveland Louis Stokes VA Medical Center, Cleveland, OH, USA
e-mail: Michael.Ignatowski2@va.gov

T. Falcone, J. Timmons-Mitchell (eds.), *Suicide Prevention*,
https://doi.org/10.1007/978-3-319-74391-2_5

Untreated, these individuals are more likely to have a poorer prognosis that includes developing chronic health conditions, have poorer health outcomes, and interact with the criminal justice system. The National Institute on Drug Abuse estimates that substance use disorders cost the United States more than $440 billion annually in costs related to health care, crime, and lost workplace productivity. One contributing factor to lost productivity is premature mortality, from associated health conditions, accidental overdose, as well as suicide [3, 4].

Substance use plays a major role in suicide risk. This link is well established, as up to 90% of individuals who do complete suicide suffer from a DSM-5 diagnosis of mental illness, substance use disorder, or both [5–7]. Substance use is second only to mood disorders as the most frequent risk factor for suicide [8]. Individuals with a substance use disorder are approximately six times more likely to report a lifetime suicide attempt than those without [9]. Rates of completed suicide among men with a substance use disorder are two–three times higher than the general population, while females with substance use disorder are six–nine times more likely to die of suicide [10, 11].

The majority of individuals with mental illness and substance use disorders do not die by suicide, so identifying additional risk factors can be important for proper assessment and care. Risk factors for suicide among substance users are similar to those of the general population and include advancing age, co-occurring affective disorders, and repeat attempts [12–15].

Though an association with suicide risk exists between substance use in general and those who abuse multiple substances, alcohol use remains one of the most studied and well-defined risks associated with acute and chronic risk [16].

Alcohol Use and Suicide

The effects of alcohol consumption on behavior are progressive and highly correlated to blood alcohol levels. Initially, alcohol produces an anxiolytic effect and may increase sociability, but at high levels, it can further reduce inhibition and impair judgment and motor function. Chronic alcohol use can detrimentally affect almost every organ in the body and is associated with mood and anxiety disorders [17].

The link between suicide and alcohol is a complex phenomenon that was already known to Emil Kraepelin over a century ago, and addiction itself was also conceptualized by Menninger as a form of chronic suicide [18, 19]. Alcohol dependence is a known major risk factor for suicidal behavior with a lifetime mortality due to suicide as high as 18% [20, 21]. As much as 40% of all patients seeking treatment for alcohol dependence reported at least one suicide attempt in their lifetime and in a review of the epidemiological literature, it was found that the lifetime risk of suicide in alcohol-dependent individuals was 2.2% and 3.4% in outpatient and inpatient settings, respectively [22–24].

A meta-analysis of 32 papers related to alcohol dependence and abuse found that the suicide risk is increased 6 times with variations of 1–60, higher for females than for males, 20 times vs. 4 times, and heavy alcohol drinkers have a 5-time higher risk of suicide than social drinkers [5].

Suicide risk for alcohol dependence was similar to that of mood disorders 7% vs. 6%, and psychological autopsy studies in multiple nations consistently showed that mood and SUD, especially alcohol, are the most prevalent disorders in suicide [25–28]. Alcohol misuse was present in the history of 56% of individuals who completed suicide, and up to 68% of males and 29% females who committed suicide met criteria for alcohol abuse or dependence [29, 30].

The association between alcohol consumption and suicide was analyzed in 13 nations, and in 10 out of 13 countries, suicide rates was positively associated with per capita consumption of alcohol [31]. There are few exceptions though. Hungary, for example, saw a 30% decline of suicide rates between 1984 and 1998 despite an increase in alcohol dependence rates of 25% between 1989 and 1996, while Portugal has a low rate of suicide despite having one of the highest rates of alcohol consumption in Europe [32, 33]. The effect of alcohol on suicide may be stronger in northern European countries, with low capita consumption and a binge drinking pattern versus southern European wine countries with a high average consumption that is more evenly distributed throughout the week [34].

Alcohol is neither a necessary nor sufficient condition for suicide but can be regarded as a contributing factor [35]. The relationship between both is complex. Alcohol may affect suicidal ideation and behavior, while suicidal ideation may affect alcohol use and alcohol use and suicide may affect each other. Alcohol use may also aggravate other factors that affect suicide, and both alcohol use and suicide might be affected by a third factor such as an underlying mood disorder [36].

Acute alcohol use is associated with suicide risk, and high rates (33–69%) of positive blood alcohol concentrations have been found among suicide completers [5, 37]. Alcohol intoxication also predicts the use of more lethal means like firearms and plays an important role in the events leading to suicide among individuals with no previous psychiatric history, because it produces disinhibition which can facilitate suicidal ideations and increase the likelihood of suicidal thoughts being put to action [37–41]. Alcohol intake may also result in a lack of behavioral inhibition and other aspects of impulsiveness like poor thinking and planning and impaired attention [42].

Impulsivity is related to suicidal and self-destructive behaviors within different psychiatric conditions like mood disorders, impulse control disorders, antisocial, and borderline personality disorders [43]. In a study of detoxified subjects with alcohol dependence, those with a history of suicidal attempts had a greater lifetime incidence of aggressive behavior and higher scores on a trait measure of aggression/impulsivity [44]. Depressed individuals with alcohol dependence have higher rates of impulsivity and suicide attempts, and it seems that the greater frequency of suicidal behavior and severity of suicidal ideation in MDD with comorbid alcohol dependence are related to more aggressive traits [45, 46].

The tendency to engage in violent behavior is also an important risk factor for suicide and might also partially account for the connection between SUD and suicide [47]. Violence may be an indicator of increased impulsivity and social isolation which increases the risk of suicide [48, 49]. It was hypothesized that individuals with difficulty to control anger were more likely to act impulsively and turn violence to themselves rather than on others [47]. Up to 75% of those who begin addiction treatment have engaged in violent behavior, and a study of 6000 adults in addiction treatment showed that those who had committed serious violent acts were twice more likely to report multiple suicide attempts [50–52]. A history of domestic violence is commonly found in men with alcohol use disorders who complete suicide [48]. Violence toward a romantic partner is a predictor of suicidal thoughts and behaviors in substance use, and a history of physical aggression toward a partner was associated with a higher level of suicidal ideation than aggression toward a non-partner [53].

There is considerable evidence on the association between aggression and serotonin deficiency [54]. Reduced serotonin transporter binding in the hippocampus was found in postmortem studies of brain tissues from patients with alcohol dependence, and binding was reduced in the 5-HT1A receptors of alcohol consumers compared to those who did not drink [55–57]. The anterior medial prefrontal cortical area of depressed patients with comorbid alcohol dependence had more severe hypofrontality than depressed patients without alcohol dependence, and this group difference disappeared after fenfluramine administration suggesting serotonin mechanisms [58]. Lower serotonin activity in the prefrontal cortex is tied to a decreased behavioral inhibition and impulsivity which might enhance suicidal behavior. Also high-lethality depressed suicide attempters with comorbid alcohol dependence have lower cerebrospinal fluid 5-HIAA levels [59].

As for comorbid psychopathology, alcoholic suicidal attempters appear to be more depressed than nonalcoholic attempters. In autopsy studies, 89% of alcohol-dependent suicides demonstrated history of another psychiatric illness, and 25% had unipolar depression [60]. In another study, 97% of patients with bipolar I disorder and comorbid drug and alcohol UD made a suicide attempt [61].

A psychological explanation for the relationship between acute alcohol use and suicidal behavior was proposed by Hufford. Alcohol increases psychological distress, hopelessness, loneliness, and depression; enhances aggressive behavior and self-aggression; changes expectation; helps propel suicidal ideation into action; and constricts attention, inhibiting effective coping strategies [37]. In a sociological interpretation, alcohol use leads to social deterioration, anomie, unemployment, debts, and social isolation [62–64].

Recognizing the extensive role alcohol can play in suicide risk is important for the care of patients. Those with alcohol use disorder should be screened for suicidal ideation and risk, and treatment for those with suicidal ideation should always take into account drinking habits. Subsequently, those at risk should be offered withdrawal management as well as psychosocial treatment, such as motivational interviewing, cognitive behavioral therapy, and 12-step treatment, and pharmacological treatments such as naltrexone and acamprosate when appropriate [65].

Opioid Use and Suicide

Abuse of illegal opioid drugs, such as heroin and legally available though often illegally obtained pain relievers such as oxycodone and fentanyl, is an ever-growing epidemic in the United States. In the 2014, 12.5 million reported misusing prescription pain relievers, and over 300,000 reported using heroin in the past year [2]. Opioids can relieve perception of pain but can also induce drowsiness and euphoria and can depress respiration. Tolerance leads to increasing doses and methods used to obtain the euphoria the opiates produce. Opiate-naive individuals or individuals who have lost tolerance due to a period of abstinence are at increased risk for respiratory depression and unintentional overdose.

In 2014 alone, overdoses claimed the lives of over 29,000 individuals in the United States, compared to less than 6000 deaths in 1999 [66]. Individuals who mix opiates with other sedating drugs such as benzodiapines or alcohol are also at higher risk.

Difficulty arises attributing deaths as intentional suicide attempts because of the high frequency of unintentional overdoses that can occur. United Kingdom statistics for heroin addict deaths in 1993 attributed to suicide was 6%, while the vast majority was attributed to unintentional overdose [67].

The suicide death number may be underestimated in this data [68]. Further complicating this data is the fact that suicide attempts in individuals with substance use disorders often involve overuse of the drugs they may typically use for recreation [69]. Concerning completed suicides that are not overdoses, individuals with opiate use disorders may also be at an increased risk for firearm death [70].

Getting individuals treatment in opiate replacement programs has shown to reduce overdose deaths, and the added support and monitoring may reduce suicide risk as well [71]. Methadone and buprenorphine are commonly used for medication-assisted treatment for opiate use disorder. Methadone is a synthetic opioid agonist that has been available for decades by licensed methadone treatment programs. A large evidence base indicates that methadone reduces risk and criminal behaviors and reduces death rates [72, 73]. Buprenorphine is a partial opioid agonist, available in a tablet, film, or implantable formulation, that binds strongly to opiate receptors, reducing the upper limits of pain relief, euphoria, as well as respiratory depression and possibility of overdose. Buprenorphine is often combined with the opioid antagonist naloxone. While naloxone has insignificant bioavailability, it serves as a deterrent for injection, as doing so would precipitate a withdrawal state instead of a euphoric high. Buprenorphine can be prescribed in an office-based setting by physicians who obtain the waiver to do so and thus is likely more readily available than methadone maintenance. Like methadone, available evidence indicates improved outcomes and reduction of illicit opiate use [74].

Another potential lifesaving measure to prevent opiate overdose death, intentional or unintentional, is the use of inhaled or injectable naloxone which can quickly reverse opioid-induced respiratory depression. Distribution of take-home naloxone rescue kits along with training for those with opiate use disorder as well as instruction for their peers and family members has the potential to help dramatically decrease overdose-related deaths [75]. Clinicians should refer individuals to treatment programs and promote access and education to naloxone rescue kits to reduce suicide risk and unintentional overdose mortality.

Cocaine Use and Suicide

Cocaine is an illicitly obtained stimulant often smoked, snorted, or injected, that enhances monoamine neurotransmitters (serotonin, norepinephrine, and dopamine), by blocking pre-synaptic reuptake. Use leads to a sympathetic response that includes increased alertness, elevate blood pressure, heart rate, respiration, and energy level as well as produce the sought-after euphoric high. In overdose, cocaine can cause life-threatening hypertension leading to myocardial infarction or stroke, as well as rhabdomyolysis and renal failure. In 2014, over 5400 deaths in the United States were attributed to intentional and unintentional cocaine overdose, higher than previous years [76].

Cocaine withdrawal symptoms result from a dopamine-depleted state in the body that occurs after stopping or reducing use, including fatigue, hunger, irritability, depression, and suicidal thoughts that can last several days following a cocaine binge [77]. Those with a prior history of depression are more likely to experience severe depression and suicidal ideation while in cocaine withdrawal [78, 79]. Depression and suicidal ideation develop in chronic heavy users in higher rates than the general population, as well as a higher incident of suicide attempts [80, 81].

A study of 749 postmortem suicides in New York City revealed that cocaine was found in 18–22% of cases, and those using cocaine were twice as likely to have taken their own life by firearm. Whether the extent of the high prevalence of suicide in the days following cocaine use is due to the withdrawal phenomenon, prior depression, or other sociodemographic factors, the withdrawal state should be viewed as an added time of elevated risk of suicide [82].

A clinician evaluating a cocaine user in withdrawal should assess for suicidal ideation and should treat this as a very real risk factor for suicide [12]. Extended observation or inpatient admission can be considered, as well as referral to substance use recovery programs. Treatments such as cognitive behavioral therapy and contingency management, which involves giving tangible rewards for positive behavior, have been shown to improve outcomes for cocaine users [83].

Conclusion

In conclusion, there is a strong association between substance use and suicide. Clinicians should recognize the importance of screening for mood disorders and suicide in patients with substance use disorders. Likewise, a careful screen for substance use should be done in patients with suicidal ideations or recent suicide attempts. Such patients should be treated and referred to appropriate services for both substance use and other comorbid psychiatric conditions.

References

1. American Psychiatric Association. Diagnostic and statistical manual of mental disorders (DSM-5). 5th ed. Arlington: American Psychiatric Publishing; 2013.
2. Center for Behavioral Health Statistics and Quality. Results from the 2015 National Survey on Drug Use and Health: detailed tables. Rockville: Substance Abuse and Mental Health Services Administration; 2016.

3. Sacks JJ, Gonzales KR, Bouchery EE, Tomedi LE, Brewer RD. 2010 national and state costs of excessive alcohol consumption. Am J Prev Med. 2015;49(5):e73–9.
4. National Drug Intelligence Center. National drug threat assessment. Washington, DC: US Department of Justice; 2011.
5. Harris EC, Barraclough B. Suicide as an outcome for mental disorders: a meta-analysis. Br J Psychiatry. 1997;170:205–28.
6. Mościcki EK. Epidemiology of completed and attempted suicide: toward a framework for prevention. Clin Neurosci Res. 2001;1(5):310–23.
7. Conwell Y, Duberstein PR, Caine ED. Risk factors for suicide in later life. Biol Psychiatry. 2002;52(3):193–204.
8. Nelson AR, Stith AY, Smedley BD, editors. Unequal treatment: confronting racial and ethnic disparities in health care (full printed version). Washington, DC: National Academies Press; 2002.
9. Kessler RC, Borges G, Walters EE. Prevalence of and risk factors for lifetime suicide attempts in the National Comorbidity Survey. Arch Gen Psychiatry. 1999;56(7):617–26.
10. Maloney E, Degenhardt L, Darke S, Mattick RP, Nelson E. Suicidal behaviour and associated risk factors among opioid-dependent individuals: a case–control study. Addiction. 2007;102(12):1933–41.
11. Darke S, Ross J, Lynskey M, Teesson M. Attempted suicide among entrants to three treatment modalities for heroin dependence in the Australian Treatment Outcome Study (ATOS): prevalence and risk factors. Drug Alcohol Depend. 2004;73(1):1–10.
12. Ilgen MA, Harris AH, Moos RH, Tiet QQ. Predictors of a suicide attempt one year after entry into substance use disorder treatment. Alcohol Clin Exp Res. 2007;31:635–42.
13. Borges G, Walters EE, Kessler RC. Associations of substance use, abuse, and dependence with subsequent suicidal behavior. Am J Epidemiol. 2000;151(8):781–9.
14. Wilcox HC, Conner KR, Caine ED. Association of alcohol and drug use disorders and completed suicide: an empirical review of cohort studies. Drug Alcohol Depend. 2004;76:S11–9.
15. Schneider B. Substance use disorders and risk for completed suicide. Arch Suicide Res. 2009;13(4):303–16.
16. Preuss UW, Schuckit MA, Smith TL, Danko GP, Buckman K, Bierut L, et al. Comparison of 3190 alcohol-dependent individuals with and without suicide attempts. Alcohol Clin Exp Res. 2002;26(4):471–7.
17. Ries RK, Fiellin DA, Miller SC, Saitz R, editors. Principles of addiction medicine. 4th ed. Philadelphia: Lippincott Williams & Wilkins; 2014.
18. Kraepelin E. Psychiatrie: ein Lehrbuch für Studirende und Aerzte. 6. vollständig umgearbeitete Auflage. Zweiter Band, Klinische Psychiatrie; Verlag von Johann Ambrosius. Leipzig: Barth; 1899.
19. Menninger KA. Man against himself. New York: Harcourt, Brace; 1938.
20. Roy A, Linnoila M. Alcoholism and suicide. Suicide Life Threat Behav. 1986;16:244–73.
21. Sher L, Zalsman G. Alcohol and adolescent suicide. Int J Adolesc Med Health. 2005;17:197–203.
22. Anderson BA, Howard MO, Walker RD, Suchinsky RT. Characteristics of substance- abusing veterans attempting suicide: a national study. Psychol Rep. 1995;77:1231–42.
23. Roy A. Distal risk factors for suicidal behavior in alcoholics: replications and new findings. J Affect Disord. 2003;77:267–71.
24. Murphy GE, Wetzel RD. The lifetime risk of suicide in alcoholism. Arch Gen Psychiatry. 1990;47:383–92.
25. Inskip HM, Harris EC, Barraclough B. Lifetime risk of suicide for affective disorder, alcoholism and schizophrenia. Br J Psychiatry. 1998;172:35–7.
26. Barraclough B, Bunch J, Nelson B, Sainsbury PA. Hundred cases of suicide: clinical aspects. Br J Psychiatry. 1974;125:355–73.
27. Rich CL, Ricketts JE, Fowler RC, Young D. Some differences between men and women who commit suicide. Am J Psychiatry. 1988;145(6):718–22.
28. Duberstein PR, Conwell Y, Caine ED. Age differences in the personality characteristics of suicide completers: preliminary findings from a psychological autopsy study. Psychiatry. 1994;57(3):213–24.

29. Conwell Y, Duberstein PR, Cox C, Herrmann JH, Forbes NT, Caine ED. Relationships of age and axis I diagnoses in victims of completed suicide: a psychological autopsy study. Am J Psychiatry. 1996;153(8):1001.
30. Kolves K, Värnik A, Tooding LM, Wasserman D. The role of alcohol in suicide: a case-control psychological autopsy study. Psychol Med. 2006;36(7):923–30.
31. Lester D. Alcoholism, substance abuse, and suicide. In: Maris RW, Berman AL, Silverman MM, editors. Comprehensive textbook of suicidology. New York: The Guilford Press; 2000. p. 357–75.
32. Rihmer Z, Belsö N, Kalmár S. Antidepressants and suicide prevention in Hungary. Acta Psychiatr Scand. 2001;88:238.
33. Lester D. Alcohol availability, alcoholism, and suicide and homicide. Am J Drug Alcohol Abuse. 1995;21:147–50.
34. Razvodovsky YE. Beverage-specific alcohol sale and suicide in Russia. Crisis. 2009;30:186–91.
35. Pompili M, Serafini G, Innamorati M, Dominici G, Ferracuti S, Kotzalidis GD, et al. Suicidal behavior and alcohol abuse. Int J Environ Res Public Health. 2010;7(4):1392–431.
36. Gossop M. Alcohol in suicide attempts and completions. Psychiatr Ann. 2005;35:513–21.
37. Hufford MR. Alcohol and suicidal behavior. Clin Psychol Rev. 2001;21:797–811.
38. Cherpitel CJ, Borges GL, Wilcox HC. Acute alcohol use and suicidal behavior: a review of the literature. Alcohol Clin Exp Res. 2004;28(Suppl):18–28S.
39. May PA, Van Winkle NW, Williams MB, McFeeley PJ, DeBruyn LM, Serna P. Alcohol and suicide death among American Indians of New Mexico: 1980–1998. Suicide Life Threat Behav. 2002;32:240–55.
40. Pirkola S, Isometsa E, Heikkinen M, Lonnqvist J. Employment status influences the weekly patterns of suicide among alcohol misusers. Alcohol Clin Exp Res. 1997;21:1704–6.
41. Brent DA, Perper JA, Allman CJ. Alcohol, firearms, and suicide among youth. JAMA. 1987;257(24):3369–72.
42. Simon TR, Swann AC, Powell KE, Potter LB, Kresnow MJ, O'Carroll PW. Characteristics of impulsive suicide attempts and attempters. Suicide Life Threat Behav. 2001;32(Suppl):49–59.
43. Sher L. Alcohol consumption and suicide. QJM. 2006;99(1):57–61.
44. Koller G, Preuss UW, Bottlender M, Wenzel K, Soyka M. Impulsivity and aggression as predictors of suicide attempts in alcoholics. Eur Arch Psychiatry Clin Neurosci. 2002;252:155–60.
45. Sher L, Oquendo MA, Li S, Huang Y, Grunebaum MF, Burke AK, et al. Lower CSF homovanillic acid levels in depressed patients with a history of alcoholism. Neuropsychopharmacology. 2003;28(9):1712.
46. Sher L, Oquendo MA, Galfalvy HC, Grunebaum MF, Burke AK, Zalsman G, et al. The relationship of aggression to suicidal behavior in depressed patients with a history of alcoholism. Addict Behav. 2005;30:1144–53.
47. Tiet QQ, Ilgen MA, Byrnes HF, Moos RH. Suicide attempts among substance use disorder patients: an initial step toward a decision tree for suicide management. Alcohol Clin Exp Res. 2006;30:998–1005.
48. Conner KR, Ilgen MA. Substance use and suicidal behaviour. In: O'Connor R, Platt S, Gordon J, editors. International handbook of suicide prevention. Chichester: Wiley-Blackwell; 2001.
49. Conner KR, Duberstein PR, Conwell Y. Domestic violence, separation, and suicide in young men with early onset alcoholism: reanalyses of Murphy's data. Suicide Life Threat Behav. 2000;30:354–9.
50. Burnette ML, Ilgen M, Frayne SM, Lucas E, Mayo J, Weitlauf JC. Violence perpetration and childhood abuse among men and women in substance abuse treatment. J Subst Abus Treat. 2008;35(2):217–22.
51. Chermack ST, Murray RL, Walton MA, Booth BA, Wryobeck J, Blow FC. Partner aggression among men and women in substance use disorder treatment: correlates of psychological and physical aggression and injury. Drug Alcohol Depend. 2008;98(1):35–44.
52. Ilgen MA, Burnette ML, Conner KR, Czyz E, Murray R, Chermack S. The association between violence and lifetime suicidal thoughts and behaviors in individuals treated for substance use disorders. Addict Behav. 2010;35(2):111–5.

53. Ilgen MA, Chermack ST, Murray R, Walton MA, Barry KL, Wojnar M, et al. The association between partner and non-partner aggression and suicidal ideation in patients seeking substance use disorder treatment. Addict Behav. 2009;34(2):180–6.
54. Badawy AA. Alcohol, aggression and serotonin: metabolic aspects. Alcohol Alcohol. 1998;33:66–72.
55. Gross-Isseroff R, Biegon A. Autoradiographic analysis of [3H]imipramine binding in the human brain postmortem: effects of age and alcohol. J Neurochem. 1988;51:528–34.
56. Chen HT, Casanova MF, Kleinman JE, Zito M, Goldman D, Linnoila M. 3H-paroxetine binding in brains of alcoholics. Psychiatry Res. 1991;38:293–9.
57. Dillon KA, Gross-Isseroff R, Israeli M, Biegon A. Autoradiographic analysis of serotonin 5-HT1A receptor binding in the human brain postmortem: effects of age and alcohol. Brain Res. 1991;554:56–64.
58. Sher L, Milak MS, Parsey RV, Carballo JJ, Cooper TB, Malone KM, et al. Positron emission tomography study of regional brain metabolic responses to a serotonergic challenge in major depressive disorder with and without comorbid lifetime alcohol dependence. Eur Neuropsychopharmacol. 2007;17(9):608–15.
59. Sher L, Oquendo MA, Grunebaum MF, Burke AK, Huang YY, Mann JJ. CSF monoamine metabolites and lethality of suicide attempts in depressed patients with alcohol dependence. Eur Neuropsychopharmacol. 2007;17(1):12–5.
60. Foster T, Gillespie K, McClelland R. Mental disorders and suicide in Northern Ireland. Br J Psychiatry. 1997;170(5):447–52.
61. Sublette ME, Carballo JJ, Moreno C, Galfalvy HC, Brent DA, Birmaher B, et al. Substance use disorders and suicide attempts in bipolar subtypes. J Psychiatr Res. 2009;43(3):230–8.
62. Skog OJ. Alcohol and suicide: Durkheim revisited. Acta Sociol. 1991;34(3):193–206.
63. Magne-Ingvar U, Öjehagen A, Träskman-Bendz L. Suicide attempters with and without reported overconsumption of alcohol and tranquillizers. Nord J Psychiatry. 1997;51(6):415–21.
64. Platt S, Robinson A. Parasuicide and alcohol: a 20 year survey of admissions to a regional poisoning treatment centre. Int J Soc Psychiatry. 1991;37(3):159–72.
65. Berglund M, Thelander S, Salaspuro M, Franck J, Andréasson S, Öjehagen A. Treatment of alcohol abuse: an evidence-based review. Alcohol Clin Exp Res. 2003;27(10):1645–56.
66. National Institute on Drug Abuse. Overdose death rates. 2015. http://www.drugabuse.gov/related-topics/trends-statistics/overdose-death-rates. Accessed 25 Nov 2016.
67. Home Office. Home Office statistical bulletin: statistics of drug addicts notified to the Home Office, UK, 1993. London: Government Statistical Service; 1994.
68. Frischer M, Bloor M, Goldberg D, Clark J, Green S, McKeganey N. Mortality among drug injectors and notified addicts. J Epidemiol Community Health. 1993;47(4):336.
69. Kwon M, Yang S, Park K, Kim DJ. Factors that affect substance users' suicidal behavior: a view from the Addiction Severity Index in Korea. Ann General Psychiatry. 2013;12(1):35.
70. Sheehan CM, Rogers RG, Boardman JD. Postmortem presence of drugs and method of violent suicide. J Drug Issues. 2015;45(3):249–62.
71. Caplehorn JR, Dalton MS, Cluff MC, Petrenas A. Retention in methadone maintenance and heroin addicts' risk of death. Addiction. 1994;89(2):203–7.
72. Connock M, Juarez-Garcia A, Jowett S, Frew E, Liu Z, Taylor RJ, et al. Methadone and buprenorphine for the management of opioid dependence: a systematic review and economic evaluation. Health Technol Assess. 2007;11(9):1.
73. Stotts AL, Dodrill CL, Kosten TR. Opioid dependence treatment: options in pharmacotherapy. Expert Opin Pharmacother. 2009;10(11):1727–40.
74. Fiellin DA, Friedland GH, Gourevitch MN. Opioid dependence: rationale for and efficacy of existing and new treatments. Clin Infect Dis. 2006;43(Suppl 4):S173–7.
75. Walley AY, Xuan Z, Hackman HH, Quinn E, Doe-Simkins M, Sorensen-Alawad A, et al. Opioid overdose rates and implementation of overdose education and nasal naloxone distribution in Massachusetts: interrupted time series analysis. BMJ. 2013;346:f174.

76. Centers for Disease Control and Prevention. CDC wonder: multiple cause of death 1999–2014. 2016. http://wonder.cdc.gov/wonder/help/mcd.html. Accessed 17 May 2016.
77. Pilotte NS. Neurochemistry of cocaine withdrawal. Curr Opin Neurol. 1997;10(6):534–8.
78. Mulvaney FD, Alterman AI, Boardman CR, Kampman K. Cocaine abstinence symptomatology and treatment attrition. J Subst Abus Treat. 1999;16(2):129–35.
79. Sofuoglu M, Dudish-Poulsen S, Brown SB, Hatsukami DK. Association of cocaine withdrawal symptoms with more severe dependence and enhanced subjective response to cocaine. Drug Alcohol Depend. 2003;69(3):273–82.
80. Narvaez JC, Jansen K, Pinheiro RT, Kapczinski F, Silva RA, Pechansky F, et al. Psychiatric and substance-use comorbidities associated with lifetime crack cocaine use in young adults in the general population. Compr Psychiatry. 2014;55(6):1369–76.
81. Friedman AS, Terras A, Zhu W, McCallum J. Depression, negative self-image, and suicidal attempts as effects of substance use and substance dependence. J Addict Dis. 2004;23(4):55–71.
82. Marzuk PM, Tardiff K, Leon AC, Stajic M, Morgan EB, Mann JJ. Prevalence of cocaine use among residents of New York City who committed suicide during a one-year period. Am J Psychiatry. 1992;149(3):371.
83. Carroll KM, Nich C, Petry NM, Eagan DA, Shi JM, Ball SA. A randomized factorial trial of disulfiram and contingency management to enhance cognitive behavioral therapy for cocaine dependence. Drug Alcohol Depend. 2016;160:135–42.

Suicide in Children and Adults with Epilepsy: A Complex Relationship

6

Jana E. Jones and Jessica M. Bordenave

Abbreviations

AEDs	Antiepileptic drugs
aHR	Adjusted hazard ratio
aOR	Adjusted odds ratio
CDC	Centers for Disease Control and Prevention
CI	Confidence interval
FDA	US Food and Drug Administration
IRR	Incidence rate ratio
KSADS	Kiddie Schedule for Affective Disorders and Schizophrenia – Present and Lifetime Version
OR	Odds ratio
PR	Prevalence ratio
SMR	Standardized mortality ratio
TLE	Temporal lobe epilepsy
WCST	Wisconsin Card Sorting Test
WHO	World Health Organization

Introduction

According to the World Health Organization (WHO), epilepsy is one of the most common neurological disorders, with approximately 50 million people worldwide diagnosed with epilepsy [1]. Epilepsy is the fourth most common neurological

J. E. Jones, Ph.D. (✉) · J. M. Bordenave, Psy.D.
Department of Neurology, University of Wisconsin School of Medicine and Public Health, Madison, WI, USA
e-mail: jejones@neurology.wisc.edu; JBordenave@uwhealth.org

T. Falcone, J. Timmons-Mitchell (eds.), *Suicide Prevention*,
https://doi.org/10.1007/978-3-319-74391-2_6

disorder after stroke, Alzheimer's disease, and migraine [2]. A recent international review and meta-analysis reported an overall lifetime prevalence of epilepsy of 7.6 per 1000 and an estimated active period prevalence of 2.83 cases per 1000 each year [3]. When examined by country income, there was a lifetime prevalence of 8.75 per 1000 and active period prevalence of 6.79 in low- and middle-income countries and a 5.18 lifetime and 2.06 active prevalence in high-income countries. In addition, 1 in 26 individuals in the United States will develop epilepsy in their lifetime [4]. The mortality of people with epilepsy in developed countries is two to three times that of the general population, with important consideration for causes due to sudden unexpected death in epilepsy (SUDEP), status epilepticus, and suicide [1].

Suicide is a potentially preventable cause of death in epilepsy, yet it accounts for a large proportion of mortality in epilepsy with rates reported to be three to five times higher compared to healthy controls in population-based studies [5–8]. In this chapter, we will review a number of the complexities involved in suicide among people with epilepsy, including the following: (a) prevalence of suicide compared to the general population in adults and children, (b) risk factors for suicidal behavior, (c) the bidirectional relationship between epilepsy and suicide, (d) the role of antiepileptic drugs (AEDs) in suicide risk, and (e) assessment of suicidal behavior as well as clinical interventions aimed at treatment and prevention of suicidality and its risk factors in epilepsy.

Prevalence Rates of Suicide and Suicidal Behavior in Epilepsy

Suicide in Adults with Epilepsy

According to the most recent reports from the Centers for Disease Control and Prevention (CDC), suicide was the 10th leading cause of death in the United States, accounting for 13.4 per 100,000 deaths in 2014 [9]. A large meta-analysis examining suicide and epilepsy mortality found that 32.5% of deaths in adults with epilepsy are due to suicide, with suicide in epilepsy accounting for an estimated 13.5% of all suicide deaths in the general population [10].

The relationship between epilepsy and suicide was first reported in 1941 by Prudhomme. A recent analysis by Tian et al. [11] examined suicide data in the general population in the United States in 17 states spanning the years 2003–2011. The researchers identified 972 suicide cases with epilepsy and 81,529 suicide cases without epilepsy. In terms of methods used for suicide, individuals with epilepsy were more likely to use some form of poison but less likely to use hanging, strangulation, suffocation, or firearms. For cases both with and without epilepsy, most suicides occurred in non-Hispanic whites between the ages of 18 and 59. When examined by age group, people with epilepsy were more likely to commit suicide than those without epilepsy, with the highest prevalence rates occurring among women aged 30–39 years old, women and men aged 40–49 years old, and men 50–59 years old. Individuals with epilepsy were less likely to commit suicide if they were younger than 30 years old or older than 70 years. In the analysis, Tian et al.

[11] also observed a trend of increasing rates of suicide in adults with epilepsy from 2005 to 2010 (13.01 to 23.20/100,00), when it peaked before declining in 2011 (20.40/100,000). The estimated average annual suicide rate among adults with epilepsy in this study suicide was 22% higher than the general population, with 16.89/100,000 persons with epilepsy compared to 13.84/100,000 in the general population.

Prevalence Rates of Suicidal Ideation and Suicidal Attempts in Adults with Epilepsy

The estimated prevalence of suicidal ideation in the general population in the United States was approximately 3–4% [12, 13] and 5–8% among adults with medical conditions such as arthritis, cancer, and stroke [14–16]. A large population-based study in Canada found a lifetime prevalence of 25% for suicidal ideation in people with epilepsy, compared to 13.3% in people without epilepsy [17]. Among a sample of people with epilepsy in England, Rai et al. [18] found 26.5% had lifetime prevalence of suicidal thoughts (12.2% in the previous year), 12.5% suicide attempts (4.1% attempts in the previous year), and 12.7% endorsed deliberate self-harm behaviors. Additionally, in a large international population-based study involving 14 countries, Scott et al. [19] reported that the presence of a physical illness was a significant risk factor for suicidal behavior, and epilepsy, in particular, was most strongly associated with suicidal ideation (odds ratio (OR) = 2.6; 95% CI, 1.3–5.1) and suicide attempts (OR = 4.5; 95% CI, 1.3–15.2).

Suicide attempts or self-harm has been studied less extensively than suicide in epilepsy, but research has shown higher rates of self-harm thoughts and behaviors in epilepsy over the general population with rates ranging from five to seven times higher [20]. Meyers et al. [20] also examined methods of self-harm behavior among individuals with epilepsy using prescribed AEDs, with carbamazepine, phenytoin, and sodium valproate reported as the most frequently utilized. In a study examining thoughts of death and self-harm in adults with epilepsy or multiple sclerosis, Dickstein et al. [21] found that 14% of adults with epilepsy reported thoughts of death or self-harm over the prior 2 weeks, with higher likelihood of the presence of depression and/or poorer perceived quality of life. Interestingly, these rates were similar in adults with multiple sclerosis. Adults with epilepsy were also at increased risk for repeated suicide attempt or self-harm behaviors over time. In this study comparing self-harm among people with and without epilepsy, Meyer et al. [20] found that adults with epilepsy had more than twice the risk of repetition of self-harm (4–11 repeated attempts over 15 years) and had a shorter time to a first attempt or self-harm repeat episode than adults without epilepsy.

Prevalence Rates of Suicide, Suicide Attempts, and Suicidal Ideation in Youth with Epilepsy

Among youth (aged 10–24 years) in the United States, suicide was the second leading cause of death, with approximately 6000 suicides completed each year [22]. In children (aged 10–14 years), suicide continued to be rare (426 suicides) [22]. Lifetime prevalence rates of suicidal behavior from the National Comorbidity Survey Replication Adolescent Supplement [23] were reported as follows: (1) suicidal ideation, 12.1%; (2) suicide plan, 4.0%; and (3) suicide attempts, 4.1%.

Among youth with epilepsy, completed suicide remained quite low, and the majority of studies reported only suicidal ideation and suicidal attempts. Among children and adolescents with physical disabilities or other chronic health conditions, Barnes et al. [24] reported that there was a 20% increase in suicidal behavior (suicidal ideation and attempts) among children and adolescents with a chronic physical condition. Youth with both a mental health and physical condition were 2.5–3.5 times more likely to have suicidal behavior. Everett Jones and Lollar [25] found that high school students in the United States with physical disabilities or long-term health issues were 2.7 times more likely to seriously consider a suicide attempt and 3.5 times more likely to make a suicide attempt compared to healthy high school students. In Denmark, Christiansen and Stenager [26] examined the association between attempted suicide in children and adolescents and a number of health conditions. These authors reported that epilepsy, asthma, insulin-dependent diabetes mellitus, and malformations were significant medical condition risk factors for suicide attempts. After adjusting for confounding variables, they further concluded that children with a psychiatric history, low socioeconomic status, previous suicide attempts, and unstable medical conditions that resulted in hospital visits were primary risk factors for suicide attempts.

Guilfoyle et al. [27] evaluated children in a new-onset epilepsy clinic ranging in ages 7–17 years at baseline and approximately at 6-month follow-up. At baseline, 24 of 132 (18%) children with epilepsy had suicidal ideation, and at 6-month follow-up, 6 continued to endorse suicidal ideation, while 18 no longer endorsed symptoms. At follow-up, 14 new cases of suicidal ideation were reported, and one was actively suicidal. Using a similar screening tool, Wagner et al. [28] reported 27% endorsed mild to moderate suicidal ideation in a sample of children with epilepsy aged 9–17 years. As part of psychiatric interview using the Kiddie Schedule for Affective Disorders and Schizophrenia – Present and Lifetime Version (K-SADS), 20% of the sample aged 5–16 years endorsed suicidal ideation [29].

Risk Factors for Suicide in Epilepsy

As noted throughout this book, suicide is a significant public health problem, and identifying modifiable risk factors for suicidal behavior is a primary focus of efforts to reduce suicides in youth and adults. In the general child and adolescent population, risk factors for suicide include psychiatric disorders, including depression, anxiety, and disruptive disorders [30, 31]. Additional risk factors for both youth and adults include victimization (e.g., sexual or physical abuse, bullying, etc.), social isolation, alcohol and substance use, sexual activity, eating disorders, past suicide attempt, and family history of suicide attempt [32, 33]. Similar to the general population, some studies have reported that additional psychosocial factors correlated with higher risk of suicidal ideation or attempts in adults with epilepsy, including previous psychiatric treatment, experience of interpersonal violence, unemployment status, substance abuse, housing problems, and maladaptive coping (escape-avoidance) [6, 20, 34]. This section will focus on two risk factors that are quite common among youth and adults with epilepsy—psychiatric comorbidity and executive dysfunction.

Psychiatric Comorbidity

Psychiatric comorbidities have been found to be prevalent among adults with epilepsy, with lifetime prevalence rates estimated at 10–34% for a mood disorder, 19–23% for anxiety, and 5–7% for panic disorder/agoraphobia [17, 18, 35]. In children with epilepsy, psychiatric comorbidity is often identified at or before the diagnosis of epilepsy and has a chronic course. Prevalence rates of mood disorders include 20–25%, anxiety disorders 13–48%, and ADHD 30% [27, 36–41]. Psychiatric comorbidities have been identified as a primary risk factor of suicide in adolescents and adults in the general population [23, 42, 43], and this risk factor has been identified in the epilepsy population as well.

A large population-based case-control study [5] found not only an increased risk of psychiatric disorders in adults with epilepsy, but the highest risk of suicide was among adults with a history of epilepsy and psychiatric comorbidities, especially mood disorders. Other studies have documented mood disorders, particularly depression and dysphoria, as significant—if not the primary—risk factors for suicide and suicidal ideation in people with epilepsy [44–46]. A case-control study examining suicide in adults with epilepsy [47] found that psychiatric disorders accounted for a ninefold increase in suicide risk. In another large population-based study, Fazel et al. [6] also found that psychiatric comorbidity increased suicide mortality rate: compared to controls without epilepsy or depression, individuals with epilepsy and a diagnosis of depression had an adjusted odds ratio (aOR) for suicide of 22.9 (95% CI, 16.6–31.6). Controls with depression but without epilepsy had an aOR for suicide of 9.9 (95% CI, 7.9–12.4), and individuals with epilepsy but not depression had an aOR of 3.1 (95% CI, 2.6–3.6). Additionally, Fazel et al. [6] found a further increased risk for suicide in individuals with epilepsy with comorbid substance misuse (aOR = 21.5; 95% CI, 16.6–27.8) compared to controls with substance misuse (aOR = 9.4; 95% CI, 7.6–11.6) and individuals with epilepsy without substance misuse (aOR = 2.2; 95% CI, 1.8–2.6).

Hecimovic et al. [48] conducted a prospective study of 193 adults with epilepsy and examined demographic and epilepsy factors, such as seizure frequency, epilepsy duration, medication toxicity, and self-perceived quality of life, in addition to depressive symptoms. While depression, medication toxicity, past suicide attempts, and quality of life scores were worse in adults that endorsed suicidal ideation compared to their non-suicidal peers, only a depression score was independently predictive of suicidal ideation. A study examining mortality in adults with refractory temporal lobe epilepsy (TLE) in Cuba found that over the course of 9 years, 3 individuals out of 117 committed suicide [49]. Two of the three were diagnosed with depression, had previous suicide attempts, and perceived poor quality of life; however, only the presence of a prodromal depressive disorder was significantly related to deaths in this study. In another study by Andrade-Machado et al. [44], the presence of a dysphoric disorder was found to be a risk factor for suicidal behavior, as 52% of individuals with an affective disorder had suicide risk, and the severity of depression was proportional to suicide risk. Quality of life was also examined, and 51% of individuals endorsed a lower quality of life score, especially among those with a dysphoric disorder. Individuals with a higher suicidal risk also had a lower quality of life compared to those without suicidal risk [44].

In a sample of children with focal and generalized epilepsy, Caplan et al. [50] reported that 20% of children reported active suicidal ideation with 37% of those individuals reporting a plan. Only 9% of healthy control children endorsed suicidal ideation. There were no suicide attempts in this sample. Children with epilepsy and a comorbid a disruptive disorder as well as anxiety and/or depression were 12 (OR, 12.4; CI: 4.05–39.38) times more likely to report suicidal ideation. Notably only 1/3 of these children were receiving treatment for their psychiatric comorbidity. Additionally, having more than one psychiatric disorder in children with epilepsy placed them at higher risk for suicidal thoughts and ideation [29].

Executive Dysfunction

Recently in the adult general population, neuropsychological studies have focused on the relationship between cognition and both suicidal ideation and attempts. Keilp et al. [51, 52] reported deficits in memory, working memory, and interference processing in suicide attempters. Keilp et al. [53] also reported that impaired attention was related to suicidal behavior. Additional studies have indicated that impulsivity and decreased decision-making ability increased the risk of suicidal behavior [54, 55]. Interestingly, Westheide et al. [56] found that executive dysfunction was only present in recent attempters who continued to report suicidal ideation.

In epilepsy populations, on a neuropsychological task of novel problem solving (Wisconsin Cart Sorting Test [WCST]), perseverative errors and other errors were associated with suicide risk and suicide attempts in adults with temporal lobe epilepsy (TLE). Additionally, adults with TLE who had more total, perseverative, and other errors were likely to have a higher risk of suicide attempts [57]. The overall model indicated a 6.3-fold increase in risk for suicide in adults with TLE with a family history of psychiatric disease, longer seizure disorder duration, current major depressive episode, left TLE, and more WCST perseverative responses and total errors. The model also explained a 7.5-fold increase in risk for suicide attempts for adults with epilepsy with family psychiatric history, current depressive episode, left TLE, and elevated WCST perseverative responses and total errors. The authors hypothesize that executive functioning plays an important role in self-control, emotional control, and other factors that might contribute to an impulsive decision to self-harm [57].

Another study examined suicidality and impulsivity in people with TLE based on a self-report measure assessing motor, non-planning, and attentional impulsivity [58]. They found that suicide risk was significantly associated with motor impulsivity (e.g., "I act on impulse," "I act on the spur of the moment", "I buy things on impulse," "I make up my mind quickly", and "I do things without thinking." [59]). There was no association, however, between suicide attempts and impulsivity scores.

Additionally, in a recent study examining risk factors for suicidal ideation in pediatric epilepsy, there were no associations between executive dysfunction, language or IQ, and suicidal ideation [29].

Epilepsy-Related Variables as Risk Factors for Suicide and Suicidal Behavior

Epilepsy carries with it potential risk factors for suicide and suicidal behavior that are specific to the disease. These include but are not limited to epilepsy syndrome, onset, duration, and seizure frequency as well as its treatments (medication vs. surgery). Additionally, the literature has indicated that there is a potential bidirectional relationship between epilepsy, depression, and suicide that may indicate an underlying pathogenesis. This section will review these potential risk factors.

Epilepsy Syndromes

Temporal lobe epilepsy (TLE) is the most common form of epilepsy, affecting approximately 50% of individuals with epilepsy [60]. In a study of 82 individuals with focal refractory epilepsy, researchers found that suicide risk was present in 33 (40%) individuals, all of whom were diagnosed with TLE. No individuals with parietal, frontal, occipital lobe, or insular epilepsy were determined to have suicidal risk [44]. Fukuchi et al. [61] found that TLE was most closely associated with death in epilepsy and suicide was only committed by individuals with TLE. Interestingly, half of suicide completions (three) occurred by jumping in front of a train during an episode of postictal psychosis.

In contrast, these findings of increased suicide risk among individuals with TLE have not always been supported. For example, Nilsson et al. [47] found no association between risk of suicide and type of epilepsy or localization/lateralization of epileptogenic focus. A large population-based study in Sweden [6] compared mortality rates of individuals with epilepsy and matched general population controls on a wide array of demographic, medical, and psychiatric variables. Significant differences between types of seizures and epilepsy syndromes were not found; instead, it was concluded that epilepsy in general is a risk factor for suicide mortality, with an aOR of 3.7 compared to population controls (95% CI, 3.3–4.2) and 2.9 compared to unaffected sibling controls (95% CI, 2.4–3.6).

Duration and Age of Onset

Research assessing the risk of suicide after diagnosis of epilepsy has found that those with newly diagnosed epilepsy are particularly vulnerable. Christensen et al. [5] determined that the highest risk of suicide was during the first 6 months following diagnosis, with a rate ratio of 5.35 (95% CI, 3.43–8.33) compared to controls. This rate was even higher (29.2; 95% CI, 16.4–551.9) for individuals with a history of comorbid psychiatric disease. Suicide risk decreased with time from epilepsy diagnosis in patients with and without a comorbid psychiatric diagnosis [5]. Fazel et al. [6] also found higher risk of suicide during the first half year after epilepsy diagnosis with an aOR of 17.9 (95% CI, 9.8–32.6), with somewhat decreased risk 6–12 months after diagnosis (aOR = 13.0; 95% CI, 6.9–24.3) and a more dramatic decreased risk for suicide a year or longer after diagnosis (aOR = 3.3; 95% CI, 2.9–3.8). In a study examining mortality in epilepsy in rural China, Ding et al. [62] found significant associations with suicide and duration of epilepsy between 10 and 20 years (adjusted hazard ratio [aHR] = 38.1; 95% CI, 2.8–520.8) and 20 and 30 years (aHR = 15.5; 95% CI, 1.3–192.1).

In contrast, a Finnish register-based cohort study [63] found that among adult patients with epilepsy, the elevated long-term risk of mortality from suicide was similar throughout the 3-interval, 18-year follow-up period ($\chi^2 = 1.89$, $p = 0.39$), with the authors suggesting that there is not a specific time period post-epilepsy diagnosis when the risk of suicide is higher. In adolescents, there was no significant increase in suicides compared to age-matched controls (HR = 0.57; 95% CI, 0.17–1.90).

Earlier age of epilepsy onset carries with it an increased risk for learning problems, psychiatric comorbidity, and longer duration of epilepsy [64, 65]. In a case-control study in Sweden, Nilsson et al. [47] found that younger onset of epilepsy (before age 18) was most strongly associated with risk of suicide, with a relative risk of 16.0 (95% CI, 4.4–58.3).

Seizure Freedom vs. Refractory Seizures

As many as 30% of people with epilepsy have seizures that are medically refractory or intractable—that is, their seizures cannot be completely controlled with antiepileptic drugs (AEDs) [1]. As previously mentioned, Andrade-Machado et al. [44] found that among individuals with refractory epilepsy, only individuals with TLE were deemed to have suicide risk, with the presence of depression increasing risk of suicide. In a cross-sectional study of suicidal ideation and attempts among individuals with epilepsy with frequent, treatment-resistant focal seizures, Hesdorffer et al. [66] found that lifetime suicidal ideation had occurred in up to 46%, recent suicidal ideation in 18%, and lifetime suicide attempts in 13%. Additionally, seizure frequency was found to be significantly associated with suicidality, as de Oliveira et al. [58] reported that individuals with epilepsy had a suicide risk with a mean of 8.26 seizures per month and individuals with epilepsy without suicide risk had a mean of 3.91 seizures per month.

Seizure freedom has also been identified to reduce the risk of suicidal behavior. Nilsson et al. [47] found that patients having seizures compared to those who were seizure free within the last year had a relative suicide risk of 2.2 (95% CI, 0.6–8.0). In addition, Baldin et al. [67] found no association with childhood-onset epilepsy, psychiatric disorders, and suicidal behavior in young adulthood. This sample was unique in that it was comprised of young adults aged 22–23 years who were seizure free and no longer on medications at the time of their follow-up evaluation.

Epilepsy Surgery

In some individuals with refractory epilepsy, surgery to resect the epileptogenic focus can lead to a significant reduction in seizures or even complete seizure freedom for many individuals. However, good seizure control after successful surgery does not eliminate psychiatric distress or risk of suicide. One study found that higher presurgical depression was predictive of higher postoperative depression, and individuals with a right-sided epileptogenic focus and resultant right temporal lobectomy had worse depression scores than left-sided surgery patients [68].

A large meta-analysis [69] of individuals with epilepsy who had undergone surgical treatment revealed that suicide in this population remained more frequent than in the general population. Hamid et al. [70] followed a cohort of 316 epilepsy patients 5 years postoperatively and observed a suicide rate of 17.4/10,000 deaths, compared to the general population rate of 1.3/10,000. Interestingly, the four patients who committed suicide were all seizure free for at least 1 year at time of death, and in the interviews before suicide, one patient had a self-report score consistent with severe depression, one had subclinical depressive symptoms, and two reported no depressive symptoms. Additionally, the patients who committed suicide had reported that surgery had a "very positive" impact on their lives and would "definitely" have surgery again.

In a large meta-analysis of research studies examining suicide in epilepsy [71], the standardized mortality ratio (SMR) for suicide was significantly elevated for individuals who had undergone temporal lobe surgery (SMR = 13.9; 95% CI, 8.93–20.74) and other types of epilepsy surgery (SMR = 6.37; 95% CI, 3.06–11.72). Across the studies examined in the meta-analysis, 34 post-surgery individuals had committed suicide: in 19 there was no information on seizure control status, 4 were seizure free, 6 had probable improved seizure control, 2 continued to have seizures, and 3 had worse seizures [71].

Suicidal Behavior and AEDs

In 1968, the first case report was published indicating a possible relationship between suicidality and AEDs, specifically diazepam [72]. Abraham [73] published a case report of topiramate-induced suicidality, and Kalinin [74] reported the possible link between suicidal behavior and AEDs. In 2008, the US Food and

Drug Administration (FDA) issued a warning that AEDs increased the risk of suicide [75]. This warning was based on meta-analysis of 199 clinical trials of 11 AEDs of which only 33 studies were included in the final analysis. Additionally, all data were based on adverse events reported during clinical trials; there was no systematic collection of suicide data. The FDA indicated a "class effect" of AEDs due to the fact that the findings were interpreted to apply across all epilepsy syndromes, psychiatric disorders, and other conditions where AEDs were indicated. According to Rudzinski and Meador [35], suicidality data were not collected prospectively or systematically, and as a result, a class effect could not be justified.

Fountoulakis et al. [76] conducted a systematic review of the literature as part of a position paper to establish recommendations for the best clinical practice for the World Psychiatric Association Section on Pharmacopsychiatry. This review contained only seven studies that met criteria for the systematic review and were included in the analysis. One study [47] did not reject nor support the FDA findings. Mula and Sander [77] indicated a low risk of suicidal behavior with levetiracetam, and Patorno et al. [78] also indicated a low risk of suicidal behavior with topiramate. No relationship was identified between AEDs and suicidal behavior in any group [79, 80]. In contrast, Andersohn et al. [81] and Pugh et al. [82] indicated that AEDs with psychiatric side effects may increase suicidality. The authors concluded that among individuals with epilepsy with mood disorders, AEDs do not increase suicidality and antidepressants may lower the risk [83, 84]. Suicidality is linked to psychiatric comorbidity rather than AEDs [85]. Additionally, Grimaldi-Bensouda et al. [86] conducted a case-control study using a large population-based database to evaluate the association between AEDs and the risk of suicide attempt. Between the years 2008 and 2012, 506 individuals with a suicide attempt were followed. Among individuals with a neurological condition, which included epilepsy, migraines, and neuropathic pain, there was no association between AEDs and suicide attempts. However, the presence of depression and anxiety increased the risk of a suicide attempt in this neurological sample.

As noted by Mula, Bell, and Sander [87], there is an increased risk of suicide associated with epilepsy, but the causes are not completely understood. Psychiatric comorbidity, type of epilepsy, and seizure control may also be contributing factors. The role AEDs play in suicidal behavior in epilepsy also remains unclear as AEDs have consistently been demonstrated to have effects on mood (see Table 6.1). Barbiturates, vigabatrin, tiagabine, and topiramate have been linked to depressive symptoms. The FDA indicated an increased risk for suicidality in topiramate, but barbiturates and vigabatrin were included in the analyses. Carbamazepine, lamotrigine, and valproate are often used as mood stabilizers, but the FDA's analyses indicated that carbamazepine and valproate had a nonsignificant protective effect against suicidal behavior and lamotrigine was implicated as increasing suicidality.

Due to the limited understanding of the underlying factors involved in suicidal behavior, epilepsy, psychiatric comorbidity, and AEDs, Mula, Bell, and Sander [87] recommended that individuals with epilepsy be closely monitored for suicidal behavior and provided practical considerations to keep in mind when working with individuals with epilepsy, including the following:

Table 6.1 Psychiatric side effects of AEDs

Drug	Depression	Anxiety	Irritability	Psychosis
Barbiturates	++	–	++[a]	–
Carbamazepine-oxcarbamazepine	–	–	+	–
Clobazam[JE1]			++	–
Ethotoin			+	+
Ethosuximide	–	–	–	+
Ezogabine			–	–
Felbamate	+	+	+	–
Gabapentin	–	–	+[a]	–
Lacosamide			+	–
Lamotrigine	–	–	+	–
Levetiracetam	–	–	+	–
Perampanel			–	–
Phenytoin	+	–	–	+
Pregabalin	+	–	–	–
Rufinamide			+	+
Tiagabine	+	–	+	–
Topiramate	++	–	+	+
Valproate	+	–	–	–
Vigabatrin	++	–	–	++
Zonisamide	+	–	+	+

Adapted from Mula, Bell, and Sander [87]
Treatment-emergent psychiatric adverse events among individuals with epilepsy during treatment with AEDs
[a]Reported mainly in children
+ Mild to moderate
++ Moderate to severe

1. Inform individuals and family members of possible psychotropic effects of AEDs.
2. Understand prior psychiatric history.
3. Screen for current symptoms of depression and anxiety.
4. Optimize AEDs with mental health as an important outcome.
5. Follow individuals with mental health issues past and current closely.
6. Refer individuals with current mental health disorders for psychiatric evaluation.

Many studies recommended future research to understand the relationship between AEDs and comorbid psychiatric disorders and suicide among individuals with epilepsy so that better treatment recommendations can be made.

Bidirectional Relationship Between Psychiatric Disorders, Epilepsy, and Suicide

Research suggested a bidirectional influence between psychiatric comorbidities and epilepsy, with a diagnosis of depression actually preceding the seizure disorder between nearly two and seven times more often in individuals with focal-onset epilepsy than in controls without epilepsy [88–90]. In a more recent population-based study in Sweden, investigators compared the risk of developing unprovoked seizures or epilepsy among individuals who had been hospitalized for a psychiatric disorder versus controls matched for year of diagnosis [91]. They found odds ratios of later developing seizures at 2.6 or higher for major depressive disorders, bipolar disorder, anxiety disorder, and suicide attempt.

A bidirectional relationship between epilepsy and suicidality itself, beyond other comorbid factors such as psychiatric distress, has also been suggested, proposing that there may be a common underlying etiology [5]. A large Iceland-based population study of adults and children found a five times greater risk of developing epilepsy in people who had a previous suicide attempt before the onset of seizures, independent of psychiatric comorbidities including depression and alcohol abuse [90].

A longitudinal study in the United Kingdom examined psychiatric disorders and suicidality before and after epilepsy diagnosis compared to matched controls [91]. The incidence rate ratio (IRR) of new cases, along with the prevalence ratio (PR), was calculated for each year for epilepsy onset, various psychiatric comorbidities, and suicidality. In this study, the IRR was significantly increased both before and after onset of epilepsy for depression, anxiety, bipolar disorder, psychosis, and suicidality, even after controlling for effects from secondary causes of epilepsy (e.g., cerebral anoxia, stroke, multiple sclerosis, and degenerative diseases) and substance abuse/dependence. These findings show that not only is epilepsy a risk factor for developing certain psychiatric disorders, but psychiatric disorders are associated with an increased risk of developing epilepsy. In considering suicide attempts/completions after onset of epilepsy, 15.2% in epilepsy cases had recurrent attempts from before the date of epilepsy onset, compared to 4.2% in controls. Further, among the post-epilepsy onset attempts, 41.7% in cases were recurrent compared to 17.9% in controls. This suggests that individuals with epilepsy were at increased risk of suicide attempt before epilepsy onset and recurrent suicide attempts after onset [91].

Hesdorffer et al. [7] conducted a retrospective population-based study examining the rates of a first suicide attempt and recurrent attempts in cases with epilepsy before they received a diagnosis of epilepsy and controling who were not diagnosed with epilepsy. They found that for those later diagnosed with epilepsy, there was a 2.9 (95% CI, 2.5–3.4) increased risk for a first suicide attempt and a 1.8 (95% CI, 1.3–2.5) increased risk for a recurrent suicide attempt compared to controls. Additionally, 32.5% of cases were diagnosed with a psychiatric disorder before a diagnosis of epilepsy, compared to 22.5% of controls. The researchers reported that the strength of association of attempted suicide was not significantly different for individuals with and without diagnosed psychiatric disorders. The authors hypothesized from these findings that there may be a common underlying biology linking epilepsy and suicide and discussed potential underlying features due to shared risk factors in both epilepsy and attempted suicide, including psychiatric disorders such as anxiety and depression, migraines with auras, and similarly impacted neurotransmitters and neurobiology.

Shared Pathogenesis

The bidirectional relationship between epilepsy and psychiatric disorders and suicide suggests that there are shared, neurobiological pathogenic pathways. Three such proposed mechanisms include (a) disturbances of neurotransmitter function in the central nervous system; (b) disturbances in endocrine functionality, especially within the hypothalamic-pituitary-adrenal (HPA) axis; and (c) inflammatory mechanisms and structural changes [92, 93].

Serotonin and norepinephrine are well-known players in mood and anxiety disorders, as well as completed suicide [93]. In animal models of epilepsy, serotonin, norepinephrine, and gamma-aminobutyric acid (GABA) have been shown to exhibit an inhibitory effect on hyperexcitability in the brain and block the development and progression of seizures in rats, mice, rabbits, cats, and rhesus monkeys [92].

In neuroimaging studies of humans, decreased serotonin receptor binding in similar regions of the brain in both major depression and epilepsy has been demonstrated [94, 95]. When comparing individuals with TLE with and without major depression, Hasler et al. [96] found similar reductions in serotonin receptor functioning in both major depression and TLE without depression, with more pronounced reduction in the same regions in individuals with depression.

Seizure disorders are associated with increased activity of glutamate, the primary excitatory neurotransmitter, which has also been found in high concentrations in cerebrospinal fluid (CSF) and the brain in individuals with mood disorders [97]. GABA, the primary inhibitory neurotransmitter, has also been implicated in both epilepsy and mood disorder processes, with lower concentrations found in the CSF and cortical regions of depressed and epileptic individuals [97, 98]. In research by Sequeira et al. [99], significant alterations in glutamate and GABA activity in the prefrontal cortex and hippocampus were identified in individuals who had completed suicide.

The HPA axis is a neuroendocrine system that regulates, among many processes, the body's reaction to stress. It has been implicated in the physiology and pathogenesis of many psychiatric disorders, including depression, anxiety, and posttraumatic stress disorder. Disturbance of this system results in higher levels of cortisol, a stress hormone, which is a biomarker for major depressive disorder and suicidality [92, 93, 100]. Animal models of epilepsy have demonstrated accelerated seizure kindling in rats treated with a cortisol hormone [101, 102]. In humans, many individuals with epilepsy report exacerbation of seizures when stressed, and elevated cortisol levels have been associated with increased seizure frequency and the postictal period following a seizure [103]. The presence of a long-standing psychiatric disorder may lower seizure threshold as a result of kindling [101]. Additionally, disruption of the HPA axis can in turn affect neurotransmitters, compounding the effect [92, 104].

Regarding inflammatory processes in the brain, common proinflammatory cytokines have been associated with both mood disorders and animal models of epilepsy. Interleukin-1β has been linked with depression and shown to have proconvulsant properties and is involved in glutamate transmission [93]. Structural changes, particularly hippocampal atrophy, enlarged amygdalar volume, and reduced gray matter volume, have also been implicated in both individuals with major depression and other mood disorders and individuals with TLE [97]. For a more in-depth discussion of the common pathogenesis processes of epilepsy, psychiatric disorders, and suicide, the reader is referred to reviews by Kanner, Mazarati and Koepp [97], and Hecimovic et al. [104].

Identifying Suicidal Behavior and Potential Interventions

Screening for Suicidal Behavior in Epilepsy

The first step in screening and prevention of suicide risk in individuals with epilepsy is evaluation and education. Many organizations worldwide have established best practice guidelines for the medical and psychiatric care and treatment of individuals with epilepsy, which include screening for depression and suicidality in all individuals with epilepsy (e.g., Scottish Intercollegiate Guidelines Network [SIGN], [105]; National Institute for Health and Care Excellence [NICE, United Kingdom], [106]). The International League Against Epilepsy (ILAE) Commission on the Neuropsychiatric Aspects of Epilepsy issued International Consensus Clinical Statements to establish guidelines regarding the assessment and management neuropsychiatric care in individuals with epilepsy [107]. Among these clinical practice statements, the commission emphasizes the importance of screening for depression, anxiety, suicidality, and other psychiatric comorbidities for all individuals with epilepsy, to avoid "watchful waiting" in those who are deemed to have "milder" episodes. Psychoeducation, therapy (particularly cognitive behavioral therapy [CBT]), consideration of all psychosocial and vocational factors, and selective serotonin reuptake inhibitors (SSRIs) are considered to be ideal clinical practice guidelines. The ILAE Commission further recommended that both surgical candidates and individuals with epilepsy who are not suitable for surgery receive comprehensive assessment by a clinical neuropsychologist and appropriate cognitive rehabilitation when possible [107].

In an interesting survey of Austrian, German, and Swiss neurologists and neuropediatricians, Strzelczyk et al. [108] examined attitudes toward counseling individuals with epilepsy about SUDEP and other epilepsy risk factors, including suicidal ideation, driving restrictions, and risks in daily life activities (i.e., drowning, falling from heights, working with machinery). Regarding suicidal ideation on AEDs, the questionnaire feedback indicated that only 3.3% of physicians counseled all of their patients on this subject, 8.5% discussed it with most patients, 19.5% with some patients, 31% rarely, and 35.1% of epilepsy neurologists reported never discussing suicidal ideation with patients or caregivers. This pattern was similar with counseling about SUDEP, with only 2.7% of neurologists discussing it with all of their patients, 8.7% with a majority, 20.8% with some patients, 44.5% with very few patients, and 23.2% never discussing SUDEP with their patients. In contrast, most physicians discuss driving restrictions and risks in daily life with all of their patients

(92.9% and 81.5%, respectively). Although the authors of this study specified suicidal ideation on AEDs in their survey, they acknowledged the established research associating only a small risk of increased suicidal thoughts and behaviors with AED treatment and emphasized that screening for depression and suicidality should be conducted in all individuals with epilepsy [108].

Screening for psychiatric disorders in epilepsy should include identifying major depressive episodes, anxiety disorders, and suicide risk. Several assessment measures exist that allow for quick screening of psychiatric symptoms within just a few minutes, lessening the time and resource burden for medical providers while still ensuring ideal clinical care for individuals with epilepsy. For depression, the Neurological Disorders Depression Inventory for Epilepsy (NDDI-E) was developed specifically for people with epilepsy to help identify the presence of major depressive episodes. This brief, six-item self-report measure can be completed in less than 3 min and assesses severity of depressive symptoms that do not overlap with common comorbid cognitive deficits and adverse effects of AEDs [92, 109]. There is a question that specifically addresses suicidality, "I'd be better off dead." A score of more than 15 is suggestive of major depression with specificity of 90% and sensitivity of 81% [109]. An elevated NDDI-E score can prompt a referral to a psychiatrist or psychologist for a more comprehensive evaluation and treatment. This measure has also been translated into a large number of languages.

The Patient Health Questionnaire (PHQ-9) is another brief screening instrument for depression, with cutoff scores for mild, moderate, moderately severe, and severe depression. Scores greater than 10 were suggestive of depression, with specificity and sensitivity of 88% [110]. It also contains a question that addresses suicidal ideation, and Altura et al. [111] found that the PHQ-9 has good sensitivity (90%) for identifying suicidal ideation in individuals with epilepsy. The ILAE Commission recommends using the PHQ or NDDI-E for use with all individuals newly diagnosed with epilepsy, as well as on an annual basis through primary care physicians or neurologists [107].

The Generalized Anxiety Disorder-7 (GAD-7) is a useful tool for brief assessment of anxiety and has been validated for use in people with epilepsy [112–114]. Like the NDDI-E, it is a self-report measure that takes less than 3 min to administer and provides score cutoffs for mild, moderate, and severe anxiety; a score greater than 10 is suggestive of a generalized anxiety disorder with a specificity of 82% and a sensitivity of 89% [92, 115]. Another study indicated that the GAD-7 can be used to screen for additional anxiety disorders, including posttraumatic stress disorder, panic disorder, and social anxiety disorder [116]. Through factor analysis, Micoulaud-Franchi et al. [112] determined that the GAD-7 and NDDI-E provide complementary information in individuals with epilepsy and recommend the routine use of both as part of the clinical evaluation.

Kanner [92] suggested two instruments for more detailed screening for suicidal ideation in epilepsy. The suicidality module of the Mini International Neuropsychiatric Interview (MINI) is composed of six yes or no items addressing suicidal plans, attempts, and active and passive suicidal ideation. The Columbia-Suicide Severity Rating Scale (C-SSRS) assessed four domains of suicidal ideation and behavior, including severity of ideation (active and passive thoughts of death), intensity of ideation (i.e., frequency, duration, controllability, deterrents, and reason for ideation), behavior (i.e., actual, aborted, and interrupted attempts, preparatory behavior, non-suicidal self-injurious behavior), and lethality [117].

Screening for suicide in youth can be completed with both parent and a young child's input. In adolescents it is more likely that the parents will be unaware of current suicidal behavior, and as a result, the adolescent should be screened separately from the parent. The Child Depression Inventory-2 [118] has a screening item for suicide on the parent-report and self-report versions. The Child Behavior Checklist [119] also utilizes one item to screen for suicidal behavior. Both of these measures have been widely used in pediatric epilepsy research. Although not validated in an epilepsy sample, Horowitz et al. [120] designed a suicide screening instrument to be used in the hospital emergency room to quickly screen for suicide in children and adolescents. The ASQ is comprised of five items, is recommended for screening for suicide risk, and is free on the National Institutes of Mental Health website (https://www.nimh.nih.gov/news/science-news/ask-suicide-screening-questions-asq.shtml).

Psychosocial Interventions to Reduce Psychiatric Comorbidity and Suicidal Risk Factors

There are very few studies examining interventions for suicidal ideation and attempts for adults and youth in general. Glenn, Franklin, and Nock [121] recently conducted a systematic review of the general literature in order to make recommendations for the treatment practices. The majority of efficacious interventions include a number of theoretical orientations including CBT, family-based therapy, interpersonal therapy, and psychodynamic therapy. There are common elements that appear to be efficacious and include the following elements [122]:

1. Target relationship or interpersonal functioning with a focus on the family
2. Include skills training
3. Intensive intervention to reduce suicidal behavior
4. Address maladaptive behavior or risk factors for suicidal behavior

Since psychiatric comorbidity appears to be the greatest risk factor for suicidal behavior, it will be important to address these disorders, particularly depression and anxiety in individuals with epilepsy. Cognitive behavior therapy has been studied extensively in the general literature with limited evidence of the efficacy of CBT in the treatment of depression in epilepsy. Gandy et al. [123] developed a 9-week CBT intervention for depression in adults with epilepsy and reported significant reductions in depressive symptoms ($p = 0.014$) as well as a reduction in suicidal ideation ($p = 0.005$). Anxiety symptoms were not significantly reduced, and QOL was not improved with intervention. Another intervention to treat depression in epilepsy was conducted using PEARLS, which was originally developed for older adults in the general population [124]. PEARLS is a cognitive behavioral intervention focusing on the elements of problem solving and behavioral activation. In a sample of adults with epilepsy, this intervention was found to be efficacious in reducing symptoms of depression [125].

There have been very few randomized controlled studies to examine the efficacy of treatment interventions in youth with epilepsy and psychiatric comorbidities. In adolescents with epilepsy and mild to moderate depression, Martinovic et al. [126] conducted a small randomized control trial of an individual cognitive behavioral therapy-based intervention and demonstrated a significant reduction in depressive symptoms of depression out to a 9-month follow-up. In a pilot study of children with epilepsy and an anxiety disorder, a computer-assisted cognitive behavioral intervention was introduced with weekly sessions over 12 weeks and was found to provide a reduction in anxiety symptoms at a 3-month follow-up [127]. However, it should be noted that neither of these intervention studies formally addressed or measured suicidal behavior before or after treatment. Additionally, we were unable to identify any treatment studies in the pediatric epilepsy literature that utilized an intervention to reduce suicidal ideation or suicidal attempts. Due to limited evidence, further research is needed to identify psychosocial interventions that address symptoms of depression, anxiety, and suicidal ideation in adults and youth with epilepsy. It will be particularly important to identify efficacious epilepsy-specific elements in psychosocial interventions that should be included in all interventions addressing psychiatric comorbidity and suicidal behavior.

Summary: Take-Home Points

Suicide and suicidal behaviors are quite elevated among youth and adults with epilepsy, with most research indicating higher rates of suicide compared to the general population. Similar to the general population, psychiatric disorders appear to be the most important risk factor for suicide and suicidal behaviors. Additionally, epilepsy-specific variables may also negatively impact the risk for suicidal behaviors in epilepsy, including syndrome, duration, and frequency of seizures. AEDs may play a role in the expression of psychiatric symptoms and suicidal behavior, but our understanding of this relationship is quite limited at this point and requires further investigation. Although epilepsy surgery frequently reduces seizure frequency, it does not seem to have the same positive effect on suicidal behaviors. In recent years, a bidirectional relationship has been identified between epilepsy, depression, and suicide indicating a common pathogenesis. With this information in mind, it is important to identify and screen for psychiatric comorbidities and suicidal risk in all adults and children with epilepsy. Although the intervention literature in epilepsy is limited, there are recommended treatments and interventions that have been established in the general population that can be adapted and applied to individuals with epilepsy. Additional research is needed to understand the relationship between epilepsy and suicide as well as the optimal interventions in the population.

References

1. World Health Organization. Atlas: epilepsy care in the world. Geneva: WHO; 2015. http://www.who.int/mental_health/neurology/Epilepsy_atlas_r1.pdf.
2. World Health Organization. Neurological disorders: public health challenges. Geneva: WHO; 2015. http://www.who.int/mental_health/neurology/neurodiso/en/.
3. Fiest KM, Sauro KM, Wiebe S, Patten SB, Kwon CS, Dykeman J, et al. Prevalence and incidence of epilepsy: a systematic review and meta-analysis of international studies. Neurology. 2017;88(3):296–303. https://doi.org/10.1212/WNL.0000000000003509.
4. Sirven JI, Shafer PQ. Epilepsy statistics. 2013. http://www.epilepsy.com/learn/epilepsy-statistics. Accessed 19 Jan 2017.
5. Christensen J, Vestergaard M, Mortensen PB, Sidenius P, Agerbo E. Epilepsy and risk of suicide: a population-based case–control study. Lancet Neurol. 2007;6(8):693–8.
6. Fazel S, Wolf A, Långström N, Newton CR, Lichtenstein P. Premature mortality in epilepsy and the role of psychiatric comorbidity: a total population study. Lancet. 2013;382(9905):1646–54.
7. Hesdorffer DC, Ishihara L, Webb DJ, Mynepalli L, Galwey NW, Hauser WA. Occurrence and recurrence of attempted suicide among people with epilepsy. JAMA Psychiat. 2016;73(1):80–6.
8. Thurman DJ, Logroscino G, Beghi E, Hauser WA, Hesdorffer DC, Newton CR, et al. The burden of premature mortality of epilepsy in high-income countries: a systematic review from the Mortality Task Force of the International League Against Epilepsy. Epilepsia. 2017;58(1):17–26. https://doi.org/10.1111/epi.13604.
9. Kochanek KD, Murphy SL, Xu JQ, Tejada-Vera B. Deaths: final data for 2014. Natl Vital Stat Rep. 2016;65(4):1–122. https://www.cdc.gov/nchs/data/nvsr/nvsr65/nvsr65_04.pdf.
10. Pompili M, Girardi P, Tatarelli R. Death from suicide versus mortality from epilepsy in the epilepsies: a meta-analysis. Epilepsy Behav. 2006;9(4):641–8. https://doi.org/10.1016/j.yebeh.2006.06.019.
11. Tian N, Cui W, Zack M, Kobau R, Fowler KA, Hesdorffer DC. Suicide among people with epilepsy: a population-based analysis of data from the US National Violent Death Reporting System, 17 states, 2003–2011. Epilepsy Behav. 2016;61:210–7.
12. Crosby A, Gfroerer J, Han B, Ortega L, Parks SE, Centers for Disease Control and Prevention (CDC). Suicidal thoughts and behaviors among adults aged ≥18 years—United States, 2008–2009. MMWR Surveill Summ. 2011;60(13):1–22.
13. Kessler RC, Berglund P, Borges G, Nock M, Wang PS. Trends in suicide ideation, plans, gestures, and attempts in the United States, 1990–1992 to 2001–2003. JAMA. 2005;293(20):2487–95.
14. Tektonidou MG, Dasgupta A, Ward MM. Suicidal ideation among adults with arthritis: prevalence and subgroups at highest risk. Data from the 2007–2008 National Health and Nutrition Examination Survey. Arthritis Care Res. 2011;63(9):1322–33.
15. Walker J, Waters RA, Murray G, Swanson H, Hibberd CJ, Rush RW, et al. Better off dead: suicidal thoughts in cancer patients. J Clin Oncol. 2008;26(29):4725–30.
16. Yang Y, Shi YZ, Zhang N, Wang S, Ungvari GS, Ng CH, et al. Suicidal ideation at 1-year post-stroke: a nationwide survey in China. Gen Hosp Psychiatry. 2017;44:38–42.
17. Tellez-Zenteno JF, Patten SB, Jetté N, Williams J, Wiebe S. Psychiatric comorbidity in epilepsy: a population-based analysis. Epilepsia. 2007;48(12):2336–44.
18. Rai D, Kerr MP, McManus S, Jordanova V, Lewis G, Brugha TS. Epilepsy and psychiatric comorbidity: a nationally representative population-based study. Epilepsia. 2012;53(6):1095–103.
19. Scott KM, Hwang I, Chiu WT, Kessler RC, Sampson NA, Angermeyer M, et al. Chronic physical conditions and their association with first onset of suicidal behavior in the world mental health surveys. Psychosom Med. 2010;72(7):712–9.
20. Meyer N, Voysey M, Holmes J, Casey D, Hawton K. Self-harm in people with epilepsy: a retrospective cohort study. Epilepsia. 2014;55(9):1355–65.

21. Dickstein LP, Viguera AC, Nowacki AS, Thompson NR, Griffith SD, Baldessarini RJ, et al. Thoughts of death and self-harm in patients with epilepsy or multiple sclerosis in a tertiary care center. Psychosomatics. 2015;56(1):44–51.
22. Centers for Disease Control and Prevention. Web-based Injury Statistics Query and Reporting System (WISQARS). http://www.cdc.gov/ncipc/wisqars. Accessed 10 Jan 2017.
23. Nock MK, Green JG, Hwang I, McLaughlin KA, Sampson NA, Zaslavsky AM, et al. Prevalence, correlates, and treatment of lifetime suicidal behavior among adolescents: results from the National Comorbidity Survey Replication Adolescent Supplement. JAMA Psychiat. 2013;70(3):300–10.
24. Barnes AJ, Eisenberg ME, Resnick MD. Suicide and self-injury among children and youth with chronic health conditions. Pediatrics. 2010;125(5):889–95.
25. Jones SE, Lollar DJ. Relationship between physical disabilities or long-term health problems and health risk behaviors or conditions among US high school students. J Sch Health. 2008;78(5):252–7.
26. Christiansen E, Stenager E. Risk for attempted suicide in children and youths after contact with somatic hospitals: a Danish register based nested case–control study. J Epidemiol Community Health. 2012;66(3):247–53.
27. Guilfoyle SM, Monahan S, Wesolowski C, Modi AC. Depression screening in pediatric epilepsy: evidence for the benefit of a behavioral medicine service in early detection. Epilepsy Behav. 2015;44:5–10.
28. Wagner JL, Smith G, Ferguson P. Self-efficacy for seizure management and youth depressive symptoms: caregiver and youth perspectives. Seizure. 2012;21(5):334–9.
29. Jones JE, Siddarth P, Gurbani S, Shields WD, Caplan R. Screening for suicidal ideation in children with epilepsy. Epilepsy Behav. 2013;29(3):521–6.
30. Chronis-Tuscano A, Molina BS, Pelham WE, Applegate B, Dahlke A, Overmyer M, et al. Very early predictors of adolescent depression and suicide attempts in children with attention-deficit/hyperactivity disorder. Arch Gen Psychiatry. 2010;67(10):1044–51.
31. Foley DL, Goldston DB, Costello EJ, Angold A. Proximal psychiatric risk factors for suicidality in youth: the Great Smoky Mountains Study. Arch Gen Psychiatry. 2006;63(9): 1017–24.
32. Dodig-Ćurković K, Ćurković M, Radić J, Degmečić D, Filaković P. Suicidal behavior and suicide among children and adolescents-risk factors and epidemiological characteristics. Coll Antropol. 2010;34(2):771–7.
33. West BA, Swahn MH, McCarty F. Children at risk for suicide attempt and attempt-related injuries: findings from the 2007 youth risk behavior survey. West J Emerg Med. 2010;11(3):257–63.
34. Gandy M, Sharpe L, Perry KN, Miller L, Thayer Z, Boserio J, et al. The psychosocial correlates of depressive disorders and suicide risk in people with epilepsy. J Psychosom Res. 2013;74(3):227–32. https://doi.org/10.1016/j.jpsychores.2012.11.001.
35. Rudzinski LA, Meador KJ. Epilepsy and neuropsychological comorbidities. Continuum. 2013;19(3):682–96.
36. Davies S, Heyman I, Goodman R. A population survey of mental health problems in children with epilepsy. Dev Med Child Neurol. 2003;45(5):292–5.
37. Fastenau PS, Johnson CS, Perkins SM, Byars AW, Austin JK, Dunn DW. Neuropsychological status at seizure onset in children risk factors for early cognitive deficits. Neurology. 2009;73(7):526–34.
38. Hermann B, Jones J, Dabbs K, Allen CA, Sheth R, Fine J, et al. The frequency, complications and aetiology of ADHD in new onset paediatric epilepsy. Brain. 2007;130(12): 3135–48.
39. Reilly C, Atkinson P, Das KB, Chin RF, Aylett SE, Burch V, et al. Screening for mental health disorders in active childhood epilepsy: population-based data. Epilepsy Res. 2014;108(10):1917–26.
40. Russ SA, Larson K, Halfon N. A national profile of childhood epilepsy and seizure disorder. Pediatrics. 2012;129(2):256–64.

41. Wagner JL, Wilson DA, Smith G, Malek A, Selassie AW. Neurodevelopmental and mental health comorbidities in children and adolescents with epilepsy and migraine: a response to identified research gaps. Dev Med Child Neurol. 2015;57(1):45–52. https://doi.org/10.1111/dmcn.12555.
42. Chesney E, Goodwin GM, Fazel S. Risks of all-cause and suicide mortality in mental disorders: a meta-review. World Psychiatry. 2014;13(2):153–60.
43. Rocco PL, Orbitello B, Ciano RP, Angarano A, Balestrieri M. Suicidal behaviour and intensity of psychiatric care in a region at high risk for suicide. Int J Psychiatry Clin Pract. 2004;8(3):153–9.
44. Andrade-Machado R, Ochoa-Urrea M, Garcia-Espinosa A, Benjumea-Cuartas V, Santos-Santos A. Suicidal risk, affective dysphoric disorders, and quality-of-life perception in patients with focal refractory epilepsy. Epilepsy Behav. 2015;45:254–60. https://doi.org/10.1016/j.yebeh.2015.01.005.
45. Blumer D, Montouris G, Davies K, Wyler A, Phillips B, Hermann B. Suicide in epilepsy: psychopathology, pathogenesis, and prevention. Epilepsy Behav. 2002;3(3):232–41.
46. Jones JE, Hermann BP, Barry JJ, Gilliam FG, Kanner AM, Meador KJ. Rates and risk factors for suicide, suicidal ideation, and suicide attempts in chronic epilepsy. Epilepsy Behav. 2003;4:31–8. https://doi.org/10.1016/j.yebeh.2003.08.019.
47. Nilsson L, Ahlbom A, Farahmand BY, Åsberg M, Tomson T. Risk factors for suicide in epilepsy: a case control study. Epilepsia. 2002;43(6):644–51.
48. Hecimovic H, Santos JM, Carter J, Attarian HP, Fessler AJ, Vahle V, Gilliam F. Depression but not seizure factors or quality of life predicts suicidality in epilepsy. Epilepsy Behav. 2012;24(4):426–9.
49. Andrade-Machado R, Benjumea-Cuartas V, Santos-Santos A, Sosa-Dubón MA, García-Espinosa A, Andrade-Gutierrez G. Mortality in patients with refractory temporal lobe epilepsy at a tertiary center in Cuba. Epilepsy Behav. 2015;53:154–60. https://doi.org/10.1016/j.yebeh.2015.08.038.
50. Caplan R, Siddarth P, Gurbani S, Hanson R, Sankar R, Shields WD. Depression and anxiety disorders in pediatric epilepsy. Epilepsia. 2005;46(5):720–30.
51. Keilp JG, Gorlyn M, Russell M, Oquendo MA, Burke AK, Harkavy-Friedman J, et al. Neuropsychological function and suicidal behavior: attention control, memory and executive dysfunction in suicide attempt. Psychol Med. 2013;43(03):539–51.
52. Keilp JG, Beers SR, Burke AK, Melhem NM, Oquendo MA, Brent DA, et al. Neuropsychological deficits in past suicide attempters with varying levels of depression severity. Psychol Med. 2014;44(14):2965–74.
53. Keilp JG, Gorlyn M, Oquendo MA, Burke AK, Mann JJ. Attention deficit in depressed suicide attempters. Psychiatry Res. 2008;159(1):7–17.
54. Jollant F, Bellivier F, Leboyer M, Astruc B, Torres S, Verdier R, et al. Impaired decision making in suicide attempters. Am J Psychiatry. 2005;162(2):304–10. https://doi.org/10.1176/appi.ajp.162.2.304.
55. Turecki G. Dissecting the suicide phenotype: the role of impulsive-aggressive behaviours. J Psychiatry Neurosci. 2005;30(6):398–408.
56. Westheide J, Quednow BB, Kuhn KU, Hoppe C, Cooper-Mahkorn D, Hawellek B, et al. Executive performance of depressed suicide attempters: the role of suicidal ideation. Eur Arch Psychiatry Clin Neurosci. 2008;258(7):414–21. https://doi.org/10.1007/s00406-008-0811-1.
57. Garcia-Espinosa A, Andrade-Machado R, Borges-Gonzalez S, Garcia-Gonzalez ME, Perez-Montoto A, Toledo-Sotomayor G. Wisconsin Card Sorting Test performance and impulsivity in patients with temporal lobe epilepsy: suicidal risk and suicide attempts. Epilepsy Behav. 2010;17(1):39–45. https://doi.org/10.1016/j.yebeh.2009.09.010.
58. de Oliveira GN, Kummer A, Salgado JV, de Araujo Filho GM, David AS, Teixeira AL. Suicidality in temporal lobe epilepsy: measuring the weight of impulsivity and depression. Epilepsy Behav. 2011;22(4):745–9.
59. Patton JH, Stanford MS. Factor structure of the Barratt impulsiveness scale. J Clin Psychol. 1995;51(6):768–74.

60. Schoenberg MR, Werz MA, Drane DL. Epilepsy and seizures. In: Schoenberg MR, Scott JG, editors. The little black book of neuropsychology: a syndrome-based approach. New York: Springer; 2011. p. 423–519.
61. Fukuchi T, Kanemoto K, Kato M, Ishida S, Yuasa S, Kawasaki J, et al. Death in epilepsy with special attention to suicide cases. Epilepsy Res. 2002;51(3):233–6.
62. Ding D, Wang W, Wu J, Yang H, Li S, Dai X, et al. Premature mortality risk in people with convulsive epilepsy: long follow-up of a cohort in rural China. Epilepsia. 2013;54(3):512–7. https://doi.org/10.1111/epi.12048.
63. Nevalainen O, Raitanen J, Ansakorpi H, Artama M, Isojärvi J, Auvinen A. Long-term mortality risk by cause of death in newly diagnosed patients with epilepsy in Finland: a nationwide register-based study. Eur J Epidemiol. 2013;28(12):981–90.
64. Aaberg KM, Bakken IJ, Lossius MI, Søraas CL, Håberg SE, Stoltenberg C, et al. Comorbidity and childhood epilepsy: a nationwide registry study. Pediatrics. 2016;138:e20160921. https://doi.org/10.1542/peds.2016-0921.
65. Nickels KC, Zaccariello MJ, Hamiwka LD, Wirrell EC. Cognitive and neurodevelopmental comorbidities in paediatric epilepsy. Nat Rev Neurol. 2016;12(8):465–76. https://doi.org/10.1038/nrneurol.2016.98.
66. Hesdorffer DC, French JA, Posner K, DiVentura B, Pollard JR, Sperling MR, et al. Suicidal ideation and behavior screening in intractable focal epilepsy eligible for drug trials. Epilepsia. 2013;54(5):879–87. https://doi.org/10.1111/epi.12128.
67. Baldin E, Hesdorffer DC, Caplan R, Berg AT. Psychiatric disorders and suicidal behavior in neurotypical young adults with childhood-onset epilepsy. Epilepsia. 2015;56(10):1623–8.
68. Quigg M, Broshek DK, Heidal-Schiltz S, Maedgen JW, Bertram EH. Depression in intractable partial epilepsy varies by laterality of focus and surgery. Epilepsia. 2003;44(3):419–24.
69. Pompili M, Girardi P, Tatarelli G, Angeletti G, Tatarelli R. Suicide after surgical treatment in patients with epilepsy: a meta-analytic investigation. Psychol Rep. 2006;98(2):323–38.
70. Hamid H, Devinsky O, Vickrey BG, Berg AT, Bazil CW, Langfitt JT, et al. Suicide outcomes after resective epilepsy surgery. Epilepsy Behav. 2011;20(3):462–4.
71. Bell GS, Gaitatzis A, Bell CL, Johnson AL, Sander JW. Suicide in people with epilepsy: how great is the risk? Epilepsia. 2009;50(8):1933–42.
72. Ryan HF, Merrill FB, Scott GE, Krebs R, Thompson BL. Increase in suicidal thoughts and tendencies: association with diazepam therapy. JAMA. 1968;203(13):1137–9.
73. Abraham G. Topiramate-induced suicidality. Can J Psychiatr. 2003;48(2):127–8.
74. Kalinin VV. Suicidality and antiepileptic drugs. Drug Saf. 2007;30(2):123–42.
75. FDA. Safety: antiepileptic drugs. http://www.fda.gov/Safety/MedWatch/SafetyInformation/SafetyAlertsforHumanmedicalProducts/ucm074939.htm.
76. Fountoulakis KN, Gonda X, Baghai TC, Baldwin DS, Bauer M, Blier P, et al. Report of the WPA section of pharmacopsychiatry on the relationship of antiepileptic drugs with suicidality in epilepsy. Int J Psychiatry Clin Pract. 2015;19(3):158–67. https://doi.org/10.3109/13651501.2014.1000930.
77. Mula M, Sander JW. Suicidal ideation in epilepsy and levetiracetam therapy. Epilepsy Behav. 2007;11(1):130–2.
78. Patorno E, Bohn RL, Wahl PM, Avorn J, Patrick AR, Liu J, et al. Anticonvulsant medications and the risk of suicide, attempted suicide, or violent death. JAMA. 2010;303(14):1401–9.
79. Arana A, Wentworth CE, Ayuso-Mateos JL, Arellano FM. Suicide-related events in patients treated with antiepileptic drugs. N Engl J Med. 2010;363(6):542–51.
80. Wen X, Meador KJ, Loring DW, Eisenschenk S, Segal R, Hartzema AG. Is antiepileptic drug use related to depression and suicidal ideation among patients with epilepsy? Epilepsy Behav. 2010;19(3):494–500.
81. Andersohn F, Schade R, Willich SN, Garbe E. Use of antiepileptic drugs in epilepsy and the risk of self-harm or suicidal behavior. Neurology. 2010;75(4):335–40.
82. Pugh MJ, Copeland LA, Zeber JE, Wang CP, Amuan ME, Mortensen EM, et al. Antiepileptic drug monotherapy exposure and suicide-related behavior in older veterans. J Am Geriatr Soc. 2012;60(11):2042–7. https://doi.org/10.1111/j.1532-5415.2012.04207.x.

83. Leon AC, Demirtas H, Li C, Hedeker D. Two propensity score-based strategies for a three-decade observational study: investigating psychotropic medications and suicide risk. Stat Med. 2012;31(27):3255–60.
84. Leon AC, Solomon DA, Li C, Fiedorowicz JG, Coryell WH, Endicott J, et al. Antiepileptic drugs for bipolar disorder and the risk of suicidal behavior: a 30-year observational study. Am J Psychiatry. 2012;169(3):285–91.
85. Andrade-Machado R, Garcia-Espinosa A, Melendrez D, Remon-Gonzalez Y, Frades-Garcia V, Quintana-Rodriguez Y. Suicidal risk and suicide attempts in people treated with antiepileptic drugs for epilepsy. Seizure. 2011;20(4):280–4. https://doi.org/10.1016/j.seizure.2010.12.010.
86. Grimaldi-Bensouda L, Nordon C, Rossignol M, Jardon V, Boss V, Warembourg F, et al. Antiepileptic drugs and risk of suicide attempts: a case–control study exploring the impact of underlying medical conditions. Pharmacoepidemiol Drug Saf. 2017;26(3):239–47. https://doi.org/10.1002/pds.4160.
87. Mula M, Bell GS, Sander JW. Suicidality in epilepsy and possible effects of antiepileptic drugs. Curr Neurol Neurosci Rep. 2010;10(4):327–32.
88. Forsgren L, Nyström L. An incident case-referent study of epileptic seizures in adults. Epilepsy Res. 1990;6(1):66–81.
89. Hesdorffer DC, Hauser WA, Annegers JF, Cascino G. Major depression is a risk factor for seizures in older adults. Ann Neurol. 2000;47(2):246–9.
90. Hesdorffer DC, Hauser WA, Olafsson E, Ludvigsson P, Kjartansson O. Depression and suicide attempt as risk factors for incident unprovoked seizures. Ann Neurol. 2006;59(1):35–41.
91. Adelöw C, Andersson T, Ahlbom A, Tomson T. Hospitalization for psychiatric disorders before and after onset of unprovoked seizures/epilepsy. Neurology. 2012;78(6):396–401.
92. Kanner AM. Suicidality and epilepsy: a complex relationship. In: Koslow SH, Ruiz P, Nemeroff CB, editors. A concise guide to understanding suicide: epidemiology, pathophysiology and prevention. Cambridge: Cambridge University Press; 2014. p. 130–7.
93. Kanner AM, Ribot R. Depression. In: Mula M, editor. Neuropsychiatric symptoms of epilepsy. Cham, Switzerland: Springer International Publishing; 2016. p. 25–41.
94. Hesselgrave N, Parsey RV. Imaging the serotonin 1A receptor using [^{11}C]WAY100635 in healthy controls and major depression. Phil Trans R Soc B. 2013;368(1615):20120004. https://doi.org/10.1098/rstb.2012.0004.
95. Toczek MT, Carson RE, Lang L, Ma Y, Spanaki MV, Der MG, et al. PET imaging of 5-HT1A receptor binding in patients with temporal lobe epilepsy. Neurology. 2003;60(5):749–56.
96. Hasler G, Bonwetsch R, Giovacchini G, Toczek MT, Bagic A, Luckenbaugh DA, et al. 5-HT 1A receptor binding in temporal lobe epilepsy patients with and without major depression. Biol Psychiatry. 2007;62(11):1258–64. https://doi.org/10.1016/j.biopsych.2007.02.015.
97. Kanner AM, Mazarati A, Koepp M. Biomarkers of epileptogenesis: psychiatric comorbidities (?). Neurotherapeutics. 2014;11(2):358–72.
98. Rajkowska G, O'Dwyer G, Teleki Z, Stockmeier CA, Miguel-Hidalgo JJ. GABAergic neurons immunoreactive for calcium binding proteins are reduced in the prefrontal cortex in major depression. Neuropsychopharmacology. 2007;32(2):471–82.
99. Sequeira A, Mamdani F, Ernst C, Vawter MP, Bunney WE, Lebel V, et al. Global brain gene expression analysis links glutamatergic and GABAergic alterations to suicide and major depression. PLoS One. 2009;4(8):e6585. https://doi.org/10.1371/journal.pone.0006585.
100. Keller J, Gomez R, Williams G, Lembke A, Lazzeroni L, Murphy GM, et al. HPA axis in major depression: cortisol, clinical symptomatology and genetic variation predict cognition. Mol Psychiatry. 2016;22(4):527–36.
101. Jones NC, O'Brien TJ. Stress, epilepsy, and psychiatric comorbidity: how can animal models inform the clinic? Epilepsy Behav. 2013;26(3):363–9.
102. Kumar G, Couper A, O'Brien TJ, Salzberg MR, Jones NC, Rees SM, et al. The acceleration of amygdala kindling epileptogenesis by chronic low-dose corticosterone involves both mineralocorticoid and glucocorticoid receptors. Psychoneuroendocrinology. 2007;32(7):834–42.

103. Maguire J, Salpekar JA. Stress, seizures, and hypothalamic–pituitary–adrenal axis targets for the treatment of epilepsy. Epilepsy Behav. 2013;26(3):352–62.
104. Hecimovic H, Salpekar J, Kanner AM, Barry JJ. Suicidality and epilepsy: a neuropsychobiological perspective. Epilepsy Behav. 2011;22(1):77–84.
105. Scottish Intercollegiate Guideline Network (SIGN). Diagnosis and management of epilepsy in adults. 2015. http://www.sign.ac.uk. Accessed 5 Jan 2017.
106. National Institute for Health and Care Excellence (NICE). The epilepsies: the diagnosis and management of the epilepsies in adults and children in primary and secondary Care. 2014. http://guidance.nice.org.uk/cg137. Accessed 5 Jan 2017.
107. Kerr MP, Mensah S, Besag F, De Toffol B, Ettinger A, Kanemoto K, et al. International consensus clinical practice statements for the treatment of neuropsychiatric conditions associated with epilepsy. Epilepsia. 2011;52(11):2133–8. https://doi.org/10.1111/j.1528-1167.2011.03276.x.
108. Strzelczyk A, Zschebek G, Bauer S, Baumgartner C, Grond M, Hermsen A, et al. Predictors of and attitudes toward counseling about SUDEP and other epilepsy risk factors among Austrian, German, and Swiss neurologists and neuropediatricians. Epilepsia. 2016;57(4):612–20. https://doi.org/10.1111/epi.13337.
109. Gilliam FG, Barry JJ, Hermann BP, Meador KJ, Vahle V, Kanner AM. Rapid detection of major depression in epilepsy: a multicentre study. Lancet Neurol. 2006;5(5):399–405.
110. Kroenke K, Spitzer RL, Williams JB. The PHQ-9: validity of a brief depression severity measure. J Gen Intern Med. 2001;16(9):606–13.
111. Altura KC, Patten SB, Fiest KM, Atta C, Bulloch AG, Jetté N. Suicidal ideation in persons with neurological conditions: prevalence, associations and validation of the PHQ-9 for suicidal ideation. Gen Hosp Psychiatry. 2016;42:22–6.
112. Micoulaud-Franchi JA, Lagarde S, Barkate G, Dufournet B, Besancon C, Trébuchon-Da Fonseca A, et al. Rapid detection of generalized anxiety disorder and major depression in epilepsy: validation of the GAD-7 as a complementary tool to the NDDI-E in a French sample. Epilepsy Behav. 2016;57:211–6. https://doi.org/10.1016/j.yebeh.2016.02.015.
113. Seo JG, Cho YW, Lee SJ, Lee JJ, Kim JE, Moon HJ, et al. Validation of the generalized anxiety disorder-7 in people with epilepsy: a MEPSY study. Epilepsy Behav. 2014;35:59–63.
114. Tong X, An D, McGonigal A, Park SP, Zhou D. Validation of the Generalized Anxiety Disorder-7 (GAD-7) among Chinese people with epilepsy. Epilepsy Res. 2016;120:31–6.
115. Spitzer RL, Kroenke K, Williams JB, Löwe B. A brief measure for assessing generalized anxiety disorder: the GAD-7. Arch Intern Med. 2006;166(10):1092–7.
116. Kroenke K, Spitzer RL, Williams JB, Monahan PO, Löwe B. Anxiety disorders in primary care: prevalence, impairment, comorbidity, and detection. Ann Intern Med. 2007;146(5):317–25.
117. Posner K, Brown GK, Stanley B, Brent DA, Yershova KV, Oquendo MA, et al. The Columbia–Suicide Severity Rating Scale: initial validity and internal consistency findings from three multisite studies with adolescents and adults. Am J Psychiatry. 2011;168(12):1266–77.
118. Kovacs M. Children's depression inventory: technical manual. 2nd ed. North Tonawanda: MHS; 2011.
119. Achenbach TM, Rescorla LA. Manual for the ASEBA school-age forms and profiles. Burlington: University of Vermont Research Center for Children, Youth and Families; 2001.
120. Horowitz LM, Bridge JA, Teach SJ, Ballard E, Klima J, Rosenstein DL, et al. Ask suicide-screening questions (ASQ): a brief instrument for the pediatric emergency department. Arch Pediatr Adolesc Med. 2012;166(12):1170–6.
121. Glenn CR, Franklin JC, Nock MK. Evidence-based psychosocial treatments for self-injurious thoughts and behaviors in youth. J Clin Child Adolesc Psychol. 2015;44(1):1–29.
122. Brent DA, McMakin DL, Kennard BD, Goldstein TR, Mayes TL, Douaihy AB. Protecting adolescents from self-harm: a critical review of intervention studies. J Am Acad Child Adolesc Psychiatry. 2013;52(12):1260–71.
123. Gandy M, Sharpe L, Nicholson Perry K, Thayer Z, Miller L, Boserio J, et al. Cognitive behaviour therapy to improve mood in people with epilepsy: a randomised controlled trial. Cogn Behav Ther. 2014;43(2):153–66.

124. Ciechanowski P, Chaytor N, Miller J, Fraser R, Russo J, Unutzer J, et al. PEARLS depression treatment for individuals with epilepsy: a randomized controlled trial. Epilepsy Behav. 2010;19(3):225–31.
125. Chaytor N, Ciechanowski P, Miller JW, Fraser R, Russo J, Unutzer J, et al. Long-term outcomes from the PEARLS randomized trial for the treatment of depression in patients with epilepsy. Epilepsy Behav. 2011;20(3):545–9.
126. Martinović Ž, Simonović P, Djokić R. Preventing depression in adolescents with epilepsy. Epilepsy Behav. 2006;9(4):619–24.
127. Blocher JB, Fujikawa M, Sung C, Jackson DC, Jones JE. Computer-assisted cognitive behavioral therapy for children with epilepsy and anxiety: a pilot study. Epilepsy Behav. 2013;27(1):70–6.

Suicide in Chronic Pain Patients: Risk Factors and Clinical Considerations

7

Jennifer K. Lehmann and Xavier F. Jimenez

Key Points

- Pain experience is affected by cognitive and emotional processes.
- Chronic pain patients are at increased risk of suicide due to psychiatric comorbidities (such as depression and substance use disorders), vulnerable periods (such as pain exacerbations, advanced age, or loss), or the combination of both.
- An actuarial approach to suicide risk in chronic pain patients is crucial to ensure safe and effective management.

Introduction

Within the United States, it is estimated that 116 million adults suffer from a chronic pain condition. Common nonmalignant pain conditions include fibromyalgia, rheumatoid arthritis, chronic headaches or migraines, neuropathy, and low-back pain. Chronic pain conditions affect every aspect of a person's life including loss of emotional and physical functioning, reduced activity levels, impaired social relationships, and potential loss of income due to an inability to work or healthcare costs [1].

Patients with chronic pain conditions are at an increased risk for suicidal behavior including suicidal ideation, suicide attempts, and death by suicide. Nearly 20% of patients with chronic pain report suicidal ideation, and between 5 and 14% of pain patients report attempting suicide [2]. Compared to the regular population,

J. K. Lehmann, M.A.
Case Western Reserve University, Cleveland, OH, USA
e-mail: lehmanj@ccf.org; jkl68@case.edu

X. F. Jimenez, M.D., M.A. (✉)
Chronic Pain Rehabilitation Section, Center for Neurological Restoration, Cleveland Clinic
Lerner College of Medicine, Neurological Institute, Cleveland Clinic, Cleveland, OH, USA
e-mail: jimenex2@ccf.org

T. Falcone, J. Timmons-Mitchell (eds.), *Suicide Prevention*,
https://doi.org/10.1007/978-3-319-74391-2_7

individuals with chronic pain conditions are at nearly double the risk of dying by suicide [3].

This chapter will attempt to identify the biological and psychosocial risk factors associated with suicidal behavior in patients with chronic pain and discuss possibilities for management and prevention.

Neurobiological Underpinnings of Pain

When thinking of pain, it is important to consider it as more than a purely sensory phenomenon. Pain is often defined as a confluence of neurological, affective, and cognitive components culminating in a given patient's specific experience. For instance, evidence shows that pain is a creation of the nervous system and not just a gauge of receptor activation at the level of tissues. Both facilitatory and inhibitory pathways augment or reduce, respectively, the sensed experience of pain. Pain inhibition involves processing via spinal-supraspinal-spinal loops [4]; implicated supraspinal structures include the prefrontal cortex, midbrain, and periaqueductal gray [5]. Such pathways are modifiable. Evidence demonstrates the activation of healthy or adaptive pain inhibition with the use of exercise, for example [6]. Of relevance to suicide is the neurobiology of chronic pain syndromes, which are believed to develop as a result of faulty pain inhibition as well [7].

The interplay of cognitions and pain modulation is complex. It is known that guarding against the possibility of pain, and anticipation of its occurrence, activates cells in the rostroventral medulla that function to amplify incoming pain signals at the level of the dorsal horn of the spinal cord. Animal models suggest that the simple facts of anticipating a pain and expecting it to be important are sufficient to trigger these "on cells," in essence activating the "amplifiers" before the pain stimulus has even begun [8]. Evidence also points to genetic variability in pain appreciation and in responses to endogenous and exogenous opioids [9–11]. Furthermore, there is compelling evidence that individuals reporting high/low pain in response to a standard stimulus demonstrate correspondingly high or low activation of somatosensory, anterior cingulate (a likely index of affective components of pain), and frontal cortices [12].

Physical Pain and Emotional Pain

Due to overlap in the neural pathways for physical and psychological pain, patients with chronic pain conditions may also suffer from debilitating psychological pain [13]. A modern conceptualization defines psychological pain as "a lasting, unsustainable, and unpleasant feeling resulting from negative appraisal of an inability or deficiency of the self" [14]. While psychological disorders are included within the conceptualization of psychological pain, psychological pain can occur independent of a psychiatric condition. Lasting psychological pain in combination with poor coping abilities can lead to a suicidal crisis [14]. The overlap between physical and emotional pain may contribute to chronic emotional pain in individuals with chronic pain disorders. If chronic pain patients have poor coping abilities in response to pain or dysfunctional attitudes, they may also be at an increased risk for suicide.

Psychological Risk Factors for Pain

Risk factors for suicide are often divided into factors that are proximal or distal to the suicidal behavior. Distal risk factors help to identify high-risk groups of individuals, such as chronic pain patients, while proximal risk factors identify precipitating events and vulnerable time periods which may contribute to a suicidal crisis. It is also imperative to identify early warning signs of a suicidal crisis. Out of the three types of risk factors, vulnerable groups, vulnerable time periods, and warning signs, each type of risk factor alone only contributes to a small piece of the puzzle of suicide risk. Indeed, each type of risk factor needs to be used in combination in order to help in the identification of patients who are vulnerable to suicide.

Vulnerable Groups

Demographic variables can be used to identify groups of patients who are vulnerable to suicidal behavior. In general, increased levels of suicidal behavior are associated with demographic variables such as older age and male sex [15]. Other patient factors such as psychiatric conditions [16] and comorbid medical conditions [17] can also be helpful in identifying high-risk groups of patients.

Psychiatric Comorbidities

Depressive disorders commonly occur in individuals with chronic pain [18]. Evidence from chronic pain clinics and community samples suggest that chronic pain conditions may lead to first symptoms of depression. In a longitudinal study of 614 patients with chronic pain, 15.5% of participants developed a first incident depressive episode during the 14-year follow-up period [19]. Additionally, of individuals meeting criteria for both MDD and a chronic physical condition, 57.1% reported that pain appeared before the onset of depressive symptoms [18]. However, longitudinal studies have also shown that depressed individuals are more likely to develop multiple physical symptoms [20] with cognitive factors mediating the development of depression as a secondary condition to chronic pain [21]. The connection between chronic pain conditions and depression is important because of the high incidence of suicidal ideation, attempt, and death in patients with depression.

Other common psychiatric comorbid conditions such as psychotic disorders, borderline personality disorder, and alcohol or drug addiction may increase suicide risk.

There is a significant risk for the misuse of opioid medications and other substances in individuals with chronic pain conditions. Individuals with poor distress tolerance [22], higher levels of depression, and increased attempts to suppress distressing or intrusive thoughts [23] are more likely to misuse prescribed opioid medications. Illicit substances may also be used by chronic pain patients as a form of pain relief. In a study of 88 chronic pain outpatients, individuals who had used illicit drugs as a form of pain relief at any time since pain onset were five times more likely to report suicidal ideation [24]. Misuse of substances in chronic pain patients is especially important considering that 17% of chronic pain deaths followed a medication overdose [25]. Medication overdoses are the number one method for suicide attempts in the chronic pain population [2].

Personality Characteristics

Trait impulsivity is linked to suicidal behavior. Although chronic pain patients are no more likely than controls to possess trait impulsivity, it may be an important risk factor for the misuse of prescribed opioid analgesics [26] and suicide by overdose [27]. In a study of 42 chronic low-back pain patients, ratings of attentional impulsiveness but not sensation seeking were associated with improper use of prescribed medication [26]. A case-cohort design study with 123,946 patients from all VHA (Veterans Health Administration) overdoses accounts for approximately 15–20% of all suicides in chronic pain patients, and risk of suicide mortality is greater among individuals receiving higher doses of opioids [25].

Chronic pain is correlated with both feelings of anger [28] and aggressive acts [29]. Patients with chronic pain display feelings of anger and chronic anger at a significantly higher rate than community non-patients, community patients, and patients with acute pain [30]. In a study of 99 patients with benign chronic pain and 109 control patients with other forms of chronic disease, overtly aggressive acts such as verbal and autoaggression were more common in chronic pain patients than in the control group [31].

Comorbid Medical Conditions

Patients with comorbid medical conditions, such as chronic pain, are at an increased risk for suicide independent of comorbid psychiatric conditions. While approximately 80–90% of suicide deaths occur in individuals with a psychiatric illness, not everyone who dies by suicide meets criteria for a psychiatric illness [32]. After controlling for psychiatric comorbidities, back pain, migraine, and psychogenic pain conditions were still associated with an increased risk of suicide [17]. The finding that certain pain conditions increase suicide risk over and above the association between pain and depression suggests that pain conditions may be enough to drive some individuals to contemplate suicide. Individuals with certain pain conditions may wish to die as a means to escape from pain [3].

Specific aspects of a patient's pain including severity and duration may also contribute to suicide risk. Some evidence has suggested that patients with more severe ratings of pain were more likely to die by suicide than patients experiencing none, mild, or moderate pain, after controlling for demographic and psychiatric characteristics [33]. However, other recent findings have shown no relationship between pain-related variables and suicidal ideation [24]. Additionally, preliminary evidence has suggested that patients who experience pain for longer durations may be at greater risk for experiencing suicidal ideation [34].

Specific types of pain conditions may be associated with different levels of risk for suicidal ideation, attempts, and completions. In a large national sample of veterans, migraines and abdominal pain were associated with an increased risk of suicide when compared with other conditions, after controlling for psychiatric and demographic factors [35]. Additionally, back pain, migraine, and psychogenic pain conditions were identified as risk factors for death by suicide [17]. Interestingly, a diagnosis of neuropathic pain was associated with a protective effect potentially due to the known source of pain in the diagnosis [35].

Vulnerable Time Periods

Stressful life events may help to explain what drives high-risk individuals to contemplate, attempt, or die by suicide [36]. A review of psychological autopsy studies revealed that nearly all adult suicides experienced at least one adverse life event within 1 year of death [37]. Interpersonal conflict or loss, unemployment, and financial problems are strongly linked with substance-misusing suicides [37]. This finding is particularly salient given that loss is a major theme in the experience of chronic pain conditions [38]. Chronic pain conditions contribute to an individual's level of stress by impacting nearly every aspect of life, and the associated stress may invoke a suicidal crisis. A qualitative study investigating the experiences of individuals with chronic back pain identified six main areas of loss: loss of abilities and roles, employment-related losses, relationship losses, loss of identity, and loss of hope [38]. Losses experienced by chronic pain patients may serve as precipitating events to a suicidal crisis.

Warning Signs

Warning signs of a suicidal crisis include increases in social isolation, agitation, and severity of depression symptoms. Cognitive dysfunctions and poor coping strategies in the face of problems may also impact judgment, inhibition, and problem-solving.

Important cognitive warning signs include hopelessness and helplessness. Hopelessness refers to the expectation that desirable outcomes will never occur, that bad outcomes will occur, and that nothing can be done to change the situation [39]. Helplessness is defined as the conviction that nothing can be done to change an undesirable situation. Recent reviews have highlighted the importance of pain-related helplessness in the experience of individuals with chronic pain [3, 24]. Negative cognitive inferential styles contribute to the development of hopelessness and helplessness. Three inferential styles or tendencies are particularly implicated: (a) attributing negative events to stable and global causes, (b) perceiving negative events as having many negative consequences, and (c) inferring negative characteristics about the self when negative events occur [40]. Cognitive states such as mental defeat and fear and cognitive styles involving catastrophizing, helplessness, and low self-efficacy may contribute to the development of hopelessness in chronic pain patients. Hopelessness is an important variable that mediates the relationship between depression and suicidal behavior [41, 42]. Particularly, hopelessness has been found to provide a more accurate estimate of suicide risk than depression severity [31]. Wenzel and Beck's model of suicidal behavior identifies hopelessness as a primary schema associated with suicide [43]. Hopelessness about pain and stressful circumstances surrounding pain conditions may ultimately drive individuals with chronic pain to consider suicide.

Sleep disturbances may impact a patient's ability for cognitive control and increase the likelihood of suicide attempts and completions. Insomnia is a common complaint of chronic pain patients [44, 45]. In a study of 100 outpatients with chronic low-back pain and without comorbid psychiatric disorders, 64% of cases endorsed experiencing insomnia due to back pain [46]. Sleep deprivation is also moderately associated with the perception of greater pain severity in patients with chronic pain [47]. In a review of the links between insomnia and depression, individuals with chronic pain were listed as a high-risk subgroup due to the elevated rates of both insomnia and suicidality in both conditions [48]. In a study of 51 outpatients with chronic pain, insomnia explained more variance in ratings of passive suicidal ideation than pain intensity [2].

Management of Suicide in Chronic Pain Patients

The clinical approach to suicidal ideation or suicidal gestures in chronic pain patients is similar to that with other populations. An actuarial approach is recommended, whereby an appreciation of aforementioned risk factors is calculated and weighed. For instance, as with other populations, previous suicide attempts are high-risk factors of completed future suicide in chronic pain patients. Similarly, loss of support, interpersonal role changes, unrelenting insomnia, and severe exacerbation of pain intensity are signs to seriously consider.

As mentioned above, comorbid substance use disorders are particularly critical to assess in chronic pain populations, as they elevate the risk of suicide dramatically. Special attention should be directed at the co-administration of opioid therapies alongside other sedating agents (particularly benzodiazepines and/or barbiturates); such medication regimens should be handled with extreme care. In fact, the Centers for Disease Control 2016 Guidelines for Prescribing Opioids for Chronic Pain have called for avoidance of such co-prescription "whenever possible" out of serious concern for accidental or intentional fatal overdose [49].

Inpatient hospitalization aimed at controlling acute pain exacerbations and/or psychiatric comorbidities while safeguarding the patient's well-being is at times warranted and should be pursued, even if at the expense of potentially damaging patient-physician rapport.

Summary

When working with chronic pain patients, one must consider the role of comorbidities (depression, particularly, but also personality disorders, substance use disorders, severe anxiety disorders, and other chronic medical conditions), personality traits (impulsivity, anger), vulnerable time periods (age, loss), and dangerous medication regimens (co-administration of opioids and sedatives). An actuarial approach to understanding suicidal risk is critical to shaping management, both behavioral and pharmacological.

References

1. Turk DC, Wilson HD, Cahana A. Treatment of chronic non-cancer pain. Lancet. 2011;377(9784):2226–35.
2. Smith MT, Edwards RR, Robinson RC, Dworkin RH. Suicidal ideation, plans, and attempts in chronic pain patients: factors associated with increased risk. Pain. 2004;111(1):201–8. https://doi.org/10.1016/j.pain.2004.06.016.
3. Tang NK, Crane C. Suicidality in chronic pain: a review of the prevalence, risk factors and psychological links. Psychol Med. 2006;36(05):575–86.
4. Swett JE, McMahon SB, Wall PD. Long ascending projections to the midbrain from cells of lamina I and nucleus of the dorsolateral funiculus of the rat spinal cord. J Comp Neurol. 1985;238(4):401–16.
5. Millan MJ. Descending control of pain. Prog Neurobiol. 2002;66:335–474.
6. Hoffman MD, Shepanski MA, MacKenzie SP, Clifford PS. Experimentally induced pain perception is acutely reduced by aerobic exercise in people with chronic low back pain. J Rehabil Res Dev. 2005;42(2):183.
7. Staud R. Abnormal endogenous pain modulation is a shared characteristic of many chronic pain conditions. Expert Rev Neurother. 2012;12(5):577–85.
8. Duncan GH, Bushnell MC, Bates RE, Dubner RO. Task-related responses of monkey medullary dorsal horn neurons. J Neurophysiol. 1987;57(1):289–310.
9. Zubieta JK, Heitzeg MM, Smith YR, Bueller JA, Xu K, Xu Y, et al. COMT val158met genotype affects µ-opioid neurotransmitter responses to a pain stressor. Science. 2003;299(5610):1240–3.
10. Uhl GR, Sora I, Wang Z. The µ opiate receptor as a candidate gene for pain: polymorphisms, variations in expression, nociception, and opiate responses. PNAS. 1999;96(14):7752–5.
11. Devor M, Raber P. Heritability of symptoms in an experimental model of neuropathic pain. Pain. 1990;42(1):51–67.
12. Coghill RC, McHaffie JG, Yen YF. Neural correlates of interindividual differences in the subjective experience of pain. PNAS. 2003;100(14):8538–42.
13. Elman I, Borsook D, Volkow ND. Pain and suicidality: insights from reward and addiction neuroscience. Prog Neurobiol. 2013;109:1–27. https://doi.org/10.1016/j.pneurobio.2013.06.003.

14. Meerwijk EL, Ford JM, Weiss SJ. Suicidal crises because of diminishing tolerance to psychological pain. Brain Imaging Behav. 2013;7(3):245–7. https://doi.org/10.1007/s11682-013-9234-3.
15. Nock MK, Kessler RC. Prevalence of and risk factors for suicide attempts versus suicide gestures: analysis of the National Comorbidity Survey. J Abnorm Psychol. 2006;115(3):616.
16. Nock MK, Hwang I, Sampson NA, Kessler RC. Mental disorders, comorbidity and suicidal behavior: results from the National Comorbidity Survey Replication. Mol Psychiatry. 2010;15(8):868–76.
17. Scott KM, Hwang I, Chiu WT, Kessler RC, Sampson NA, Angermeyer M, et al. Chronic physical conditions and their association with first onset of suicidal behavior in the world mental health surveys. Psychosom Med. 2010;72(7):712–9.
18. Ohayon MM, Schatzberg AF. Chronic pain and major depressive disorder in the general population. J Psychiatr Res. 2010;44(7):454–61.
19. Gerrits MM, van Oppen P, van Marwijk HW, Penninx BW, van der Horst HE. Pain and the onset of depressive and anxiety disorders. Pain. 2014;155(1):53–9.
20. Larson SL, Clark MR, Eaton WW. Depressive disorder as a long-term antecedent risk factor for incident back pain: a 13-year follow-up study from the Baltimore Epidemiological Catchment Area sample. Psychol Med. 2004;34(02):211–9.
21. Rudy TE, Kerns RD, Turk DC. Chronic pain and depression: toward a cognitive-behavioral mediation model. Pain. 1988;35(2):129–40.
22. RK MH, Weiss RD, Cornelius M, Martel MO, Jamison RN, Edwards RR. Distress intolerance and prescription opioid misuse among patients with chronic pain. J Pain. 2016;17(7):806–14.
23. Garland EL, Brown SM, Howard MO. Thought suppression as a mediator of the association between depressed mood and prescription opioid craving among chronic pain patients. J Behav Med. 2016;39(1):128–38.
24. Racine M, Choinière M, Nielson WR. Predictors of suicidal ideation in chronic pain patients: an exploratory study. Clin J Pain. 2014;30(5):371–8.
25. Ilgen MA, Kleinberg F, Ignacio RV, Bohnert AS, Valenstein M, McCarthy JF, et al. Noncancer pain conditions and risk of suicide. JAMA Psychiat. 2013;70(7):692–7.
26. Marino EN, Rosen KD, Gutierrez A, Eckmann M, Ramamurthy S, Potter JS. Impulsivity but not sensation seeking is associated with opioid analgesic misuse risk in patients with chronic pain. Addict Behav. 2013;38(5):2154–7.
27. Cheatle MD. Depression, chronic pain, and suicide by overdose: on the edge. Pain Med. 2011;12(s2):S43–8.
28. Greenwood KA, Thurston R, Rumble M, Waters SJ, Keefe FJ. Anger and persistent pain: current status and future directions. Pain. 2003;103(1–2):1–5.
29. Bruns D, Disorbio JM, Hanks R. Chronic nonmalignant pain and violent behavior. Curr Pain Headache Rep. 2003;7(2):127–32.
30. Fishbain DA, Bruns D, Lewis JE, Disorbio JM, Gao J, Meyer LJ. Predictors of homicide–suicide affirmation in acute and chronic pain patients. Pain Med. 2011;12(1):127–37.
31. Margari F, Lorusso M, Matera E, Pastore A, Zagaria G, Bruno F, et al. Aggression, impulsivity, and suicide risk in benign chronic pain patients–a cross-sectional study. Neuropsychiatr Dis Treat. 2014;10:1613.
32. Cavanagh JTO, Carson AJ, Sharpe M, Lawrie SM. Psychological autopsy studies of suicide: a systematic review. Psychol Med. 2003;33(3):395–405.
33. Wolfe F, Häuser W, Hassett AL, Katz RS, Walitt BT. The development of fibromyalgia–I: examination of rates and predictors in patients with rheumatoid arthritis (RA). Pain. 2011;152(2):291–9.
34. Wilson KG, Kowal J, Henderson PR, McWilliams LA, Péloquin K. Chronic pain and the interpersonal theory of suicide. Rehabil Psychol. 2013;58(1):111.
35. Ilgen MA, Bohnert AS, Ignacio RV, McCarthy JF, Valenstein MM, Kim HM, et al. Psychiatric diagnoses and risk of suicide in veterans. Arch Gen Psychiatry. 2010;67(11):1152–8.
36. Overholser JC, Braden A, Dieter L. Understanding suicide risk: identification of high-risk groups during high-risk times. J Clin Psychol. 2012;68(3):349–61.

37. Foster T. Adverse life events proximal to adult suicide: a synthesis of findings from psychological autopsy studies. Arch Suicide Res. 2011;15(1):1–5.
38. Walker J, Sofaer B, Holloway I. The experience of chronic back pain: accounts of loss in those seeking help from pain clinics. Eur J Pain. 2006;10(3):199.
39. Liu RT, Kleiman EM, Nestor BA, Cheek SM. The hopelessness theory of depression: a quarter-century in review. Clin Psychol. 2015;22(4):345–65.
40. Abela JR, Seligman ME. The hopelessness theory of depression: a test of the diathesis-stress component in the interpersonal and achievement domains. Cognit Ther Res. 2000;24(4):361–78.
41. Beck U. Risk society: towards a new modernity. London: Sage; 1992.
42. Overholser JC, Fisher L, Braden A, Peak N. Despair beyond repair? Severity of hopelessness in depressed psychiatric inpatients. J Dep Ther. 2015;1(1):1–10.
43. Wenzel A, Beck AT. A cognitive model of suicidal behavior: theory and treatment. Appl Prev Psychol. 2008;12(4):189–201.
44. Marty M, Rozenberg S, Duplan B, Thomas P, Duquesnoy B, Allaert F. Quality of sleep in patients with chronic low back pain: a case-control study. Eur Spine J. 2008;17(6):839–44.
45. Ancoli-Israel S. The impact and prevalence of chronic insomnia and other sleep disturbances associated with chronic illness. Am J Manag Care. 2006;12(8 Suppl):S221–9.
46. Bahouq H, Allali F, Rkain H, Hmamouchi I, Hajjaj-Hassouni N. Prevalence and severity of insomnia in chronic low back pain patients. Rheumatol Int. 2013;33(5):1277–81.
47. Schrimpf M, Liegl G, Boeckle M, Leitner A, Geisler P, Pieh C. The effect of sleep deprivation on pain perception in healthy subjects: a meta-analysis. Sleep Med. 2015;16(11):1313–20.
48. Winsper C, Tang NK. Linkages between insomnia and suicidality: prospective associations, high-risk subgroups and possible psychological mechanisms. Int Rev Psychiatry. 2014;26(2):189–204.
49. Dowell D, Haegerich TM, Chou R. CDC guideline for prescribing opioids for chronic pain—United States, 2016. JAMA. 2016;315(15):1624–45.

Part III

Medical Services

Primary Care Behavioral Health (PCBH) Model and Suicide

8

Alexander D. Smith, Meghan D.M. Fondow, and Elizabeth A. Zeidler Schreiter

The Forefront of Suicide Prevention

On average, it has been estimated that passive and active suicidal ideation are present in 2.4–3.3% of the general patient population in primary care [1, 2]. Yet, greater than half of patients who endorse suicidal ideation in the past month have not received mental health services during that time [1]. While the overall percentage of primary care patients with suicidal ideation is significant but small, a large proportion of people who die by suicide sought care in primary care within a month (45%) and a year (77%) preceding their death [3, 4]. Additionally, people who died by suicide had significantly less contact with mental health services the month (19%) and year (32%) prior to their deaths [4]. Despite patients often seeing a Primary Care Provider (PCP) prior to death by suicide, many of these patients were without mental health diagnoses, suggesting room for improvement in assessment in primary care [3]. As a result of patients being more likely to have contact with a provider in primary care as opposed to specialty mental health, it is imperative to review our current systems to develop a more thorough understanding of how the assessment and treatment of suicidal ideation can be enhanced within the primary care setting. The first step is to ensure that appropriate screening is occurring to identify patients who pose suicide risk.

Screening for Suicide Risk

The US Preventive Services Task Force (USPSTF) released an updated review of the literature which has maintained their conclusion from 2004 that there has been insufficient evidence demonstrating the benefits and costs for screening for

A. D. Smith, Psy.D. (✉) · M. D. M. Fondow, Ph.D. · E. A. Zeidler Schreiter, Psy.D.
Access Community Health Centers, Madison, WI, USA
e-mail: alex.smith@accesshealthwi.org; meghan.fondow@accesshealthwi.org; elizabeth.zeidlerschreiter@accesshealthwi.org

T. Falcone, J. Timmons-Mitchell (eds.), *Suicide Prevention*,
https://doi.org/10.1007/978-3-319-74391-2_8

suicidality among adolescents or adults within primary care [5]. This suggests that screening for suicidality does not provide accurate identification of those who are at risk for attempting or dying by suicide. Although multiple screening tools are utilized in primary care, such as the Columbia-Suicide Severity Rating Scale (C-SSRS) and the Edinburgh Postnatal Depression Scale (EPDS), one of the most heavily researched and widely used measure for depression and suicide risk in primary care is the Patient Health Questionnaire-9 (PHQ-9) [6–8]. Research on the PHQ-9 offers insight into the shortcomings of relying on screening tools as the primary method for suicide prevention in this setting.

PHQ-9

The PHQ-9 is a nine-item questionnaire that is intended to assess for symptoms commonly associated with depression. Item 9 on the questionnaire targets the frequency of patients' thoughts about death and/or self-harm [9]. This item has been found to have a specificity of 0.84 and sensitivity of 0.69 among patients who presented with depression in primary care [10]. Patients who responded "more than half the days" or "nearly every day" to Item 9 accounted for 53% of suicide attempts and 54% of deaths by suicide over the following year. Of note, patients who reported frequent thoughts of suicide were identified as being at low risk of imminent suicidal behavior, but risk increased over several days and continued for many months [11]. The findings of these studies support the utility of the PHQ-9 as a screening measure for suicidality in primary care.

Although the PHQ-9 can be a useful tool, it is important to be aware of its limitations. One study determined that approximately one fifth of the sampled population who attempted or died by suicide had never reported suicidal ideation on the PHQ-9. Furthermore, they found that one fourth of those who attempted suicide and had completed the questionnaire within 1 week of their attempt had responded "not at all" to Item 9 [11]. This study serves as a warning to providers that they should interpret patients' responses with caution for screening alone is insufficient in identifying suicide risk. Caution should also be taken when solely relying on depression screening tools to assess suicide risk. Nock et al. [12] reported that, although depression was predictive of the development of suicidal ideation, depression alone was not predictive of suicidal ideation transitioning to a plan to die by suicide. They found that marked anxiety or agitation or poor impulse control was more likely to be predictive of suicidal ideation evolving into a suicide plan or attempt. These studies suggest that further research is needed to create and/or identify screeners that are more effective at identifying patients who are at risk of attempting or dying by suicide in primary care.

PHQ-9 Versus EPDS

The Edinburgh Postnatal Depression Scale (EPDS) is a ten-item screening tool for postpartum depression, and Item 10 queries about thoughts of self-harm [13]. When considering differences between the PHQ-9 and EPDS, it is important to note that a study conducted using a sample of pregnant women in Peru, who were administered both screening tools, reported that the PHQ-9 identified a greater number of participants with suicidal ideation compared to the EPDS (15.8% vs. 8.8%) [14]. The authors concluded that the factors likely contributing to these differences were time frame (PHQ-9 inquires about suicidal ideation in the past 2 weeks compared to 1 week on the EPDS) and inclusion/exclusion of passive suicidal ideation (PHQ-9 asks about both passive and active self-harm vs. only active self-harm on the EPDS). These results suggest that providers should consider inquiring about passive suicidal ideation as well as history of suicidal ideation, even if patients do not endorse thoughts of self-harm, when administering the EPDS; otherwise, valuable information could be missed. Despite its potential limitations, the EPDS is a valuable tool and has been found to identify significant rates of suicidal ideation both during (4.1%) and after (3.4%) pregnancy with 1.1% of patients, who endorsed suicidal ideation, being identified as high risk [15]. Another study discovered that 9% of the women who completed the EPDS endorsed recent suicidal ideation [16].

PHQ-9 Versus C-SSRS

The Columbia-Suicide Severity Rating Scale (C-SSRS), which is also available in an electronic format (eC-SSRS) and in over 100 country-specific languages, is a suicide risk assessment tool that evaluates the severity and frequency of suicidal ideation and behaviors [17, 18]. Instead of a 2-week timeframe, as used by the PHQ-9, the C-SSRS assesses for suicidal ideation in the past month and suicidal behaviors in the previous 3 months [17]. Although the C-SSRS is frequently utilized in clinical trials and within primary care, little to no research on the effectiveness of the C-SSRS in managing suicide risk in primary care appears to exist. Yet, there is promising evidence supporting its use.

Some researchers view the C-SSRS as being a better screening tool for suicidality than the PHQ-9. Posner et al. [18] identify one limitation of the PHQ-9 as not providing a distinction between higher and lower risk indicators because Item 9 includes passive suicidal ideation, which the authors believe contributes to the low poor predictive value of the PHQ-9. It is suspected that this influences the high rate of false-positive findings with the PHQ-9 as compared to the C-SSRS [19, 20]. Another criticism of the PHQ-9 is that it does not specifically assess for suicidal ideation or behavior unlike the C-SSRS [18, 20]. The C-SSRS was developed with the intention of gathering additional information to allow for a more thorough assessment of risk including preparatory behaviors, aborted and interrupted suicide attempts, and actual suicide attempts [20]. A prospective study conducted by Mundt et al. [21] using the eC-SSRS discovered that patients were 4–9 times more likely to report suicidal behavior during the time of the study if they endorsed lifetime suicidal ideation with intent to act and/or prior suicidal behavior at baseline, and Posner et al. [17] found that the item on the C-SSRS inquiring about worst-point lifetime suicidal ideation was predictive of suicide attempts among adolescents. These findings are valuable and potential benefits of using the C-SSRS in assessing suicide risk compared to the PHQ-9. Furthermore, the C-SSRS has been found to be more effective at detecting suicide attempts (more than 40%) as compared to chart reviews (18%) within emergency department settings [22]. Given the potential gains associated with adopting the C-SSRS as a standard screening tool in primary care, there is a need for increased research due to the limited research on its use in this setting.

Insights from the Literature

Research suggests that further investigation and development is needed to create and implement screening tools that have higher rates of positive predictive value. Primary care is an important setting to evaluate these tools given the likelihood of a patient-provider interaction prior to acting on suicidal thoughts. However, this is a difficult task given the complexity of identifying those who are at risk of dying by suicide. Therefore, the USPSTF has upheld their recommendation that healthcare organizations that screen for depression should have systems in place to provide proper diagnosis, treatment, and follow-up care [5]. Studies have shown that screening tools increase rates of detection for adults and adolescents, such as Wintersteen who found that utilization of screening questions increased the rate of detection of suicide risk and referral of adolescents to outpatient specialty mental health services by approximately 392% [23]. Although screening tools offer potential promise in identifying patients of high suicide risk, it is essential for PCPs and medical support staff to be knowledgeable about how to address suicide risk.

Need for Training in Primary Care

Education and Training on Suicide in Medical School

According to the findings of Sudak et al. [24], a majority of family practice, pediatrics, and internal medicine training directors recognize a need for a standardized curriculum covering the assessment and treatment of depression and suicide. However, the training by specialization varies widely. They discovered that less than half of pediatrics and internal medicine training directors recognized their didactic training on suicide as being sufficient. Family practice training directors' satisfaction was much higher at around 80% [24], and Hooper et al. [25] found that physicians who were specialized in family medicine were more likely to assess for suicide risk compared to physicians who were not. This suggests a need for standardizing curriculum across specialties in order to increase providers' confidence in addressing suicide risk.

PCPs and Suicide Risk Assessment

PCPs generally have low rates of suicide risk assessment for at-risk patients. Feldman et al. [26] reported that PCPs only inquired about suicide 27% of the time when patients, who did not request psychotropic medications, presented with depressive symptoms. PCP inquiry increased when patients specifically requested medication to treat their mental health-related symptoms; however, PCPs were not as likely to assess for suicide risk when patients requested a specific brand of medication as opposed to a general request for medication. In another study, Hopper et al. [25] found approximately one third of physicians conducted a suicide risk assessment even though 98% of them identified a patient as being depressed with moderate levels of severity. While physicians were more likely to investigate suicide risk with patients who were perceived as having a more severe symptom presentation, they found that over 60% did not indicate that they would assess for suicide risk even though they categorized the patient as being "depressed" or "very depressed." Incorporating screeners has been one attempt to facilitate a discussion between PCPs and their patients about depression and suicide.

Even when screening tools, such as the PHQ-9, are used, PCPs often continue to exhibit reluctance to engage in discussion about suicide. In fact, further inquiry about suicide happens with approximately 11% of patients who endorse thoughts of self-harm or suicidality on the PHQ-9, and it is less likely to occur when the patient is male [27]. Even more concerning is that PCPs are more prone to have a discussion about suicide when patients endorse the lowest levels of suicidal ideation on the PHQ-9 or if the patient is female, even when the prevalence rates of reported suicidal ideation among men and women on Item 9 of the PHQ-9 in this study were equal. One factor that may contribute to limited to no exploration of suicide among males is that male patients are less likely to initiate suicide-related conversation compared to female patients [27]. Increasing provider awareness of this predisposition is critical since men die by suicide 3.5 times more often than women [28].

Individual Factors Influencing Suicide Assessment and Treatment

Researchers have attempted to identify potential PCP-related factors that impact assessment and treatment of suicidality. Graham et al. [29] sought to better understand the relationships between PCPs' gender, level of training, and self-perceived competence relating to suicide treatment. They discovered that gender was not predictive of PCPs' willingness to treat suicidality. Yet, PCPs who identified as female were predictive of having low self-perceived competence. Also, PCPs identifying as female, who viewed mental health consultation as being essential, were the only group to have a low level of self-perceived competence. However, their level of self-perceived competence increased with training. PCPs who identified as male, viewed mental health providers as inessential, had low levels of training, and had high levels of self-perceived competence did not experience a significant increase in their level of self-perceived competence after training. Though individual differences in PCPs exist, self-perceived competence and gender do not appear to impact their willingness to treat suicidality unlike receiving a higher level of training, which has been associated with increased willingness [27, 29]. A limitation of these studies is that they did not explore PCPs' actual level of competence in treating suicidality.

A study that did analyze the likelihood that a PCP would assess for suicide risk reported that being White, young, male, and specializing in family medicine is significantly correlated with the likelihood that a PCP will assess for suicide risk [25]. In another study, practicing in an academic setting or having personal experience with depression was found to be associated with higher rates of inquiry about suicide among providers [26]. These two studies suggest that PCPs' perceived willingness and self-perceived competence in addressing suicide risk might not truly reflect what occurs in clinical practice.

Two Myths Regarding Suicide

Another reason for additional training is to dispel common provider myths related to suicide. One belief among some physicians is that asking about suicide will "plant" the idea into the patient's mind. Researchers have categorized this belief as a myth. Dazzi et al. [30] reviewed 13 journal articles published between 2001 and 2013 on this topic to determine if there is an iatrogenic effect associated with screening for suicide. They did not find any evidence to suggest that suicide screening has an iatrogenic effect on adolescent or adult populations. In fact, they reported that inquiring about suicide might actually reduce, as opposed to increase, suicidal ideation. Therefore, inquiring about suicidality in primary care may result in a reduction in suicide risk among patients.

A second myth is that antidepressants should not be prescribed to patients who endorse suicidality due to an increased potential for suicidal behavior. The FDA modified the black box warning in 2007 to specify that the warning about the potential for increased suicidal thinking and behavior applies to people aged 24 years and younger. Furthermore, they note that adults aged 65 and older experience a reduced suicide risk with an antidepressant trial [31]. Valuck et al. [32] found that antidepressants provide a protective effect for suicide attempt. However, it is important to note that they found suicide risk was at its highest whenever an antidepressant trial was initiated. Additional factors that increased risk were discontinuation of an antidepressant prior to 56 days and titration. A review of the current literature suggests that antidepressants can help to mitigate suicide risk, but caution should be taken whenever an antidepressant trial is initiated, abbreviated, or titrated.

Benefits of Training

Overall, the research provides evidence supporting increased training for providers on the assessment and treatment of depression and suicidality. Interventions targeted at enhancing PCPs' and nurses' knowledge about depression care have been shown to heighten identification of patients with recent suicidal ideation [33]. Training has also been shown to enhance providers' willingness to address suicide irrespective of a PCPs' level of self-perceived confidence [29]. Most importantly, providing PCPs with trainings on how to identify and treat depression and restricting access to lethal means have been found to reduce suicide rates [34].

Supplementary training for PCPs facilitates improvement in the ability to attune to verbal and nonverbal indications suggestive of an at-risk patient, which extends beyond patient report and their responses to screening tools. Still, even with the appropriate training, PCPs' time is limited creating an obstacle to appropriately address suicide risk. One strategy to assist with the process and reduce further barriers is integrating behavioral health providers within the medical setting with a model such as the Primary Care Behavioral Health model.

Primary Care Behavioral Health Model

The Primary Care Behavioral Health (PCBH) model is an integrated model of care where behavioral health providers are referred to as behavioral health consultants or BHCs [35]. In this model of care, the BHC serves dual roles as consultant to the primary customer (the medical provider) and a behavioral health provider delivering direct behavioral health services to patients. The focus of behavioral health work is related to patient functioning across the life span. Therefore, BHCs' primary aim is to assist PCPs in managing patients' behavioral needs [35]. BHCs work alongside PCPs and medical support staff to ensure availability when needed. This differs from many other forms of behavioral health integration in that BHCs are not behavioral health providers operating within a primary care setting separately from the PCPs, which is considered co-located care, and BHCs are able to see a higher percentage of patients compared to other integrated collaborative care models [36]. BHCs are able to see twice as many patients as other integrated models of care since BHC visits are typically 30 min or less as compared to other models where visits are 1 hour [35]. PCPs and BHCs see patients in the same exam rooms to emphasize that patient care is being managed using a team-based approach. For this reason, the PCBH model lends itself well to supporting PCPs and medical support staff in assessing and treating patients in crisis.

Rationale

Based on a review of the literature, Gunn and Blount [37] report that 25–30% of primary care visits have a presenting issue related to a mental health or substance abuse concern. They also note that PCPs prescribe 60–70% of psychotropic medications; however, PCPs frequently do not have the necessary time or training to adequately address patients' mental health-related issues. This information suggests that PCPs would benefit from assistance in identifying and treating the psychiatric problems of their patients. There has been evidence backing its usefulness and effectiveness in supporting medical providers.

BHC intervention in as little as two to three visits has been associated with clinically meaningful improvements in the areas of well-being, symptom management, and functioning [38]. Gains received from BHC intervention have been reported as being maintained for an average of 2 years post-intervention [39]. Relating to suicidality, Bryan et al. [40] found that suicidal ideation diminished over the course of 2 to 8 BHC visits among a sample of 497 primary care patients. In addition to the patient-related gains associated with the PCBH model, this model has been found to create positive systemic changes. For instance, a study conducted by Serrano and Monden [41] found that improvements were made in depression screening, documenting behavioral goals, prescribing practices with antidepressants, and diminishing unnecessary referrals to specialty mental health services. Although further research is warranted, these studies aid in supporting the viability of the PCBH model in primary care.

How It Works

Unlike specialty mental health services where appointments often range from 45 to 50 min in length, a typical BHC visit ranges from 15 to 30 min [35]. The PCBH model utilizes a population-based care perspective meaning that the goal is to improve the overall health of the population through preventative and direct care for behaviorally based problems and through systemic change of the primary care system [35]. One fundamental component of population-based care is maintaining targeted visits to allow for increased availability to providers for warm handoffs. This involves limiting the number of BHC follow-up appointment slots based on provider needs. Patients are typically seen for four or fewer visits, and Robinson and Reiter [35] estimate that less than 15–20% of their patients are seen for more than four visits. Assessments are generally limited to the referral problem, and interventions are targeted and brief. This allows for BHCs to see a higher volume of patients and assist PCPs in addressing patients' underlying behavioral issues. Besides patient-related assessment and intervention, there are several ways in which BHCs support PCPs beyond mental health-related interventions.

For instance, BHCs are well positioned to provide direct and indirect training to both PCPs and medical support staff. According to Hunter and Goodman [36], the PCBH model stands apart from other models since it is the only one where consultative interactions are utilized to transfer behavioral intervention skills to PCPs as one of the primary goals. Therefore, BHCs can assist in not only managing patients who present with suicide risk but also training providers in being able to assess and intervene when a patient endorses suicidality. This includes nursing and medical support staff who encounter patients who endorse suicidality when triaging either in person or via telephone. As previously mentioned, training providers has been shown to increase detection and reduce incidents of suicide [33, 34], which is likely a result of providers reporting heightened perception of competence and willingness in treating suicidal ideation [29], and is a current need in primary care [24, 29].

In addition to training providers, BHCs assist in care coordination between community agencies. For example, when patients pose an imminent suicide risk, BHCs will assist the PCP in coordinating with emergency services, if needed, and/or the hospital to facilitate an admission. BHCs will follow up with the patient and hospital to determine the care plan going forward. Assisting PCPs with care coordination increases efficiency of workflows while continuing to provide quality care to patients.

To be able to successfully provide these services, BHCs are required to have several skills. They should be able to rapidly identify problems and adapt assessments and treatments in a manner that best serves the patients and PCPs within the context of patients' lives. To do this, BHCs piece together and address a variety of factors (e.g., psychological trauma, food insecurity, homelessness, chaotic lives) to improve the quality of patient care. This requires BHCs to have the ability to conduct a functional analysis during a visit to pinpoint a presenting issue and establish measurable outcomes to monitor patients' progress. They are required to be knowledgeable about the relationship between medical and psychological systems and have a basic awareness of psychotropic medications. BHCs should also have general knowledge about and ability to treat psychiatric conditions, chronic physical health conditions (e.g., diabetes, chronic pain), and substance abuse. Communication skills are necessary to provide PCPs with a succinct overview of patients' presenting issues, symptoms, and barriers to treatment as well as recommendations for intervention to inform PCPs' treatment plans. BHCs are also required to know how to appropriately document within patients' electronic health records (EHRs) [35, 36]. Working within the PCBH model requires BHCs to have effective time management skills, an ability to work in a fast-paced environment, a willingness to work as part of a team, and self-awareness to prevent burnout.

Suicide Management in the PCBH Model

Screening

Bryan et al. [42] recommend screening patients for suicide risk during their initial contact with a BHC. Screening should be brief and targeted, taking into account health literacy levels and language. Therefore, the PHQ-9, C-SSRS, and EPDS are potential screening tools to be considered for use in primary care. If patients' responses indicate a positive screening, the next step is to determine the nature and content of the ideation, as it is important to distinguish suicidal ideation (e.g., "I have thought about ending my life") from non-suicidal morbid ideation (e.g., "It wouldn't be the worse thing in the world if I didn't wake up tomorrow") [42]. Further assessment is warranted if a patient endorses suicidal ideation and can be addressed during a PCP or BHC visit with the patient.

Risk Assessment

Given that the PCBH model emphasizes a time-efficient approach, it is important to organize the suicide risk assessment in a way that places top priority to predictors of suicidal behavior with the strongest empirical support. In addition to gathering information related to current or recent suicidal ideation, a key component of the suicide risk assessment is inquiry into patients' suicide histories, including past thoughts, plans, and attempts, as well as self-injurious and rehearsal behaviors. Even if it is determined that the patient has non-suicidal morbid ideation, it is imperative to ask patients about their unique histories of suicidal ideation, any current or previous plans to die by suicide, and past suicide attempts. This information is beneficial for advising the patient's care team regarding potential suicide risk and may have implications for the PCP's treatment plan (e.g., avoid treating patient with medication that has a greater potential for lethality if used in excess).

Bryan et al. [42] suggest that it is the BHC's objective to obtain a "snapshot" of the patient's suicide history for patients with multiple attempts. They recommend that the patient should be asked, in order, about their first suicide attempt, "most serious" attempt, and most recent attempt. Notably, increased attention should be given to patients with multiple suicide attempts [43] as well as those who continue to wish they were dead in response to living through a previous attempt because of their elevated suicide risk [43, 44].

After attaining a brief suicide history, it is important to gather information about the patient's current suicidal ideation including if they presently have a plan. A patient with a plan is at a higher risk of acting on suicidal ideation, especially when there is availability of means to follow through with it. Therefore, it is critical to determine if they have the opportunity to make an attempt (e.g., access to a firearm) as well as their confidence in following through with it. Providers should also establish the duration and intensity of the patient's suicidal thoughts and assess for preparatory and rehearsal behaviors related to their current plan. Additional information that should be assessed includes factors perpetuating or contributing to their suicidal ideation, mental health history (e.g., severe depressive episodes, comorbid disorders), substance use history/current use, stressful life events, level of social support, coping strategies, and protective factors (e.g., positive life events, good education, good social support) [42, 45]. The suicide risk assessment aids in classifying patients as low, moderate, high, or imminent risk.

Having an algorithm to identify patients' level of risk is important to informing PCPs of the next steps for treatment. Bryan et al. [46] suggest an algorithm for classifying suicide risk. *Low-risk* patients are those who endorse no recent suicidal ideation and less than two suicide attempts. *Moderate-risk* patients endorse (1) recent suicidal ideation without a plan and less than two suicide attempts or (2) no recent suicidal ideation and two or more suicide attempts. *High-risk* patients endorse (1) recent suicidal ideation with a plan, less than two suicide attempts, and no recent preparations or practice or (2) recent suicidal ideation without a plan and two or more suicide attempts. *Imminent-risk* patients are those who report (1) recent suicidal ideation with a plan and recent preparations or practice and less than two suicide attempts or (2) recent suicidal ideation with a plan and two or more suicide attempts. Based on a patient's level of suicide risk, the recommended interventions vary.

Intervention

Once a suicide risk assessment has been conducted, a clinical determination is made based on the information collected as how to manage risk. In addition to the patient's level of risk, the PCP's level of comfort in treating a patient's mental health-related symptoms should be considered. The following are recommendations for addressing suicidality based on a patient's identified level of risk.

Low-risk patients are most often managed in clinic. Typically, there are little to no changes in treatment [46]. However, BHCs and PCPs should continue to monitor any potential changes in the level of suicide risk during follow-up appointments and ensure that screening tools, such as the PHQ-9, are administered at subsequent visits. BHCs will also work with patients to develop self-awareness (e.g., "I have thoughts of suicide whenever I feel helpless or crave substances") and strategies, such as relaxation techniques, to enhance self-management of symptoms. Intervention for *moderate-risk* patients generally consists of providing patients with crisis line telephone numbers, educating on stress management (including relaxation and mindfulness exercises), encouraging behavioral activation, establishing close follow-up in the form of telephone contact and/or scheduled appointments, considering pharmacological intervention, and potentially referring the patient to specialty mental health services in the community [42, 46]. Safety planning with patients and coordinating with the PCP are critical with *high-risk* patients. This includes developing a crisis response plan with the patient and providing them with local and national crisis line telephone numbers. When BHCs are unable to directly meet with the patient because the patient declines services, BHCs can offer support to the PCP in coordinating care with the necessary community agencies. This entails contacting a hospital diversion program, if available in the community, or an emergency department to advocate for patient in being evaluated for admission, if the patient expresses willingness. High-risk patients do not meet the necessary threshold for involuntary hospitalization; therefore, it is critical to have a crisis response plan in place and attempt to involve their family in monitoring for changes in symptoms. In addition to a crisis response plan, the PCP or a BHC should provide means restriction counseling [46]. Means restriction counseling has been shown to be an effective method of lowering the death by suicide rate [34, 47]. These patients require close follow-up and will often be scheduled to see a BHC or PCP the same week or will be contacted to check in via telephone. The primary goal of the medical team is to work together to assist in stabilizing the patient. *Imminent-risk* patients require intensive treatment. They should be encouraged to present to the emergency department for immediate treatment if willing to go. If a patient is willing to go voluntarily to the emergency department, the BHC or PCP will coordinate with the hospital to prepare them for the patient's intended arrival. If a patient meets the criteria for an involuntary hospitalization and is unwilling to go on their own accord, the BHC and PCP must work together to ensure that the patient is psychiatrically hospitalized to prevent harm to self. This requires BHCs to be familiar with the legal process for an involuntary hospitalization as it varies by state. Patients should follow up as soon as possible with their PCP and a BHC following discharge from an inpatient hospital stay to reassess suicide risk, coordinate care, and establish a crisis response plan [46].

Documentation

Documentation goes directly into a patient's EHR when working in the PCBH model in primary care. BHCs' progress notes are typically visible by all providers. When documenting suicide risk of patients, there are components that should be entered into the progress note such as the results of suicide screening, information obtained during the risk assessment, interventions used during the visit, any consultations with PCPs or other professionals, and follow-up plan [42]. It is also advised to document any changes in risk factors and patient adherence to recommendations [42]. Moreover, suicidal ideation and suicide attempts should be documented using diagnostic codes within patients' EHRs. Although mentioned in the progress note, suicidal ideation and suicide attempts are recorded as a diagnostic code for only 3% and 19% of patients, respectively [48]. Ensuring that documentation is properly completed assists with continuity of care.

The PCBH Model in Practice

This section provides a general synopsis of our current practices across three primary care clinics to supplement the current literature on addressing suicide risk within the PCBH model. The following information provides insight into how we address suicide utilizing a team-based approach as well as the nuances of our program.

Screening/Prevention

In addition to PCPs and BHCs ability to assess and treat suicidality, medical support staff also plays a fundamental role in managing psychiatric emergencies in clinic as well as over the telephone. It is not uncommon for medical support staff to receive telephone calls from patients who report exacerbated symptoms of depression or suicidal ideation. These patients are often seeking same-day appointments or assistance in managing their distress. Therefore, BHCs at our clinics assist in creating algorithms, known as care algorithms, for medical support staff to follow while triaging these calls. Care algorithms consist of specific questions that medical support staff should ask patients when concern for suicide risk is present [35]. Patients' responses to questions about suicide then inform the explicit steps that should be taken by medical support staff in managing the situation. BHCs are easily accessible at our clinics to assist in fielding telephone calls and making clinical recommendations whenever patients present with suicide risk. We also offer in-house staff trainings to enhance medical support staff's comfort level and ability to provide such services.

When a patient is in clinic, a PCP, nurse-midwife, member of the medical support staff, or BHC will administer the PHQ-9 or EPDS. Prior to the beginning of the shift, medical support staff will review the scheduled patients' EHRs to identify patients with a diagnosis of depression. They will then discuss their findings with the PCP during their "huddle" to determine if screening is warranted. Additionally, a PCP or member of the medical support staff may provide a patient with a screening measure whenever a patient presents as visibly depressed or anxious or the content of their conversation is suggestive of depression. Patients' responses on screening tools help to prompt providers to discuss depression with them as well as offer BHC services. We have found that the administration of these screenings has been helpful in facilitating conversations between PCPs and patients about both depression and suicide. This is essential because patients have the right to decline BHC services, and it is important that providers are comfortable addressing suicidality. BHCs will also administer the PHQ-9 and/or EPDS for multiple reasons including it is an initial visit, the patient has a history of depression or suicidal ideation, the patient is requesting or beginning a trial a psychotropic medication, or there have been other clinical indications identified. Patients with high scores who do not endorse suicidality on screening tools are still directly asked about suicidal ideation given that they may have felt uncomfortable endorsing thoughts of self-harm on the PHQ-9 or EPDS.

Risk Assessment and Intervention

In terms of suicide risk assessment and intervention, our approach does not vary significantly from the previously outlined recommendations made by Bryan et al. [46]. However, a noticeable difference from the suggested interventions outlined in Bryan et al. [46] is that we will often offer patients, who are identified as being of moderate or higher suicide risk, assistance in connecting with a hospital diversion program. These are local programs that accept voluntary admissions and provide close supervision, a safe environment, 24-hour support, and medication assistance in a less restrictive environment than an inpatient hospital setting. Our patients, who have taken advantage of these services, typically report high satisfaction with their experiences and describe their stay as being a respite from their present stressors; however, the space at these facilities are limited. BHCs will assist in coordinating care to ensure that patients will receive a bed once one is available. Follow-up after being discharged from a hospital diversion program is highly recommended.

Another intervention that we rely upon at our clinics is the use of a consulting psychiatrist. BHCs will refer patients based on the severity, chronicity, and complexity of the presenting psychiatric and potential substance abuse issues to the consulting psychiatrist for further diagnostic clarification and/or treatment recommendations. For example, patients who present with suicide risk, except for those who are identified as being an imminent suicide risk, may be referred to consulting psychiatry by a BHC for a written or 1-hour face-to-face consult. Regardless of the type of consult, the psychiatrist produces a report with recommendations for the PCP since the PCP is responsible for patients' medication management. Patients are typically able to see our consulting psychiatrist in less than 3 weeks, which is critical given the lack of psychiatry services in our community, especially for patients with Medicare. This service allows for PCPs to feel increased confidence and comfort in managing a patient's psychotropic medications in the context of suicidality.

For further information on the consulting psychiatry portion of our program, see Zeidler Schreiter et al. [49, 50].

Care Management

It has been found that care management calls have been associated with a 50% improvement in depression scores and have little associated cost [51]. Similarly, our care management services have been effective in supporting potentially high-risk patients from disengaging with their healthcare providers. At our clinics, BHC's provide care management services based on patients' scores on the PHQ-9 and EPDS in an effort to monitor at-risk patients. Patients are added to our care management lists when they obtain a total score of 15 or higher (moderately severe to severe) on the PHQ-9 or obtain a total score of 10 or higher (suggestive of postpartum depression or anxiety) on the EPDS. Patients' scores on the PHQ-9 and EPDS are recorded in their EHRs. This allows for care management lists to be populated every quarter. BHCs contact these patients to check regarding mood, assess for suicidality, and encourage patients in following up with their PCP and/or a BHC.

Summary

Primary care is at the forefront of prevention and treatment of suicidality. This is particularly true given that patients express increased willingness to seek out treatment for mental health-related symptoms in primary care versus specialty mental health as first-line care. Patients who die by suicide are also more likely to be seen by a PCP prior to death compared to a mental health professional. Despite these findings, PCPs do not always have the necessary time or knowledge to address patients' mental health-related issues. Screening tools have been adopted to try to fulfill this gap in care; however, they have significant limitations despite their potential benefits. Even when screening tools are utilized in an appropriate manner, further inquiry regarding suicidality does not always occur. There has been an identified need to increase PCPs' training on assessing and managing suicide risk. One model of care that allows for direct and indirect training as well as enhanced support to PCPs and medical support staff is the Primary Care Behavioral Health (PCBH) model.

The PCBH model is an integrated model of care that is able to address this need. BHCs' primary role is to support PCPs and medical support staff in managing patients' behavioral health needs, including assessment and treatment of suicidality. Although further research is needed, there is evidence to support the effectiveness of the PCBH model in addressing depression and suicidality in primary care. Additionally, BHCs directly and indirectly provide training to PCPs and medical support staff regarding crisis management, including how to manage suicide risk. Accurately determining a patient's level of suicide risk helps BHCs, PCPs, and medical support staff to provide timely and effective services.

References

1. Olfson M, Weissman MM, Leon AC, Sheehan DV, Farber L. Suicidal ideation in primary care. J Gen Intern Med. 1996;11(8):447–53. https://doi.org/10.1370/afm.719.
2. Schulberg HC, Bruce ML, Lee PW, Williams JW, Dietrich AJ. Preventing suicide in primary care patients: the primary care physician's role. Gen Hosp Psychiatry. 2004;26(5):337–45. https://doi.org/10.1016/j.genhosppsych.2004.06.007.
3. Ahmedani BK, Simon GE, Stewart C, Beck A, Waitzfelder BE, Rossom R, et al. Health care contacts in the year before suicide death. J Gen Intern Med. 2014;29(6):870–7. https://doi.org/10.1007/s11606-014-2767-3.
4. Luoma JB, Martin CE, Pearson JL. Contact with mental health and primary care providers before suicide: a review of the evidence. Am J Psychiatry. 2002;159(6):909–16. https://doi.org/10.1176/appi.ajp.159.6.909.
5. O'Connor E, Gaynes BN, Burda BU, Soh C, Whitlock EP. Screening for and treatment of suicide risk relevant to primary care: a systematic review for the U.S. Preventive Services Task Force. Ann Intern Med. 2013;158(10):741–54. https://doi.org/10.7326/0003-4819-158-10-201305210-00642.
6. Bauer AM, Chan YF, Huang H, Vannoy S, Unützer J. Characteristics, management, and depression outcomes of primary care patients who endorse thoughts of death or suicide on the PHQ-9. J Gen Intern Med. 2013;28(3):363–9. https://doi.org/10.1007/s11606-012-2194-2.
7. Kroenke K, Spitzer RL, Williams JB, Löwe B. The patient health questionnaire somatic, anxiety, and depressive symptom scales: a systematic review. Gen Hosp Psychiatry. 2010;32(4): 345–59. https://doi.org/10.1016/j.genhosppsych.2010.03.006.
8. Yeung AS, Jing Y, Brenneman SK, Chang TE, Baer L, Hebden T, et al. Clinical Outcomes in Measurement-based Treatment (COMET): a trial of depression monitoring and feedback to primary care physicians. Depress Anxiety. 2012;29(10):865–73. https://doi.org/10.1002/da.21983.
9. Kroenke K, Spitzer RL, Williams JB. The PHQ-9: validity of a brief depression severity measure. J Gen Intern Med. 2001;16(9):606–13. https://doi.org/10.1046/j.1525-1497.2001.016009606.
10. Uebelacker LA, German NM, Gaudiano BA, Miller IW. Patient Health Questionnaire depression scale as a suicide screening instrument in depressed primary care patients: a cross-sectional study. Prim Care Companion CNS Disord. 2011;13(1). https://doi.org/10.4088/PCC.10m01027.
11. Simon GE, Rutter CM, Peterson D, Oliver M, Whiteside U, Operskalski B, et al. Does response on the PHQ-9 Depression Questionnaire predict subsequent suicide attempt or suicide death? Psychiatr Serv. 2013;64(12):1195–202. https://doi.org/10.1176/appi.ps.201200587.
12. Nock MK, Hwang I, Sampson NA, Kessler RC. Mental disorders, comorbidity and suicidal behavior: results from the National Comorbidity Survey Replication. Mol Psychiatry. 2010;15(8):868–76. https://doi.org/10.1038/mp.2009.29.
13. Cox JL, Holden JM, Sagovsky R. Detection of postnatal depression: development of the 10-item Edinburgh Postnatal Depression Scale. Br J Psychiatry. 1987;150:782–6. https://doi.org/10.1192/bjp.150.6.782.
14. Zhong QY, Gelaye B, Rondon MB, Sánchez SE, Simon GE, Henderson DC, et al. Using the Patient Health Questionnaire (PHQ-9) and the Edinburgh Postnatal Depression Scale (EPDS) to assess suicidal ideation among pregnant women in Lima, Peru. Arch Womens Ment Health. 2015;18(6):783–92. https://doi.org/10.1007/s00737-014-0481-0.
15. Kim JJ, La Porte LM, Saleh MP, Allweiss S, Adams MG, Zhou Y, et al. Suicide risk among perinatal women who report thoughts of self-harm on depression screens. Obstet Gynecol. 2015;125(4):885–93. https://doi.org/10.1097/AOG.0000000000000718.
16. Howard LM, Flach C, Mehay A, Sharp D, Tylee A. The prevalence of suicidal ideation identified by the Edinburgh Postnatal Depression Scale in postpartum women in primary care: findings from the RESPOND trial. BMC Pregnancy Childbirth. 2011;11:57. https://doi.org/10.1186/1471-2393-11-57.

17. Posner K, Brown GK, Stanley B, Brent DA, Yershova KV, Oquendo MA, et al. The Columbia-Suicide Severity Rating Scale: initial validity and internal consistency findings from three multisite studies with adolescents and adults. Am J Psychiatry. 2011;168(12):1266–77. https://doi.org/10.1176/appi.ajp.2011.10111704.
18. Posner K, Subramany R, Amira L, Mann JJ. From uniform definitions to prediction of risk: the Columbia Suicide Severity Rating Scale approach to suicide risk assessment. In: Cannon KE, Hudzik TJ, editors. Suicide: phenomenology and neurobiology. Cham: Springer; 2014. p. 59–84.
19. Viguera AC, Milano N, Laurel R, Thompson NR, Griffith SD, Baldessarini RJ, et al. Comparison of electronic screening for suicidal risk with the Patient Health Questionnaire Item 9 and the Columbia Suicide Severity Rating Scale in an outpatient psychiatric clinic. Psychosomatics. 2015;56(5):460–9. https://doi.org/10.1016/j.psym.2015.04.005.
20. Katzan IL, Viguera AC, Burke T, Buchanan J, Posner K. Improving suicide screening at the Cleveland Clinic through electronic self-reports: PHQ-9 and the Columbia-Suicide Severity Rating Scale (C-SSRS). Poster session presented at: The International Academy of Suicide Research 2013 World congress on suicide; 2013 Jun 10–13; Montreal, Canada.
21. Mundt JC, Greist JH, Jefferson JW, Federico M, Mann JJ, Posner K. Prediction of suicidal behavior in clinical research by lifetime suicidal ideation and behavior ascertained by the electronic Columbia-Suicide Severity Rating Scale. J Clin Psychiatry. 2013;74(9):887–93. https://doi.org/10.4088/JCP.13m08398.
22. Arias SA, Zhang Z, Hillerns C, Sullivan AF, Boudreaux ED, Miller I, et al. Using structured telephone follow-up assessments to improve suicide-related adverse event detection. Suicide Life Threat Behav. 2014;44(5):537–47. https://doi.org/10.1111/sltb.12088.
23. Wintersteen MB. Standardized screening for suicidal adolescents in primary care. Pediatrics. 2010;125(5):938–44. https://doi.org/10.1542/peds.2009-2458.
24. Sudak D, Roy A, Sudak H, Lipschitz A, Maltsberger J, Hendin H. Deficiencies in suicide training in primary care specialties: a survey of training directors. Acad Psychiatry. 2007;31(5):345–9. https://doi.org/10.1176/appi.ap.31.5.345.
25. Hooper LM, Epstein SA, Weinfurt KP, DeCoster J, Qu L, Hannah NJ. Predictors of primary care physicians' self-reported intention to conduct suicide risk assessments. J Behav Health Serv Res. 2012;39(2):103–15. https://doi.org/10.1007/s11414-011-9268-5.
26. Feldman MD, Franks P, Duberstein PR, Vannoy S, Epstein R, Kravitz RL. Let's not talk about it: suicide inquiry in primary care. Ann Fam Med. 2007;5(5):412–8. https://doi.org/10.1370/afm.719.
27. Vannoy SD, Robins LS. Suicide-related discussions with depressed primary care patients in the USA: gender and quality gaps. A mixed methods analysis. BMJ Open. 2011;1(2):e000198. https://doi.org/10.1136/bmjopen-2011-000198.
28. Centers for Disease Control and Prevention. Web-based Injury Statistics Query and Reporting System (WISQARS). 2014. http://www.cdc.gov/injury/wisqars/index.html. Accessed 25 Nov 2016.
29. Graham RD, Rudd MD, Bryan CJ. Primary care providers' views regarding assessing and treating suicidal patients. Suicide Life Threat Behav. 2011;41(6):614–23. https://doi.org/10.1111/j.1943-278X.2011.00058.x.
30. Dazzi T, Gribble R, Wessely S, Fear NT. Does asking about suicide and related behaviours induce suicidal ideation? What is the evidence? Psychol Med. 2014;44(16):3361–3. https://doi.org/10.1017/S0033291714001299.
31. US Food and Drug Administration. Revision to product labeling. 2007. http://www.fda.gov/downloads/drugs/drugsafety/informationbydrugclass/ucm173233.pdf. Accessed 25 Nov 2016.
32. Valuck RJ, Orton HD, Libby AM. Antidepressant discontinuation and risk of suicide attempt: a retrospective, nested case-control study. J Clin Psychiatry. 2009;70(8):1069–77. https://doi.org/10.4088/JCP.08m04943.
33. Nutting PA, Dickinson LM, Rubenstein LV, Keeley RD, Smith JL, Elliott CE. Improving detection of suicidal ideation among depressed patients in primary care. Ann Fam Med. 2005;3(6):529–36. https://doi.org/10.1370/afm.371.

34. Mann JJ, Apter A, Bertolote J, Beautrais A, Currier D, Haas A, et al. Suicide prevention strategies: a systematic review. JAMA. 2005;294(16):2064–74. https://doi.org/10.1001/jama.294.16.2064.
35. Robinson PJ, Reiter JT. Behavioral health consultation and primary care: a guide to integrating services. 2nd ed. New York: Springer; 2016.
36. Hunter CL, Goodie JL. Operational and clinical components for integrated-collaborative behavioral healthcare in the patient-centered medical home. Fam Syst Health. 2010;28(4):308–21. https://doi.org/10.1037/a0021761.
37. Gunn WB, Blount A. Primary care mental health: a new frontier for psychology. J Clin Psychol. 2009;65(3):235–52. https://doi.org/10.1002/jclp.20499.
38. Bryan CJ, Morrow C, Appolonio KK. Impact of behavioral health consultant interventions on patient symptoms and functioning in an integrated family medicine clinic. J Clin Psychol. 2009;65(3):281–93. https://doi.org/10.1002/jclp.20539.
39. Ray-Sannerud BN, Dolan DC, Morrow CE, Corso KA, Kanzler KE, Corso ML, et al. Longitudinal outcomes after brief behavioral health intervention in an integrated primary care clinic. Fam Syst Health. 2012;30(1):60–71. https://doi.org/10.1037/a0027029.
40. Bryan CJ, Corso KA, Corso ML, Kanzler KE, Ray-Sannerud B, Morrow CE. Therapeutic alliance and change in suicidal ideation during treatment in integrated primary care settings. Arch Suicide Res. 2012;16(4):316–23. https://doi.org/10.1080/13811118.2013.722055.
41. Serrano N, Monden K. The effect of behavioral health consultation on the care of depression by primary care clinicians. WMJ. 2011;110(3):113–8.
42. Bryan CJ, Corso KA, Neal-Walden TA, Rudd MD. Managing suicide risk in primary care: practice recommendations for behavioral health consultants. Prof Psychol Res Pr. 2009;40(2):148–55. https://doi.org/10.1037/a0011141.
43. Rudd MD. Fluid vulnerability theory: a cognitive approach to understanding the process of acute and chronic suicide risk. In: Elliott CE, editor. Cognition and suicide: theory, research, and therapy. Washington, DC: American Psychological Association; 2006. p. 355–67.
44. Brown GK, Steer RA, Henriques GR, Beck AT. The internal struggle between the wish to die and the wish to live: a risk factor for suicide. Am J Psychiatry. 2005;162(10):1977–9. https://doi.org/10.1176/appi.ajp.162.10.1977.
45. Suresh Kumar PN, George B. Life events, social support, coping strategies, and quality of life in attempted suicide: a case-control study. Indian J Psychiatry. 2013;55(1):46–51. https://doi.org/10.4103/0019-5545.105504.
46. Bryan CJ, Corso KA, Macalanda J. An evidence-based approach to managing suicidal patients in patient-centered medical home. Cogn Behav Pract. 2014;21(3):269–81. https://doi.org/10.1016/j.cbpra.2014.04.006.
47. Shenassa ED, Rogers ML, Spalding KL, Roberts MB. Safer storage of firearms at home and risk of suicide: a study of protective factors in a nationally representative sample. J Epidemiol Community Health. 2004;58(10):841–8. https://doi.org/10.1136/jech.2003.017343.
48. Anderson HD, Pace WD, Brandt E, Nielsen RD, Allen RR, Libby AM, et al. Monitoring suicidal patients in primary care using electronic health records. J Am Board Fam Med. 2015;28(1):65–71. https://doi.org/10.3122/jabfm.2015.01.140181.
49. Zeidler Schreiter EA, Pandhi N, Fondow M, Fahey L. Access Community Health Centers Integrated Primary Care Consulting Psychiatry Toolkit. 2014. http://www.hipxchange.org/Access. Accessed 25 Nov 2016.
50. Zeidler Schreiter EA, Pandhi N, Fondow MD, Thomas C, Vonk J, Reardon CL, et al. Consulting psychiatry within an integrated primary care model. J Health Care Poor Underserved. 2013;24(4):1522–30. https://doi.org/10.1353/hpu.2013.0178.
51. Simon GE, VonKorff M, Rutter C, Wagner E. Randomised trial of monitoring, feedback, and management of care by telephone to improve treatment of depression in primary care. BMJ. 2000;320(7234):550–4. https://doi.org/10.1136/bmj.320.7234.550.

Suicide Risk Assessment Tools and Management in Emergency Department

9

Karolina Mlynek, Christopher Sola, and Naveed Khokhar

Introduction

Suicide is the leading cause of death globally, with nearly 1 million people dying by each year, averaging one suicide every 40 seconds [1]. Compounding the issue, for every death from suicide, approximately 33 people attempt suicide [2], and every attempt affects many other people, including family members, friends and, co-workers. A single attempt may affect as many as 30–60 people [3], and individuals affected by suicide ("survivors of suicide loss") are at higher risk for suicide themselves [4]. In the United States, 42,773 people died by suicide in 2014 [5], averaging 117 suicides per day, making suicide the tenth leading cause of death across all age groups [6, 7], claiming twice as many lives as homicide each year. Nearly 650,000 ED visits yearly relate directly to suicidal behavior [8]. The estimated economic burden of suicide and suicidal behaviors is $41–44 billion annually [9].

Compounding the issue, in addition to the thousands of people who die by suicide every year in the United States, many more attempt suicide but do not die. For every suicide death, there are approximately [10]:

- Three hospitalizations for each suicide attempt
- Ten emergency department visits for a suicide attempt
- Thirty-three attempts that do not lead to hospitalizations or emergency department visits

K. Mlynek, M.D., M.B.A. (✉) · C. Sola, D.O. · N. Khokhar, M.D.
Department of Psychiatry, Cleveland Clinic, Cleveland, OH, USA
e-mail: mlynekk2@ccf.org; solac@ccf.org; khokhan@ccf.org

T. Falcone, J. Timmons-Mitchell (eds.), *Suicide Prevention*,
https://doi.org/10.1007/978-3-319-74391-2_9

Table 9.1 Most common predisposing factors for suicide

Previous suicide attempts
Mental disorders
Age, sex, gender, race
Sense of isolation
Occupation
Health
Family history and genetics
Other risk factors

Predisposing Factors

The etiology of suicidal behavior is multifactorial, and there is a deficiency in adequately recognizing the signs of suicide risk in patients, making it hard to predict [11]. The importance of screening and acknowledging the predisposing factors is particularly important in emergency department, where many at-risk individuals initially present. Table 9.1 reviews the risk factors that should be taken into consideration when screening individuals in an ED setting [12, 13]. It is vital to keep these risk factors in mind when evaluating these patients, because although there is no foolproof way to predict who may eventually attempt or die by suicide, these are associated with greater risk.

Previous Suicide Attempts

A history of prior suicide attempts is the strongest single prognostic factor of future suicide attempt [14, 15].

Mental Disorders

Psychiatric disorders are highly correlated with future suicide attempts and completion; more than 90% of individuals who attempt suicide and up to 95% of those completing suicide have some kind of underlying mental health disorder [16, 17]. Increasing severity of mental health disorder and multiple psychiatric comorbidities, including anxiety disorders, depression, bipolar disorder, alcohol or other substance misuse, and psychosis [18], personality disorders—especially cluster B (antisocial, borderline, histronic, and narcissistic) personality disorders, often characterized by impulsivity and aggressiveness [17]—and eating disorders all confer an increased risk of suicide attempt. The highest risk of completed suicide is associated with a prior attempt in patients with schizophrenia, bipolar disorder, and major depression [19].

Age, Sex, Gender, and Race

The risk of suicide generally increases with age [7], though emergency department visits for attempted suicide and self-harm are particularly common among adolescents, young adults, African-Americans, and females [8]. Although women tend to have more suicide attempts, men complete suicide 3.5–4 times more frequently, which is the result of the tendency of men to utilize more immediately lethal methods (firearms), compared to women, who more frequently employ methods (most common, poison) that allow time to seek help [20].

Sense of Isolation

Absence of support and living alone increase the risk of suicide, as does marital status. Never having been married confers the highest risk, than those who are widowed, separated, divorced, married without children, and married with children, in descending order of risk [21]. The risk associated with being widowed is highest in the first week after bereavement and decreases over the first few months thereafter, but remains elevated throughout the first year following the loss [22]. The anniversary of an important relationship loss also confers increased risk [12].

Occupation

Generally, suicide tends to be greater in the unskilled and unemployed workers. However, among highly skilled workers, physicians may be at increased risk of suicide [23, 24]. The rate of suicide in military veterans exceeds that of the general population in the United States [25]. The Centers for Disease Control and Prevention (CDC) estimates that suicide in military veterans accounts for roughly 20% of all the deaths in the United States [20].

Health

Suicide risk rises with major physical and chronic illnesses, including chronic pain. Table 9.2 summarizes the most common illnesses associated with increased risk of suicidal ideation and attempt [4, 26].

Table 9.2 Illnesses associated with increased risk of suicide

Malignancies
Risk tends to peak in the first few months after diagnosis but remains high in the first 5 years
Degenerative diseases
Huntington disease, multiple sclerosis, and Parkinson's disease
Traumatic injuries
Traumatic brain injury and spinal cord injury
Other CNS disorders
Epilepsy and migraine
Sleep disturbances and insomnia
Recent surgery

Family History and Genetics

There is a familial risk of suicidal behaviors. The risk of suicide attempt is increased in relatives of people who died by suicide, and the risk of completed suicide is higher in relatives of individuals who had a history of suicide attempts [27]. Both genetic and environmental factors may play a role involved in this increased risk. Statham et al. estimate the heritability of suicide to be in the range of 30–50% [28]. However, despite the evidence of heritability, the identification of specific genes associated with increased suicide risk is rather vague and has inconclusive results [29]. Advancing paternal age, associated with genetic mutations during spermatogenesis, may increase the risk of suicide attempts in one's offspring [30].

Other Risk Factors

The risk of suicide increases in patients with *easy access to firearms*, *violent behavior* [31], and *homelessness*, particularly in those with psychiatric disorders [32]. It is also higher in *minority sexual orientation*, which is often associated with social stigma, prejudice, and discrimination [33]. Table 9.3 summarizes protective factors that play an important role in suicide risk reduction [1, 34].

Offering the same ideas arranged differently, some have suggested the following five-domain "overlap model" matrix of the categorical risk factors to consider, including *psychiatric diagnosis*, *personality* (aggression, impulsivity, hopelessness) traits, *psychosocial* events/stressors, *genetic* factors, and *biological* (neurochemical/biochemical) factors [17]. Figure 9.1 summarizes the overlap matrix model [17].

Common Presentation in Emergency Department

Suicidal patients that present to emergency department typically fit into one of four common categories [15]:

1. Patients with initial medical complaints that try to conceal the suicidal ideation and attempt
2. Patients who report suicidal ideation without an active plan to self-harm

Table 9.3 Suicide: protective risk factors

Good family, social and community support system
Cultural and religious beliefs that discourage suicide
Skills in problem-solving and conflict resolution
Pregnancy and parenthood
Constrained access to means of suicide
Easy and reliable access to healthcare
Extraversion and optimism
Solid reasons for living

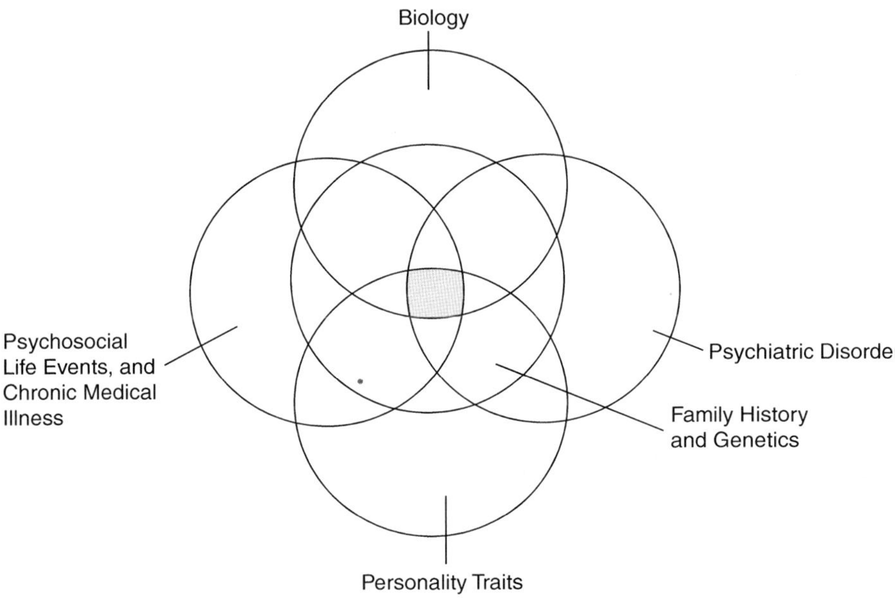

Fig. 9.1 Overlap model (five domains)

3. Overtly suicidal patients who were actively attempting to kill themselves
4. Patients declared dead in ED

Suicide Risk: Assessment Tools

There is no universally accepted suicide risk assessment tool recognized as the gold standard for use in acute crises. Table 9.4 summarizes available risk assessment tools used in the United States and abroad. We included only the tools relevant to the emergency department setting, where quick and reliable screening is essential.

Developed in 1983, the SAD PERSONS scale is a clinical assessment tool for medical students to assess the suicide risk in patients [39]. Table 9.5 summarizes components of this ten-item scale, in which each letter corresponds to a likely risk factor for suicide [39]. One point is awarded for each factor present, and scores are interpreted on the following scale:

0–2: No risk of suicide
3–4: Send home but check frequently
5–6: Consider hospitalization
7–10: Definitely hospitalize

Table 9.4 Risk assessment tools relevant to the emergency department setting

SAD PERSONS scale
Modified SAD PERSONS scale
Violence and suicide assessment scale
Columbia—suicide severity rating scale (C-SSRS)
SAFE-ED patient safety screener
Safe-T test: the suicide assessment five-step evaluation and triage
Beck hopelessness scale[a]
Beck depression inventory II (BDI-II)[a]
Beck scale for suicidal ideation[a]
Manchester self-harm rule[b]
ReACT self-harm rule[b]
Suicide assessment scale (SUAS)[c]
High-risk construct scale[d]
Smartphone tools for suicide prevention

[a]The Beck inventories are available *for purchase only* through the Pearson clinical website. They can be found at: http://www.pearsonclinical.com/psychology.html. Those tests take approximately 5–10 min to complete and can be either self-administered or administered by a trained professional
[b]Manchester self-harm rule and ReACT self-harm rule were studied in the United Kingdom [35, 36]
[c]Suicide assessment scale (SUAS) was utilized in Sweden [37]
[d]High-risk construct scale was utilized in Canada [38]

Table 9.5 SAD PERSONS assessment scale factors [39]

S = sex (male)
A = age (<19 or >45)
D = depression
P = previous suicide attempt
E = ethanol abuse
R = rational thinking loss
S = social support lacking
O = organized plan
N = no spouse
S = sickness (chronic)

This scale, although easy to memorize and use, unfortunately often failed to identify patients who required psychiatric admission or community psychiatric aftercare, and it was not predictive of future self-injurious behaviors [40].

Modified version of the SAD PERSONS scale (MSPS) is shown in Table 9.6 [41].

Although the mnemonic is easy to recall, the scoring system is more complicated and more difficult to score accurately without a form, which may not always be easily accessible in the emergency room setting. Scores are interpreted as follows:

0–5: May be safe to discharge (depending upon circumstances)
6–8: Probably requires psychiatric consultation
>8: Probably requires hospital admission

Table 9.6 Modified SAD PERSONS assessment scale factors [41]

S = sex (male) [1]
A = age (<19 or >45) [1]
D = depression or *hopelessness* [2]
P = previous suicide attempt or *psychiatric care* [1]
E = ethanol abuse or *drug use* [1]
R = rational thinking loss (organic brain syndrome or psychosis) [2]
S = *separated, divorced, or widowed* [1]
O = organized plan or *serious attempt* [2]
N = no social support [1]
S = *stated future intent* (determined to repeat attempt or ambivalent) [2]

This modified version of the scale has high sensitivity (94%) but lower specificity (71%) [42].

Table 9.7 shows a violence and suicide assessment scale items [43].

This scale may be a valuable instrument for clinicians in emergency departments as a framework for a clinical interview [43]. Feinstein and Plutchik demonstrated that scores correlated with clinical judgment; that is, higher-scoring patients were more likely to require admission to an inpatient ward [43]. This scale mainly assessed an overall risk of violence but did take into account suicidal ideation, lack of social support, substance abuse, and refusal to cooperate. Additionally, the scales predicted the need for suicide precautions and violence on the wards.

Table 9.7 Violence and suicide assessment scale [43]

Current violent thoughts (during interview)
4 Expresses intense wish to kill someone specific
3 Reveals command hallucinations to injure someone
2 Expresses ambivalent wish to kill someone specific
1 Expresses nonspecific feelings of rage and hostility
0 Reveals no homicidal ideas
Recent violent behaviors (during the past several weeks)
4 Showed serious assaultive behavior (attempt to strangle, stab, or shoot someone)
3 Beat up someone badly (fractured bones or required hospitalization)
2 Slapped, punched, or pushed someone (without serious outcomes)
1 Broke things in the house
0 Showed good control of his (her) behavior
Past history of violent/antisocial/disruptive behaviors (lifetime history)
4 Has committed violent acts in the past
4 Has been arrested for assaultive behavior
3 Carries weapons (gun, knife, razor, chain, etc.)
3 Has access to weapons
2 Has been arrested for automobile infractions
2 Has a criminal record
2 Chronic problems with authority (truancy, running away from home, family fights)

(continued)

Table 9.7 (continued)

2 Has a history of impulsive or unpredictable behavior (loses temper easily, overeats, sexual promiscuity, etc.)
2 Frequent changes of living situation as a child
0 Has no past history of violence
Recent suicidal behaviors (during the past several weeks)
4 Made a serious suicidal attempt (tried to kill self—gunshot, hanging, jumping, ingestion)
3 Made a suicidal gesture (superficially cut wrist)
3 Made a specific suicide plan
3 Attempt made with little chance of discovery by others
2 Had no interest or hope for the future
0 Has no suicidal plans or attempts
Past history of suicide (lifetime history)
4 Mother, father, or sibling has committed suicide or made a suicide attempt
3 Has/had diagnosis of major affective disorder or psychosis
3 Has made one or more previous suicide attempts
2 Current attempt is an "anniversary" reaction
2 Has a serious medical illness or disability
0 Has no past history of suicidal ideas or attempts
Support systems/stresses
3 No family, friends, social agency, or psychiatric available
2 Has questionable connection with family, friends, social agency, or psychiatrist
2 Has had many recent life stresses (job, family, children, health)
1 Has a family which is marginally willing or able to help
0 Has a family strongly committed and able to help
Ability to cooperate
3 Refuses to cooperate with interview and treatment plan
2 Unable to cooperate with interview and treatment plan
1 Wants help but motivation is weak
0 Actively seeks treatment, willing and able to cooperate
Substance abuse
3 Is intoxicated
3 Is in withdrawal
3 Is a compulsive long-term drug abuser (alcohol and other drugs)
2 Is an occasional drug abuser (alcohol and other drugs)
1 Recreational use of drug
0 No abuse of any drugs
Reactions during interview
4 Assaultive behavior against a person (or object) in the environment
3 Challenges authority (curses, yells, screams)
2 Shows approach-avoidance behavior toward interviewer
1 Shows motoric activity (pacing, smoking, fidgeting)
1 Seems very impatient
0 Calm, seated, responsive to questions

Columbia: Suicide Severity Rating Scale (C-SSRS)

Columbia—suicide severity rating scale (C-SSRS) shown in Table 9.8 is a fairly new assessment tool and has been considered the gold standard for evaluation of suicide assessment since 2012 [44, 45]. However, recent critical examination suggests that it does not address the full spectrum of suicidal ideation and behavior. There are also several versions of this scale that seem to be inconsistent, and its

Table 9.8 Columbia—suicide severity rating scale (C-SSRS)

C-SSRS screener with triage points		
Suicide ideation definitions and prompts	**Past month**	
Ask questions that are in bolded and underlined	**Yes**	**No**
Ask questions 1 and 2		
1. *Wish to be dead*: Person endorses thoughts about a wish to be dead or not alive anymore, or wish to fall asleep and not wake up *Have you wished you were dead or wished you could go to sleep and not wake up?*		
2. *Suicidal thoughts*: General nonspecific thoughts of wanting to end one's life/commit suicide, "I've thought about killing myself" without general thoughts of ways to kill oneself/associated methods, intent, or plan" *Have you actually had any thoughts of killing yourself?*		
If YES to 2, ask questions 3, 4, 5, and 6. If NO to 2, go directly to question 6		
3. *Suicidal thoughts with method* (*without specific plan or intent to act*): Person endorses thoughts of suicide and has thought of a least one method during the assessment period. This is different than a specific plan with time, place, or method details worked out. "I thought about taking an overdose but I never made a specific plan as to when where or how I would actually do it…and I would never go through with it" *Have you been thinking about how you might do this?*		
4. *Suicidal intent* (*without specific plan*): Active suicidal thoughts of killing oneself and patient reports having *some intent to act on such thoughts*, as oppose to "I have the thoughts but I definitely will not do anything about them" *Have you had these thoughts and had some intention of acting on them?*		
5. *Suicide intent with specific plan*: Thoughts of killing oneself with details of plan fully or partially worked out and person has some intent to carry it out *Have you started to work out or worked out the details of how to kill yourself? Do you intend to carry out this plan?*		
6. *Suicide behavior question*: *Have you ever done anything, started to do anything, or prepared to do anything to end your life?* Examples: Collected pills, obtained a gun, gave away valuables, wrote a will or suicide note, took out pills but didn't swallow any, held a gun but changed your mind or it was grabbed from your hand, or went to the roof but didn't jump or actually took pills, tried to shoot yourself, cut yourself, tried to hang yourself, etc. *If YES, ask*: *How long ago did you do any of these?* Over a year ago? Between 3 months and a year ago? Within the last 3 months?		

categories are ambiguous and imprecisely defined [44]. Different versions of this screener are available at: http://www.cssrs.columbia.edu/scales-practice-cssrs.html.

Triage Protocol for C-SSRS Screening (Items 1–5 linked to last item answered YES):

Item 1—mental health referral at discharge

Item 2—mental health referral at discharge

Item 3—care team consult (psychiatric nurse) and possible patient safety monitor/procedures

Item 4—psychiatric consultation and patient safety monitor/procedures

Item 5—psychiatric consultation and patient safety monitor/procedures

Item 6—if over a year ago, mental health referral at discharge

If between 1 week and 1 year ago—care team consult (psychiatric nurse) and patient safety monitor

If 1 week ago or less—psychiatric consultation and patient safety monitor

Disposition: mental health referral at discharge

Care team consult (psychiatric nurse) and possible patient safety monitor/procedures

Psychiatric consultation and patient safety monitor/procedures

ED-SAFE Patient Safety Screener

A multicenter study evaluated assessment of, and intervention for suicidal patients in eight different emergency departments across the United States and consisted of three phases: treatment-as-usual, introduction of universal suicide screening performed by nurses (Table 9.9) [46], and a secondary risk assessment tool provided by physicians (Table 9.10) [46]. The screening tool proved quick and efficient and resulted in almost universal screening for suicide risk, with 95% of nurses screening for suicidal ideation in phase 3 and 80% of physicians conducting the secondary risk assessment by the end of the study [47].

Table 9.9 Initial screening (completed by nursing)

Over the past 2 weeks
1. Have you felt down, depressed, or hopeless? ☐ Yes ☐ No ☐ Unable to complete
2. Have you had thoughts of killing yourself? ☐ Yes ☐ No ☐ Unable to complete
3. Have you ever attempted to kill yourself? ☐ Yes ☐ No ☐ Unable to complete
4. If yes to item 3, ask when did this happen? ☐ Within the past 24 h (including today) ☐ Within the last month (but not today) ☐ Between 1 and 6 months ago ☐ More than 6 months ago

Table 9.10 Secondary risk assessment (completed by physician)

"Yes" to any of questions below means that mental health professional should be consulted
1. Did the patient screen positive on BOTH PSS items-active ideation with a past attempt? ☐ Yes ☐ No ☐ Refused ☐ Patient unable to complete
2. Has the individual begun a suicide plan? ☐ Yes ☐ No ☐ Refused ☐ Patient unable to complete
3. Has the individual recently had intent to act on his/her ideation? ☐ Yes ☐ No ☐ Refused ☐ Patient unable to complete
4. Has the patient ever had a psychiatric hospitalization? ☐ Yes ☐ No ☐ Refused ☐ Patient unable to complete
5. Does the patient have a pattern of excessive substance use? ☐ Yes ☐ No ☐ Refused ☐ Patient unable to complete
6. Is the patient irritable, agitated, or aggressive? ☐ Yes ☐ No ☐ Refused ☐ Patient unable to complete

Safe-T Test: The Suicide Assessment Five-Step Evaluation and Triage

The suicide assessment five-step evaluation and triage test is conveniently available as both a pocket card and a smartphone application. This tool assesses both protective factors and risk factors for suicidal ideation. Protective assessment of risk level is based on clinical judgment, after evaluation of the first three steps [48, 49]. The card can be downloaded at http://www.sprc.org or http://www.stopsuicide.org. Table 9.11 shows a suicide assessment five-step evaluation and triage for clinicians [50].

Smartphone Tools for Suicide Prevention

Many suicide prevention apps are currently available on the healthcare market. It is important to keep in mind that while those can be helpful, none of them provide a comprehensive, evidence-based support for patients at risk. Physicians should recommend those smartphone tools with caution, since seemingly helpful content may actually be harmful, and physicians may derive a false sense of security by recommending an application that is ultimately not helpful [51].

Importantly, even in the context of a very thorough assessment of suicide risk in the emergency department, it remains impossible to reliably predict who will attempt or commit suicide and who will not. Even the most precise scales are unable to account for patients who spontaneously end their lives. Good clinical judgment, close follow-up, and effective treatments can help diminish the risk [42]. Hospital professionals may benefit from further suicide assessment training that can improve knowledge and skills necessary to not only prevent suicide but also to provide a spectrum of choices for effective treatment about suicide. The use of an assessment tool may formalize the process and minimize the inadvertent omission of some portion of a thorough risk assessment, but despite offering a quantifiable risk measurement, caution should be employed when selecting such a tool [42].

Table 9.11 Safe-T test

1. Identify risk factors
Suicidal behavior: history of prior suicide attempts, aborted suicide attempts, or self-injurious behavior
Current/past psychiatric disorders: especially mood disorders, psychotic disorders, alcohol/substance abuse, ADHD, TBI, PTSD, cluster B personality disorders, conduct disorders (antisocial behavior, aggression, impulsivity). Comorbidity and recent onset of illness increase risk
Key symptoms: anhedonia, impulsivity, hopelessness, anxiety/panic, global insomnia, command hallucinations
Precipitants/stressors/interpersonal: triggering events leading to humiliation, shame, or despair (e.g., loss of relationship, financial or health status—real or anticipated). Ongoing medical illness (esp. CNS disorders, pain). Intoxication. Family turmoil/chaos. History of physical or sexual abuse. Social isolation
Change in treatment: discharge from psychiatric hospital, provider, or treatment change
Access to firearms
Note the risk factors that can be modified to reduce risk
2. Identify protective factors
Internal: ability to cope with stress, religious beliefs, frustration tolerance
External: responsibility to children or beloved pets, positive therapeutic relationships, social supports
Note the protective factors that can be enhanced
3. Conduct suicide analysis
Ideation: frequency, intensity, duration—in last 48 h, past month, and worst ever
Plan: timing, location, lethality, availability, preparatory acts
Behaviors: past attempts, aborted attempts, rehearsals (tying noose, loading gun) vs. non-suicidal self-injurious actions
Intent: extent to which the patient [1] expects to carry out the plan and [2] believes the plan/act to be lethal vs. self-injurious. Explore ambivalence: reasons to die vs. reasons to live
Homicide inquiry: when indicated, esp. in character-disordered or paranoid males dealing with loss or humiliation. Inquire in four areas listed above
For youths: ask parent/guardian about evidence of suicidal thoughts, plans, or behaviors and changes in mood, behaviors, or disposition
4. Define risk level/intervention
Assessment of risk level is based on clinical judgment, after completing steps 1–3
Reassess as patient or environmental circumstances change
Determine risk. Choose appropriate intervention to address and reduce risk
5. Document
Assessment of risk, rationale, intervention, and follow-up
Risk level and rationale; treatment plan to address/reduce current risk (e.g., medication, setting, psychotherapy, ECT, contact with significant others, consultation); firearms instructions, if relevant; follow-up plan. For youths, treatment plan should include roles for parent/guardian

Table 9.12 Risk factors useful in quick stratification of suicide risk in emergency department

Depression
Suicidal ideation and previous suicide attempts
Panic attacks
History of violence
Alcohol abuse
Drug withdrawal
Psychotic symptoms/prior psychiatric treatment
Anxiety

Preventive Measures in Emergency Department

Emergency departments are crucial places for recognition and potential prevention of suicidal population; 39% of patients who die by suicide (39%) were seen in ED in the year preceding it [47]. A comprehensive evaluation of suicidal ideation and behavior should include a review of known risk factors and warning signs. Many emergency department patients presenting with such warning signs are overlooked and misdiagnosed with something less threatening [15]. Somatic complaints may represent an indirect cry for help from patients who are suicidal [15]. Asking about the items presented in Table 9.12 can help physicians identify some of the underlying causes of often vague symptoms and quickly stratify patient's risk.

Depression (35%) and previous suicide attempts (13%) are prevalent among ED patients. Ask first about depression history, following up with direct questions about suicidal ideation, intent, or plan [52]. Asking directly—despite frequent concern by caregivers—is not associated with increased risk for suicide attempt or completion [12].

Clinicians demonstrating a sincere interest in patient's feelings and concerns are more likely to succeed in determining whether a patient is suicidal or not. A distressed patient is less likely to open up to an interviewer that he perceives as disinterested or indifferent.

Alcohol and substance use further complicate the picture, and chronic substance users present more frequently to the emergency department for stabilization. Acutely intoxicated patients often express suicidal ideation, only to deny any such thought when sober, and suicide attempts are both more likely [53] and more lethal [54] when a patient is acutely intoxicated. From a psychiatric perspective, it is best to observe intoxicated patients in the emergency department until they are clinically and legally (for substances where legal standards exist, such as alcohol) sober, so that they are able to participate in the suicide risk assessment [15, 48].

At-risk patients require constant observation to ensure their safety. This typically requires individual (1:1) staffing and removing all potentially harmful objects (e.g., IV lines, belts, shoelaces, metal utensils, loose sheets, and sharp medical instruments)

from the patient's room and is important, as is searching all patient belongings to identify and remove potentially harmful objects [48]. Mechanical restraints should be used with caution (only if less invasive means to keep the patient safe are unlikely to be successful), and pharmacological interventions should target the lowest effective dose for the shortest required time. Brief counseling about reducing access to lethal medications and firearms may be beneficial [48]. Once the patient's safety is ensured, treatment and management of an underlying cause can begin.

Managing At-Risk Patients

Management of suicidal patients is multidimensional and guided by understanding of underlying diagnoses, so thorough assessment of underlying medical and psychiatric illness is vital. No specific routine diagnostic testing has demonstrated clinical benefit, though toxicological screening may guide clinical decision-making. In acute situations, using psychotropic medications in the emergency setting may result in rapid resolution of the crisis. Acute use of antidepressants is not recommended, as these take several weeks to achieve therapeutic effect, though continuing antidepressants to avoid a discontinuation syndrome may help to alleviate one potential source of patient stress.

Once the patient is safe and medically stabilized, the next step is deciding the appropriate setting for further treatment. Triage is important as not all patients with suicidal ideation require inpatient hospitalization, which may be required if no other measured can assure patient's safety. Physicians should not offer a "no-suicide contract" or "safety contract," as these are unenforceable and unreliable and may provide a false sense of security [55]. Involuntary hospitalization rules vary from state to state, so it is important for physicians to familiarize themselves with their state regulations.

Consideration for outpatient management is limited to cases in which the risks of completing suicide are judged to be minimal, often based on the protective factors listed above, as when the patient has a reliable support network to remain safe. Collateral information gathered from members of that support system is essential for proper evaluation of support network. Psychotherapeutic interventions targeting decreased hopelessness and cognitive distortions and psychosocial interventions increasing available support are vital in the treatment of those high-risk individuals most prone to suicide [17].

If the suicidal patient threatens to leave ED and is considered a danger to himself or others, each US state has laws designed to permit pursuit of involuntary hospitalization and possible commitment. Laws vary from state to state [15].

Treatment for Suicidal Ideation and Suicide Attempts in Emergency Department

In the emergency department, the only required treatment for a suicide attempt is to medically stabilize the patient, which may require inpatient hospitalization in an intensive care unit or a general medical floor. In that instance, arranging for 1:1

staffing and requesting a psychiatric consultation to help with ongoing management is indicated.

At this time, there is only one medication, clozapine, approved by the FDA for suicide risk reduction in patients with schizophrenia but includes a host of potential complications (side effects, interactions with many other medications, required blood draws), so it is not routinely utilized to this end [56].

Lithium also has the literature support for decreasing suicidality, although it has not been approved by the FDA as yet [57]. Ketamine, an N-methyl-d-aspartate (NMDA) receptor antagonist, has a rapid-onset antidepressant effect and may quickly suppress suicidal ideation. Currently it is not used in the United States [58].

There is no one-size-fits-all intervention from a psychiatric perspective, as suicide is heterogeneous. Stabilizing the underlying psychiatric issue and addressing psychosocial stressors, when possible, are the first steps in the emergency department.

References

1. World Health Organization. Preventing suicide: a global imperative. 2014. http://www.who.int/mental_health/suicide-prevention/exe_summary_english.pdf?ua=.
2. Bolton JM, Gunnell D, Turecki G. Suicide risk assessment and intervention in people with mental illness. BMJ. 2015;351:h4978.
3. Berman AL. Estimating the population of survivors of suicide: seeking an evidence base. Suicide Life Threat Behav. 2011;41(1):110–6.
4. US Surgeon General, National Action Alliance for Suicide Prevention. National strategy for suicide prevention: goals and objectives for action, 2012. Washington, DC: HHS; 2012. http://www.surgeongeneral.gov/library/reports/national-strategy-suicide-prevention/index.html.
5. Centers for Disease Control and Prevention. Web-based injury statistics query and reporting system (WISQARS). http://www.cdc.gov/ncipc/wisqars. Accessed 20 Sept 2016.
6. TH MC Jr, Castro VM, Roberson AM, Snapper LA, Perlis RH. Improving prediction of suicide and accidental death after discharge from general hospitals with natural language processing. JAMA Psychiatry. 2016;73(10):1064–71. https://doi.org/10.1001/jamapsychiatry.2016.2172.
7. American Foundation for Suicide Prevention. Suicide statistics. https://afsp.org/about-suicide/suicide-statistics/. Accessed 17 Oct 2016.
8. Ting SA, Sullivan AF, Boudreaux ED, Miller I, Camargo CA. Trends in US emergency department visits for attempted suicide and self-inflicted injury, 1993-2008. Gen Hosp Psychiatry. 2012;34:557–65.
9. Crosby AE, Ortega L, Stevens MR, Centers for Disease Control and Prevention (CDC). Suicides—United States, 2005–2009. MMWR Suppl. 2013;62(3):179–83.
10. Suicide Prevention Resource Center. Suicidal thoughts and suicide attempts. http://www.sprc.org/scope/attempts.
11. Joint Commission. New sentinel event alert on preventing suicide in health care settings. 2016. http://jointcommission.new-media-release.com/2016_sea_suicide/. Accessed 1 Nov 2016.
12. Blumenthal SJ. Suicide: a guide to risk factors, assessment, and treatment of suicidal patients. Med Clin North Am. 1988;72(4):937–71.
13. Riba M, Ravindranath D, Winder G. Clinical manual of emergency psychiatry. 2nd ed. Arlington: American Psychiatric Association Publishing; 2015.
14. Haukka J, Suominen K, Partonen T, Lönnqvist J. Determinants and outcomes of serious attempted suicide: a nationwide study in Finland, 1996–2003. Am J Epidemiol. 2008;167(10):1155–63.
15. Buzan RD, Weissberg MP. Suicide: risk factors and therapeutic considerations in the emergency department. J Emerg Med. 1992;10(3):335–43.

16. Hirschfeld RM, Russell JM. Assessment and treatment of suicidal patients. N Engl J Med. 1997;337(13):910.
17. Blumenthal SJ, Kupfer DJ. Generalizable treatment strategies for suicidal behavior. Ann N Y Acad Sci. 1986;487:327–40.
18. Bostwick JM, Pankratz VS. Affective disorders and suicide risk: a reexamination. Am J Psychiatry. 2000;157(12):1925–32.
19. Tidemalm D, Långström N, Lichtenstein P, Runeson B. Risk of suicide after suicide attempt according to coexisting psychiatric disorder: Swedish cohort study with long term follow-up. BMJ. 2008;337:a2205.
20. Karch DL, Dahlberg LL, Patel N, Davis TW, Logan JE, Hill HA, et al. Surveillance for violent deaths—National Violent Death Reporting System, 16 states, 2006. MMWR Surveill Summ. 2009;58(1):1–44.
21. Heikkinen ME, Isometsä ET, Marttunen MJ, Aro HM, Lönnqvist JK. Social factors in suicide. Br J Psychiatry. 1995;167(6):747–53.
22. Ajdacic-Gross V, Ring M, Gadola E, Lauber C, Bopp M, Gutzwiller F, et al. Suicide after bereavement: an overlooked problem. Psychol Med. 2008;38(5):673–6.
23. Milner A, Spittal MJ, Pirkis J, LaMontagne AD. Suicide by occupation: systematic review and meta-analysis. Br J Psychiatry. 2013;203(6):409–16.
24. Schernhammer ES, Colditz GA. Suicide rates among physicians: a quantitative and gender assessment (meta-analysis). Am J Psychiatry. 2004;161(12):2295–302.
25. Pietrzak RH, Goldstein MB, Malley JC, Rivers AJ, Johnson DC, Southwick SM. Risk and protective factors associated with suicidal ideation in veterans of operations enduring freedom and Iraqi freedom. J Affect Disord. 2010;123(1):102–7.
26. Turecki G, Brent DA. Suicide and suicidal behaviour. Lancet. 2016;387(10024):1227–39.
27. Brent DA, Melhem N. Familial transmission of suicidal behavior. Psychiatr Clin North Am. 2008;31(2):157–77.
28. Statham DJ, Heath AC, Madden PA, Bucholz KK, Bierut L, Dinwiddie SH, et al. Suicidal behaviour: an epidemiological and genetic study. Psychol Med. 1998;28(4):839–55.
29. Turecki G. The molecular bases of the suicidal brain. Nat Rev Neurosci. 2014;15(12):802–16.
30. D'Onofrio BM, Rickert ME, Frans E, Kuja-Halkola R, Almqvist C, Sjölander A, et al. Paternal age at childbearing and offspring psychiatric and academic morbidity. JAMA Psychiatry. 2014;71(4):432–8.
31. Conner KR, Cox C, Duberstein PR, Tian L, Nisbet PA, Conwell Y. Violence, alcohol, and completed suicide: a case-control study. Am J Psychiatry. 2001;158(10):1701–5.
32. Nilsson SF, Hjorthøj CR, Erlangsen A, Nordentoft M. Suicide and unintentional injury mortality among homeless people: a Danish nationwide register-based cohort study. Eur J Pub Health. 2014;24(1):50–6.
33. Haas AP, Eliason M, Mays VM, Mathy RM, Cochran SD, D'Augelli AR, et al. Suicide and suicide risk in lesbian, gay, bisexual, and transgender populations: review and recommendations. J Homosex. 2011;58(1):10–51.
34. Qin P, Mortensen PB. The impact of parental status on the risk of completed suicide. Arch Gen Psychiatry. 2003;60(8):797–802.
35. Cooper J, Kapur N, Dunning J, Guthrie E, Appleby L, Mackway-Jones K. A clinical tool for assessing risk after self-harm. Ann Emerg Med. 2006;48(4):459–66.
36. Steeg S, Kapur N, Webb R, Applegate E, Stewart SL, Hawton K, et al. The development of a population-level clinical screening tool for self-harm repetition and suicide: the ReACT Self-Harm Rule. Psychol Med. 2012;42(11):2383–94.
37. Niméus A, Alsén M, Träskman-Bendz L. The suicide assessment scale: an instrument assessing suicide risk of suicide attempters. Eur Psychiatry. 2000;15(7):416–23.
38. Cochrane-Brink KA, Lofchy JS, Sakinofsky I. Clinical rating scales in suicide risk assessment. Gen Hosp Psychiatry. 2000;22(6):445–51.
39. Patterson WM, Dohn HH, Patterson J, Patterson GA. Evaluation of suicidal patients: the SAS PERSONS scale. Psychosomatics. 1983;24(4):343–5.

40. Saunders K, Brand F, Lascelles K, Hawton K. The sad truth about the SAD PERSONS scale: an evaluation of its clinical utility in self-harm patients. Emerg Med J. 2014;31(10):796–8.
41. RS H, Rothstein RJ. Assessment of suicide potential by nonpsychiatrists using the SAD PERSONS score. J Emerg Med. 1988;6(2):99–107.
42. Ronquillo L, Minassian A, Vilke GM, Wilson MP. Literature-based recommendations for suicide assessment in the emergency department: a review. J Emerg Med. 2012;43(5):836–42.
43. Feinstein R, Plutchik R. Violence and suicide risk assessment in the psychiatric emergency room. Compr Psychiatry. 1990;31(4):337–43.
44. Giddens JM, Sheehan KH, Sheehan DV. The Columbia-Suicide Severity Rating Scale (C-SSRS): has the "gold standard" become a liability? Innov Clin Neurosci. 2014;11(9):66–80.
45. http://www.cssrs.columbia.edu/scales-practice-cssrs.html.
46. Boudreaux ED, Miller I, Goldstein AB, Sullivan AF, Allen MH, Manton AP, et al. The Emergency Department Safety Assessment and Follow-up Evaluation (ED-SAFE): method and design considerations. Contemp Clin Trials. 2013;36(1):14–24.
47. Betz ME, Arias SA, Miller M, Barber C, Espinola JA, Sullivan AF, et al. Change in emergency department providers' beliefs and practices after use of new protocols for suicidal patients. Psychiatr Serv. 2015;66(6):625–31.
48. Betz ME, Boudreaux ED. Managing suicidal patients in the emergency department. Ann Emerg Med. 2016;67(2):276–82.
49. SAMHSA. Suicide Assessment Five-step Evaluation and Triage (SAFE-T). http://store.samhsa.gov/shin/content//SMA09-4432/SMA09-4432.pdf. Accessed 29 Sept 2016.
50. https://www.integration.samhsa.gov/images/res/SAFE_T.pdf.
51. Larsen ME, Nicholas J, Christensen H. A systematic assessment of smartphone tools for suicide prevention. PLoS One. 2016;11(4):e0152285.
52. Allen MH, Abar BW, McCormick M, Barnes DH, Haukoos J, Garmel GM, et al. Screening for suicidal ideation and attempts among emergency department medical patients: instrument and results from the Psychiatric Emergency Research Collaboration. Suicide Life Threat Behav. 2013;43(3):313–23.
53. Bagge CL, Littlefield AK, Conner KR, Schumacher JA, Lee HJ. Near-term predictors of the intensity of suicidal ideation: an examination of the 24 h prior to a recent suicide attempt. J Affect Disord. 2014;165:53–8.
54. Liotta M, Mento C, Settineri S. Seriousness and lethality of attempted suicide: a systematic review. Aggress Violent Behav. 2015;21:97–109.
55. Sadock BJ, Sadock VA, Ruiz P, Kaplan HI. Kaplan & Sadock's comprehensive textbook of psychiatry. 8th ed. Philadelphia: Lippincott Williams and Wilkins; 2005.
56. Meltzer HY, Alphs L, Green AI, Altamura AC, Anand R, Bertoldi A, et al. International suicide prevention trial study group clozapine treatment for suicidality in schizophrenia: International Suicide Prevention Trial (InterSePT). Arch Gen Psychiatry. 2003;60(1):82–91. Erratum in: Arch Gen Psychiatry.2003;60(7):735.
57. Cipriani A, Hawton K, Stockton S, Geddes JR. Lithium in the prevention of suicide in mood disorders: updated systematic review and meta-analysis. BMJ. 2013;346:f3646.
58. Rajkumar R, Fam J, Yeo EY, Dawe GS. Ketamine and suicidal ideation in depression: jumping the gun? Pharmacol Res. 2015;99:23–35.

The Darkness at the End of Life: Suicide in Palliative Care Settings

10

Fernando Espí Forcén and Juan R. Jaramillo

Introduction

In palliative care settings, the evaluation and management of suicide risk carry special challenges. Suicide and the desire for a hastened death in patients with terminal diseases have carried controversies in society with a good amount of media attention. A person's right to die with dignity is now largely embraced by society. However this idea can shadow the imperative need to do proper evaluations for depression and suicidal ideation in patients with cancer and other terminal illnesses. Perhaps due to this gray area, there are still complex questions as to how to evaluate and manage patients with suicidal ideation in palliative care settings. Even in patients with poor prognosis due to a severe terminal illness, a death by suicide can be very tragic for the patient and their loved ones. In this chapter, we will attempt to elucidate the major aspects concerning suicide with patients in palliative care settings.

Historical Aspects

Throughout the history of humanity, disagreements about treatments and approaches in palliative care settings have been a matter of controversy. Historically and consistent with our contemporary values, suicide has not been approved by society. However, people have generally shown positive attitudes toward withdrawing care in patients with terminal illnesses and toward the prevention of unnecessary suffering. Evidence of compassionate care in the human species can be found as early as in *Homo heidelbergensis*, in *Homo neanderthalensis*, and in our species *Homo*

F. Espi Forcen, M.D., Ph.D. (✉)
Department of Psychiatry, Rush University Medical Center, Chicago, IL, USA

J. R. Jaramillo, M.D.
Department of Psychiatry, Owensboro Health Regional Hospital, Owensboro, KY, USA

T. Falcone, J. Timmons-Mitchell (eds.), *Suicide Prevention*,
https://doi.org/10.1007/978-3-319-74391-2_10

sapiens during the Paleolithic period. There is now archeological evidence that children born with severe disabilities or individuals with physical impairments received care. This is supported by the findings of osteogenic regeneration of the bone in the areas that caused the disability [1].

In Ancient Greece, both the Pythagorean and Hippocratic schools of medicine disapproved the practice of euthanasia and assisted suicide. As such, a sentence in the Hippocratic Oath specifically advises against the administration of lethal toxins to any patient. This statement in the Hippocratic Oath has been used as an argument against the practice of physician-assisted suicide. Founder of the Academy, Plato also disapproved the practice of active euthanasia. In his *Laws*, he suggests that doctors administering lethal doses to patients might be the subject of punishment. Nonetheless he also states that patients with incurable diseases should receive treatment toward the alleviation of their suffering. In the *Republic* he argues that patients unable due to their suffering to live a normal life should not receive treatment for the prolongation of life. Epicurus states that each of us is free to put an end to our life if we are suffering from unbearable pain, provided this misfortune is neither brief nor intermittent [2].

In the more individualistic age of Hellenism and the Roman Empire, a death in luxury or without suffering could be styled euthanasia. The doctor had neither a place in those acts of dying nor in cases of natural death. He shunned death as a failure of his art. An article written by Van Hooff explains that sometimes a doctor was called in to assist in voluntary death, a role that was not forbidden by the Hippocratic Oath. Van Hooff argues that an appeal to this oath by opponents of euthanasia in the modern sense of the word therefore is mistaken [3].

With the popularity of Christianity within the Roman Empire, society largely disapproved the practice of euthanasia in any form as it was considered a sinful behavior. The manual *Ars moriendi* was originally written between 1414 and 1418 and soon distributed in its Latin version all over Europe. Slightly later it was translated into the main European languages, including German, Dutch, English, Swedish, Italian, Catalan, and Spanish, turning into a very popular manual for friars to help people cope with death. The manual was used by Dominican friars to assist the dying toward salvation. For that, the dying were provided with the mission to fight five temptations: lack of faith, despair, impatience, pride, and greed. Later editions of the book came with some illustrations executed by Master E.S. in 1450. In one of these illustrations, the moribund is depicted as a cachectic person on his bed, and next to him there is man slaying his throat. This man represents the temptation of suicide that the moribund must fight. People in the Middle Ages were aware of the possibility of suicide in an attempt to prevent the physical suffering that could come with death. In order to have a good death, it was important to accept and experience this suffering the same way that Jesus accepted the suffering during the Passion [4].

Saint Thomas More is sometimes (and erroneously) quoted as being the first prominent Christian to approve euthanasia. In his book *Utopia* (1516), where the Utopian priests encourage euthanasia when a patient was terminally ill and suffering pain. "...if a disease is not only distressing but also agonising without cessation, then the priests and public officials exhort this man...to free himself from this bitter life...or else to permit others to free him..." It must be noted, however, that what More describes is a fictional society, without Christian beliefs, a more secular society where all religions are benignly accepted and none is followed [5].

In 1870, Dr. Samuel Williams was one of the first doctors to publicly advocate for the use of morphine to alleviate patients' pain even if that would accelerate their death. This practice is related to what we know today as comfort care measures in the United States or passive euthanasia in Europe [6].

Terminology

Whereas in other areas of psychiatry, a less complex distinction between passive and active suicidal ideation has been helpful enough to describe clinical settings. In palliative care, clinicians often face complex situations worth it for the use of different terminology. For example, one patient with stage IV cancer may have suicidal ideation as the result of a worsening depressive disorder, whereas another patient with no significant psychiatric symptoms similar prognosis may not want to prolong physical suffering knowledgeable of the irreversibility of their prognosis. As such, it is worth defining some terminology that concerns this topic.

- *Suicidal ideation:* Also called suicidal thinking, it concerns a person having thoughts of suicide. Suicidal ideation can also range in severity and vary from a more simple passive wish to die or be dead to more active suicidal ideation. This can be often related to depression, anxiety, hopelessness, and adjustment or to other medical causes, such as difficulty to tolerate pain, uncertainty about the prognosis, or existential despair.
- *Suicidal intent or plan:* In this case the patient expressed different ways in which he or she would commit suicide. The patient may describe a plan or potential methods such as overdosing, hanging, running across the traffic, or jumping off a bridge.
- *Desire for hastened death:* Often patients with terminal illnesses can suffer from depression and despair leading to a wish to die sooner. This desire can be more passive. Other times, they may ask to withhold treatments. In some occasions, desire for hastened death may come with an active plan for suicide [7, 8].
- *Physician-assisted suicide:* In six states of the Unites States, physicians can prescribe a lethal drug to patients so that they can end their lives on their own. This concept is different from euthanasia or "mercy killing" as the physician just prescribes the medication but does not administer it. Despite the little variation, in the United States, while physician-assisted suicide is legal in some states, euthanasia or "mercy killing" would be considered a criminal act. Despite alluding to the word "suicide" in its definition, physician-assisted suicide is not considered a form of suicide; otherwise it would be illegal. Arguments to support physician-assisted

suicide are the defense of personal autonomy and reduced suffering. Arguments against this practice are the deviance from the Hippocratic Oath and different spiritual beliefs in defense of life. Another argument against this practice is the belief that many patients requesting assisted suicide could have inadequately treated pain, undiagnosed depression, or cognitive distortions that if appropriately addressed and treated could change the patient's perception [9, 10].

- *Comfort care:* Depending on the context, this concept can be also used as synonym of palliative care and hospice care. In the hospital, comfort care measures can imply the withdrawal of active treatment toward the alleviation of pain and suffering even if this withdrawal may imply that the patient's life could end up sooner. Often, pain medication can be increased to alleviate patient's pain, and as such, patients may die sooner than naturally expected [11]. Comfort care is considered ethical when continuation of active treatment would come at expense of prolonging unnecessary suffering at the cost of little to no benefit. In some European countries like Spain, the term passive euthanasia is used to describe comfort care. However, in the concept of passive euthanasia entails a physician's knowledge that the alleviation of pain with opioids and other substances will probably accelerate patient's death. As such, the use of the morphine drip in a patient during the last few days or hours of life may be considered comfort care in the United States and passive euthanasia in Spain. In both cases, the action would be the same one (start a morphine drip to alleviate suffering), but the cognition of the physician would be different. In comfort care, the action would imply alleviation of suffering with the hope of not accelerating natural death, and in passive euthanasia, the physician would acknowledge that the morphine drip would carry an obvious acceleration of patient's death that would end his or her suffering.
- *Euthanasia:* In these settings, the physician would administer the patient a fatal overdose that would end his or her life. The main difference with physician-assisted suicide would be that in this case the physician would administer the lethal dose to the patient instead of the patient self-administering the drug [12]. In the United States, euthanasia is illegal, and the practice is subject to the criminal law. In some European countries, the term passive euthanasia is used to describe comfort care or interchangeable with assisted suicide. In the Netherlands, for example, the physician would typically administer sedative sodium thiopental intravenously to induce a deep coma followed by a pancuronium to cause a cardiorespiratory arrest.
- *Palliative chemotherapy:* This is a relatively new concept in the field of oncology. It concerns the use of chemotherapy and active treatment in patients with advanced cancer. The aim is to decelerate the growth of cancer and prolong life. In these settings, patients would continue to get active treatment despite poor prognosis. Nonetheless, palliative chemotherapy carries other risks. Patients would have to deal with the side effects of chemotherapy. Furthermore a recent study at Cornell University found that patients receiving palliative chemotherapy are thought to be less likely to die where they would have wanted, to complete do-not-resuscitate orders and to acknowledge that they were terminally ill [13].

Ethical Aspects

Still there continues to be a number of controversies in respect to the legal and ethical issues around assisted suicide in the medical field and the judicial system. Individuals who oppose legalization often claim that depression, distorted beliefs of becoming a burden to others, and other potentially treatable physical and psychological conditions play a major role in an individual's decision to request assisted suicide. Advocates of assisted suicide defend the freedom of a person and the autonomy to decide when and how to end one's life. That way it would be prevented that some patients do this in secrecy or impulsively without clear understanding of the alternatives and other treatment options. Despite assisted suicide being legalized already in six states of the United States [14], the practice is still rare. Nonetheless, over the recent years, it has been increasing. In 2014, a 24-year-old woman with treatment-resistant depression obtained permission to be euthanized by a team of physicians and psychiatrists with the idea that her condition would not improve. This case led to multiple debates as to where to set the limits of which conditions and in what circumstances patients should be eligible to obtain permission for assisted suicide.

In the assessment and evaluations of patients who desire hastened death or request assisted suicide, it is essential to be empathic and nonjudgmental. That way patients will be able to discuss the circumstances leading to their requests in an honest and frank manner. In the same manner, physicians will be able to detect treatable conditions such as depression, hopelessness, pain, and other psychological factors that may permit the discussion of different treatment alternatives the patient may not be aware of.

Important Factors to Consider in the Suicide Risk Evaluation

When evaluating a patient who expressed suicidal ideation and desire for hastened death or assisted suicide, it is important to first evaluate for all the treatable risk factors that may lead a patient to suicide in palliative care setting. The clinician must evaluate for physical and psychiatric reasons that may cause suffering and despair. Some of the most important reasons can be pain, depression, hopelessness, fear of being a burden to others, delirium, psychiatric and social issues, and/or spiritual concerns.

- Pain and other physical symptoms: A number of studies show that cancer pain is one of the leading causes of suicide. Untreated pain may cause significant despair and impulsive behaviors. Often patients evaluated for suicidal ideation report having no longer suicidal thoughts once their pain is adequately controlled. Intolerable pain should be one of the first symptoms a clinician should evaluate for. Other physical symptoms such as fatigue, severe nausea and vomiting, dizziness, sleep problems, and shortness of breath can precipitate suicidal thoughts. It is important to assess for potential physical symptoms and treat them.

- Cognitive disorders and delirium: Due to metabolic abnormalities, different medical complications causing hypoxia, liver failure, kidney failure, dehydration, infections, or excessive opioid use in pain management can impair a patient's cognition, judgment, and decision-making ability. Delirium due to medical conditions or treatments is characterized by an alteration in patient's attention or arousal with other cognitive-associated problems. Impulsive behaviors can often happen, and as such a patient may express a desire to end their lives or an intention to act on it. The role of the psychiatrist in these setting is important to diagnose and detect delirium and educate the team members on the phenomenology of delirium and how it can affect a patient's decision-making. Cognitive impairment and delirium are especially frequent in patients with advanced cancer and more debilitated patients. It is considered a risk factor for suicide, probably via helplessness and impulsivity.
- Depressive and anxiety symptoms: In psychiatry, the idea that depression and anxiety play a major role in suicide is largely embraced. Patients with cancer and terminal illnesses have an increased incidence of depression as compared to the general population. A significant number of patients with desire for hastened death meet criteria for depressive disorder. In fact, depression is considered the main risk factor for desire for hastened death. Hopelessness and helplessness are other symptoms of depression. Patients in palliative care settings often lose hope as they feel there is no more curative treatment being offered to them. According to the studies carried by Aaron Beck and colleagues, a higher score in the hopelessness subscale in the Beck Depression Inventory is correlated to higher risk for ending their lives. Overall patients with depression and hopelessness are considered to be at highest risk for suicide [15]. Acute anxiety and sleep deprivation are considered important risk factors for imminent suicide. Anxiety is related to poor judgment and impulsive behaviors which may also increase suicide risk. Patients often don't have history of anxiety or depression but suffer from these symptoms in the form of adjustment disorder with anxiety and depressive symptoms. Cancer itself can be very debilitating causing symptoms that overlap with depressive symptoms such as lack of concentration and attention, decreased energy, sleep and appetite problems, lack of interest and ability to feel pleasure, and irritable or depressed mood. Thus the diagnosis of depression in patients with cancer can often be challenging, and different criteria may apply. In patients with debilitating cancer and prominent physical symptoms, often the diagnosis of mood or anxiety disorder due to general medical condition is used.
- Fear of losing control or becoming a burden to others: Oregon residents who took advantage of the Death with Dignity Act in 2015 were those with decreasing ability to participate in activities that made life enjoyable, loss of autonomy, and loss of dignity. Loss of autonomy implies a loss of control over one's body and the fear of becoming a burden to loved ones. This is often a major reason for desire for hastened death and request of assisted suicide [16, 17].
- Social support: A lack of family and social support and lack of resources may enhance the fear of becoming a burden and increase the rates of requests for

assisted suicide. A number of studies have found correlations between lower levels of social support and higher desire for death in patients with cancer [18].

- Psychiatric history: History or presence of psychiatric disorders enhances the risk of desire for hastened death and suicidal ideation. Especially in patients with personality disorder, a cancer diagnosis may challenge their defenses increasing the risk for impulsivity and suicidal behaviors [14, 19].
- Spiritual and existential concerns: Religion and spiritual well-being has been considered a protective factor against suicide and desire for hastened death. Loss of meaning and purpose in life as well as incomplete tasks or regrets and anxiety about what may happen after death may cause existential despair and a desire for hastened death [14, 19].

Evaluating for Suicide Risk in Palliative Care Settings

The assessment of suicide in patients with cancer and terminal illnesses can be challenging. First of all, it will be important to evaluate and consider all the risk factors mentioned in the prior section. Thus, the clinician must evaluate for untreated pain, as this is often a major reason patients report suicidal ideation. In patients with suicidal ideation and concomitant intolerable pain, the appropriate treatment of pain may cease their suicidal thinking. It is also imperative to evaluate for other physical symptoms such as nausea, vomiting, fatigue, shortness of breath, dizziness, and immobility, among others. Again, the treatment of these symptoms and educating the patient on the plan of care to alleviate these physical symptoms can be anxiety relieving and already a treatment for their suffering and despair.

After evaluating for treatable pain and somatic symptoms, the clinician must evaluate the cognition of the patient. Delirium is also a risk factor for suicide, but the management would be different. Delirium often presents with impaired memory and attention, and as such, even if the patient may have stated earlier a desire for hastened death or suicidal thinking, he or she may not remember about that at the time of the evaluation. In these situations, it is important to not be confrontational and continue with a reasonable assessment for delirium and other risks. In patients with delirium, it is essential to obtain collateral information from family members, nurses, primary team, and other caretakers and staff.

Once a patient has been evaluated for untreated pain and physical symptoms and delirium, the clinician can proceed evaluating for mood and anxiety symptoms. First, it will be important to collect a more detailed history about the nature of suicidal ideation and the context in which the patient made such statement. For that it is important to obtain collateral information from the team. When did the patient mention about suicide? What did he or she say exactly? Did they mention a plan? Have they had any suicidal gesture or behaviors? The same questions should be asked to the patient. Following, an open-ended empathic psychiatric interview will allow us to learn more about the patient's particular circumstances. It is important to differentiate desire for hastened death from suicidal ideation or intention. It is also relevant to explore if patient meets criteria for a psychiatric disorder such as adjustment disorder, anxiety, or depressive disorder. It is crucial to evaluate for personality disorders and explore which are the patient's defenses. Maladaptive defenses such as splitting, acting out, projection, or projective identification are often present in patients with borderline, narcissistic, antisocial, and histrionic personality disorder but can be present in any patient. As part of the general psychiatric interview, the clinician must evaluate for presence of severe psychiatric disorders such as bipolar disorder and schizophrenia and other mood and psychotic disorders. It is essential to do a general risk assessment including prior history of suicidal ideation or desire for hastened death, history of suicidal gestures or behaviors, history of suicidal attempts, history of violent, impulsive or aggressive behaviors, past psychiatric history, history of prior psychiatric treatments, and psychiatric admission.

Another aspect to consider in the evaluation of patients reporting risk of suicide is the quality of their relationships. Patients with little social support are at higher risk for suicide. It is important to do a thorough psychosocial assessment, including relationship patterns, recent losses in life, and recent disappointments in relationships with people with whom they had intimacy in their life such as family members, partners, close friends, etc. Offering support and advice in these settings or even contacting family members with whom the patient had a recent altercation can be helpful. The clinician must also evaluate for financial concerns in regard to the hospital bills and the cost of treatment. In the recent years, financial stress has become an important distressful burden patients with cancer and in palliative care settings have to deal with.

Finally, patients often face existential concerns. They have to deal with the anxiety of not being alive, the anxiety of being dead, and the anxiety of disappearing from earthly living. Anxiety and existential despair can come from the anxiety of not knowing what comes after death. From an ontic, naturalistic, and experiential point of view, what comes after death is unknown to us. For this type of existential anxiety, it is important to be present with the patient and accompany and support him or her when dealing with this universal uncertainty.

Managing Patients with Suicide Risk

In the management of patients at risk for suicide, it is crucial to prioritize safety measures. Sharp objects should be removed, suicide and escape precautions should be started as per protocol, and a one-to-one sitter can be assigned to the patient for monitoring and prevention of suicidal behaviors.

It is imperative to start treatment for symptomatic control of pain and other physical symptoms as well as delirium and/or anxiety symptoms. As such, analgesics can be used for the treatment of pain. For that the consultant must collaborate with the primary team. Often, it is helpful to consult the pain team for reevaluation of pain and further ideas in regard to the patient's uncontrolled pain. In depression and pain, some antidepressants like venlafaxine and duloxetine can be helpful, especially in patients with neuropathic pain secondary to chemotherapy or diabetes [20,

21]. For the alleviation of physical symptoms, other treatments can be considered; for instance, nausea and vomiting can be often controlled with benzodiazepines like lorazepam or antipsychotics like olanzapine as well as other antiemetic agents [22, 23]. Sleep problems, irritability, appetite loss, and anxiety can be also treated with antipsychotics in palliative care settings, to prevent enhancing delirium risk in these patients. In cases of anxiety and depression, antidepressants can be used. Other times, antipsychotic and antiemetic and at times antidepressant medications can cause akathisia and other extrapyramidal symptoms that may increase the risk for impulsive and suicidal behaviors. There is a need to monitor for side effects from medications [24, 25].

The supportive therapeutic intervention at the time of the interview can be informative and therapeutic for the patient. Every patient has particular circumstances, and for that, an empathic listener that provides advice and support can be tremendously helpful. In supportive bedside psychotherapy, different techniques from different schools can be used. As such, one patient may benefit from socratic questioning of cognitive distortions about relationships and regrets, another patient may benefit from mere empathic listening of their suffering and concern, and even a psychodynamic interview can be helpful in these settings to identify and enhance adaptive defenses and encourage the patient to face current challenges in a similar way that he or she may have done in the past.

Finally it is important to maximize the hospital resources. Some hospitals include comprehensive integrative medicine departments with music therapy, pet therapy, and other useful resources. Today, most hospitals have a chaplaincy department. Patients with spiritual needs and concerns show great benefit from chaplain visits. Muscle relaxation, visual imagery, and hypnosis are now trendy techniques used regularly by psychiatrists and other clinicians toward the alleviation of pain and anxiety in hospital settings.

Specific Therapies

Today there are multiple therapies meant toward the treatment of patients with cancer in palliative care. Interpersonal therapy, family therapy, grief therapy, cognitive behavioral therapy, dialectic behavioral therapy, acceptance and commitment therapy, and even some dynamic interventions have been shown to be helpful in the treatment of patients with terminal illnesses and their families. For this chapter, we will focus on two therapies that were conceptualized toward the specific treatment of patients with cancer and terminal illnesses: dignity therapy and meaning-centered psychotherapy.

– *Dignity therapy*: This form of therapy was designed by Harvey Chochinov. It assists individuals in addressing their own priorities in psychosocial and spiritual aspects of life. It invites patients to address memories, issues, and reflections about what they would wish to offer to those they are about to live behind. Typically patients share life stories and values and speak about how they wished to be remembered and their most important accomplishments, hopes and dreams for their loved ones, and advice and guidance for the most important people in their lives. The sessions are tape-recorded. Then the therapist creates a verbatim and writes a cohesive narrative prior to meet again with the patient to ensure accuracy and completeness. The patient is then given a copy of this document referred as the "generativity document." The patient will then decide when he or she wants to share this document with their loved ones [26].

- *Meaning-centered psychotherapy*: This treatment has been developed by William Breitbart and Shannon Poppito at Memorial Sloan Kettering Cancer Center in New York. The approach of this therapy was inspired by Viktor Frankl's work and seminal book *Man's Search for Meaning* [27]. After surviving a concentration camp in World War II, Frankl arrived to the conclusion that a man has a will to meaning, an inherent drive to connect to something greater than one's needs and, through this, to find meaning and self-transcendence. Meaning-centered psychotherapy is divided in seven sessions in which both the therapists and the patient discuss concepts and sources of meaning, cancer and meaning, storytelling and life project, limitations in life, responsibility, creativity, and experiencing nature and humor toward the enhancement of the patient's quality of life and transcendence [28].

Compassionate Care and Final Remarks

In the evaluation and treatment of patients with suicidal risk or desire for hastened death, compassionate care is essential. In palliative care settings, patients deal not only with pain and physical and depressive symptoms but also with the existential anxiety of dying and, as such, facing the uncertainty of the unknown. With cancer and other severe illness diagnoses, a fear of losing autonomy and becoming a burden can be very prominent. Due to a lack of control over their lives, care, and situation, a patient may express desire for hastened death, become suicidal, or request assisted death in an attempt to regain control over their illnesses and their future. In the management of this patient, it is important to be compassionate and creative to face the uniqueness of every person. For example, just supplying ear plugs to a patient who cannot sleep at night due to noise in the hospital may help him rest appropriately and regain strength, something that will improve mood and anxiety symptoms and decrease desire for hastened death risk. Sometimes we may provide empathic comfort to our patients by helping them understand that they are not different from us, as it is the fate of all humans to deal with mortality. It is crucial to provide compassionate care to patients with delirium, who are unable to appropriately communicate their needs. In patients with delirium, the team must be especially sensitive when assessing for pain, physical symptoms, impulsivity, and suicide risk. At the same time, it is of essential to take care of the patients' families and loved ones. Educating them on the treatment plan and listening to their concerns can be very helpful in the patients' care, as they often participate in their recoveries by caring for them and reorienting and assisting them to drink and eat to regain strength. No matter the circumstances, if patients leave us, it is important to honor their memories by caring for their loved ones and console them as they cope with their loss. Taking care of patients with cancer and terminal illnesses can be as challenging as rewarding. Often clinicians who work in palliative care settings experience an increased sense of fulfillment in their lives and an enhanced sense of living and being in this world [29].

References

1. Hublin J-J. The prehistory of compassion. PNAS. 2009;106(16):6429–30.
2. Papadimitriou JD, Skiadas P, Mavrantonis CS, Polimeropoulos V, Papadimitriou DJ, Papacostas KJ. Euthanasia and suicide in antiquity: viewpoint of the dramatists and philosophers. J R Soc Med. 2007;100(1):25–8.
3. Van Hooff AJ. Ancient euthanasia: 'good death' and the doctor in the Graeco-Roman world. Soc Sci Med. 2004;58(5):975–85.
4. Espi Forcen F, Espi Forcen C. Ars moriendi: coping with death in the late middle ages. Palliat Support Care. 2016;14(5):553–60.
5. More T. Utopia. London: Penguin Classics; 2003.
6. Dowbiggin I. The modern art of dying: a history of euthanasia in the United States. J Hist Behav Sci. 2006;42(3):282–4.
7. Hudson PL, Kristjanson LJ, Ashby M, Kelly B, Schofield P, Hudson R, et al. Desire for hastened death in patients with advanced disease and the evidence base of clinical guidelines: a systematic review. Palliat Med. 2006;20(7):693–701.
8. Breitbart W, Rosenfeld B, Pessin H, Kaim M, Funesti-Esch J, Galietta M, et al. Depression, hopelessness, and desire for hastened death in terminally ill patients with cancer. JAMA. 2000;284(22):2907–11.
9. MacDonald R. Physician-assisted suicide. JAMA. 1995;274(24):1911–2. https://doi.org/10.1001/jama.1995.03530240020027.
10. Emanuel EJ, Onwuteaka-Philipsen BD, Urwin JW, Cohen J. Attitudes and practices of euthanasia and physician-assisted suicide in the United States, Canada, and Europe. JAMA. 2016;316(1):79–90.
11. Blinderman CD, Billings JA. Comfort care for patients dying in the hospital. N Engl J Med. 2015;373(26):2549–61.
12. McCarrick PM. Active euthanasia and assisted suicide. Kennedy Inst Ethics J. 1992;2(1):79–100.
13. Wright AA, Zhang B, Keating NL, Weeks JC, Prigerson HG. Associations between palliative chemotherapy and adult cancer patients' end of life care and place of death: prospective cohort study. BMJ. 2014;348:g1219.
14. Chochinov HM, Breitbart W. Handbook of psychiatry in palliative medicine. 2nd ed. New York: Oxford University Press; 2009.
15. Beck AT, Brown G, Berchick RJ, Stewart BL, Steer RA. Relationship between hopelessness and ultimate suicide: a replication with psychiatric outpatients. Am J Psychiatry. 1990;147(2):190–5.
16. Goodwin P. The Oregon death with dignity act. Am Fam Physician. 1995;52(2):398–400.
17. Ganzini L, Goy ER, Dobscha SK. Why Oregon patients request assisted death: family members' views. J Gen Intern Med. 2008;23(2):154–7.
18. Rodin G, Zimmermann C, Rydall A, Jones J, Shepherd FA, Moore M, Fruh M, Donner A, Gagliese L. The desire for hastened death in patients with metastatic cancer. J Pain Symptom Manage. 2007;33(6):661–75.
19. Holland JC, Breitbart WS, Jacobsen PB, Loscalzo MJ, McCorkle R, Butow PN. Psycho-oncology. 3rd ed. New York: Oxford University Press; 2015.
20. Tasmuth T, Härtel B, Kalso E. Venlafaxine in neuropathic pain following treatment of breast cancer. Eur J Pain. 2002;6(1):17–24.

21. Smith EM, Pang H, Cirrincione C, Fleishman S, Paskett ED, Ahles T, et al. Effect of duloxetine on pain, function, and quality of life among patients with chemotherapy-induced painful peripheral neuropathy: a randomized clinical trial. JAMA. 2013;309(13):1359–67.
22. Malik IA, Khan WA, Qazilbash M, Ata E, Butt A, Khan MA. Clinical efficacy of lorazepam in prophylaxis of anticipatory, acute, and delayed nausea and vomiting induced by high doses of Cisplatin: a prospective randomized trial. Am J Clin Oncol. 1995;18(2):170–5.
23. Licup N. Olanzapine for nausea and vomiting. Am J Hosp Palliat Med. 2010;27(6):432–4.
24. Espi Forcen F, Root JC, Alici Y. Antipsychotic-induced akathisia in cancer settings. Psychooncology. 2017;26(7):1053–6. https://doi.org/10.1002/pon.4247.
25. Espi Forcen F, Matsoukas K, Alici Y. Antipsychotic-induced akathisia in delirium: a systematic review. Palliat Support Care. 2016;14(1):77–84.
26. Chochinov HM, Hack T, Hassard T, Kristjanson LJ, McClement S, Harlos M. Dignity therapy: a novel psychotherapeutic intervention for patients near the end of life. J Clin Oncol. 2005;23(24):5520–5.
27. Frankl V. Man's search for meaning. Boston: Beacon Press; 2006.
28. Breitbart W, Poppito SR. Individual meaning-centered psychotherapy for patients with advanced cancer: a treatment manual. New York: Oxford University Press; 2014.
29. Espi Forcen F. Accompanying patients who face the ultimate fear: a fellowship in psycho-oncology. Palliat Support Care. 2017;15(4):504–5. https://doi.org/10.1017/S1478951516000651.

Part IV

Prevention

Suicide Prevention: A Primer for Healthcare Professionals

11

Michael F. Hogan

Introduction

Suicide is the tenth leading cause of death in the United States, with more than 40,000 deaths annually. Many individuals are deeply affected by suicide loss in their families and by close friends. Suicide is probably the worst outcome of mental healthcare not only for those who die but also for their families and their therapists. But the costs of self-harm greatly exceed the impact of suicide alone. There are almost 500,000 emergency department (ED) visits annually after self-harm; costs for ED visits and hospitalizations associated with these injuries among young adults in 2010 were estimated at $2.6 billion [1]. The number and rate of suicide deaths continue to rise. In 2001, there were 30,622 deaths from suicide (a rate of 10.75 deaths/100,000 population); by 2014, there were 42,773 deaths, and the rate had increased to 13.41/100,000 [2].

This chapter will broadly address developments in suicide care, summarizing new evidence about detecting and managing suicidal patients. Helping healthcare professionals and organizations achieve clinical competence in suicide care is beyond the scope of the chapter, though resources for developing skills will be suggested. This primer on suicide care is necessary because all mental health practitioners and a majority of mainstream health professionals are likely to encounter suicidal patients and because most clinical training programs do not adequately prepare them to provide suicide care [3]. There are several reasons for this gap. First, many evidence-based and best-practice approaches to identifying and working with suicidal patients are relatively new, having been developed and tested recently. As a result, most training programs have not yet incorporated these methods. Second, suicide care has not been seen as a core responsibility of most

M. F. Hogan, Ph.D.
National Action Alliance on Suicide Prevention, Washington, DC, USA

Case Western Reserve University School of Medicine, Cleveland, OH, USA

T. Falcone, J. Timmons-Mitchell (eds.), *Suicide Prevention*,
https://doi.org/10.1007/978-3-319-74391-2_11

healthcare organizations. Managing suicidal patients was traditionally central to mental health crisis care and to inpatient psychiatric units but an afterthought for most other settings such as primary care.

Suicide Prevention Is Emerging as a Healthcare Priority

To illustrate how suicide prevention in healthcare is changing, the first National Strategy for Suicide Prevention [4] did not define suicide prevention as a core responsibility of healthcare services. This goal was added to the updated 2012 National Strategy [5].

Another example of an improved focus on suicide prevention for healthcare settings is how suicide prevention has been addressed by accrediting bodies. In 1996 The Joint Commission (TJC) published its first Sentinel Event Alert (SEA) addressing suicide prevention. It applied to inpatient psychiatric care and was later amended to address all in-hospital care. In 2016, TJC issued a new SEA, indicating that all ambulatory and inpatient healthcare settings should proactively take steps to identify suicidal patients, take immediate steps for their safety, and secure access to appropriate treatment [6]; its aim is to "assist all health care organizations providing both inpatient and outpatient care to better identify and treat individuals with suicidal ideation" (p. 1). Coming from the leading accreditor of hospitals, the alert is a significant step toward establishing suicide prevention as a healthcare priority.

In this same year, the Council on Accreditation (COA) added new standards focused on identifying and managing suicidal patients, and the Commission on Accreditation of Rehabilitation Facilities (CARF) issued a Quality Practice Notice on suicide prevention [7] to its accreditation customers. These changes illustrate how the bar of suicide care is being raised and why attention to the topic is important and is becoming more important for health and behavioral health practitioners.

The field of suicide prevention, like work on other public health priorities, has emphasized primary prevention and community mobilizing efforts such as building awareness among "gatekeepers," community personnel like teachers or police officers who might then better identify people at risk of suicide and refer them to care. While most treatment settings were not expert at suicide care, there is some evidence these traditional prevention methods are effective. The Garrett Lee Smith Memorial Act, enacted in 2004, created a youth suicide prevention grant program for states, colleges, and American Indian/Alaska Native communities. The program is administered by the Substance Abuse and Mental Health Services Administration (SAMHSA); grant activities have emphasized screening, strengthening community partnerships, and building awareness for suicide warning signs in schools and communities by training frontline personnel to identify and refer at-risk youth to care. Results suggest that counties implementing these activities had lower suicide attempts and deaths among youth compared to matched counties. However, reductions in suicide were seen only among youth and did not persist after the programs ended, suggesting that broader and more sustained efforts are needed [8, 9].

Most Current Care for Suicidal Patients Is Inadequate

The increasing suicide rate, new knowledge about effective methods that are not widely used, and data on patterns of suicide among people under care have raised questions about the adequacy of "usual care" for suicidal individuals. Many individuals who die by suicide were engaged in care or had recent contact with health providers. About 45% of those who died by suicide saw a primary care physician in the 30 days before they died [10, 11].

These patterns suggest that suicidal individuals are often not detected. Simon et al. [12] examined the relationship between elevated responses to question 9 of the widely used PHQ-9 screening questionnaire ("thoughts that you would be better off dead, or hurting yourself in some way" in the past 2 weeks) and suicide deaths. They found a tenfold increase in suicide within the next year for patients reporting frequent thoughts of self-harm, suggesting that routine screening could detect suicidal individuals who could then be treated. The findings do not suggest that accurate prediction of when future suicide attempts might occur is possible. But if it is feasible to predict which individuals are at elevated risk in the near term, then better care and surveillance might help them. Improved screening and assessment can thus help fill the first critical gap in the health system's response to suicide.

A second area of concern is whether getting suicidal people engaged in routine mental healthcare—traditionally a high priority for the field of suicide prevention—is sufficient. The data suggest otherwise. Several states have recently linked data on participation in mental health and addiction care with death records; up to a quarter of all individuals who died by suicide had received mental healthcare in the year or two prior to their death [13–15], while on average only 2–3% of the population is served in these systems. Suicide risk is greatly elevated for people with major mental illness (e.g., depression, schizophrenia, bipolar illness) [16]. However, the state data coupled with obvious gaps in care (inadequate training of mental health professionals and limited use of the newer clinical approaches to be discussed below) suggest that the rate of suicide among patients receiving mental health services can be substantially reduced.

The routine standard of care within mental health services is to hospitalize patients at high risk of suicide. Once patients' risk is judged to be reduced, they are discharged with guidance to engage in follow-up care. However, while inpatient mental health settings provide treatment for mental disorders, they usually do not directly treat suicidal thoughts or feelings. Additionally, only about half of such patients complete a follow-up outpatient visit within a week [17], even though the risk of suicide is over three times as likely the first week after discharge from a psychiatric facility [18] and remains significantly above the base rate throughout the year [19]. Establishing suicide prevention as a priority will require significant changes by health systems and mental health programs in terms of policies, protocols, and staff training.

Can Improved Healthcare Prevent Suicide?

Following the 2001 Institute of Medicine's *Crossing the Quality Chasm* report [20], the Henry Ford Health System (HFHS) began efforts to prevent suicide among its patients. The goal of the "perfect depression care" initiative was "zero defect" mental healthcare [21]. Stimulated by the call for fundamental changes to improve patient safety, HFHS used deaths by suicide as one measure. Prevention experts Crosby and Stone [22] summarized the approach: "This model relied on suicide assessment for all behavioral health patients ... strategies included means restriction, provider education, follow-up via phone calls, and peer support services" (p411). The HFHS program reduced the suicide rate among patients receiving behavioral healthcare from an average of 96/100,000 in 1999–2000 to an average of 24/100,000 in 2001–2010, a reduction of about 75% [23], signaling that sustained and robust healthcare improvements might impact suicide.

Formal steps to improve suicide care within healthcare organizations received a boost with formation of the National Action Alliance for Suicide Prevention (Alliance) in 2010. The Alliance is a public-private group initially launched by Health and Human Services Secretary Sebelius and Department of Defense Secretary Gates and supported by the Substance Abuse and Mental Health Services Administration (SAMHSA). The work of the Alliance is largely done through task forces. One of the first, the Clinical Care and Intervention Task Force, examined the research on detecting and managing suicidality and considered efforts to reduce suicide in healthcare settings. The task force concluded that there was strong evidence for successfully detecting and managing suicidality in healthcare. In addition to looking at HFHS, the task force reviewed results of the National Suicide Prevention Lifeline, which showed that supportive contacts (by phone, text, or letter) reduce suicide among vulnerable individuals [24], and the Central Arizona Programmatic Suicide Deterrent System Project, which emphasized staff training and leadership.

After considering the available research and these exemplars, the task force concluded that improved suicide care was feasible. They found that three common factors were key to the successes of these programs: "*Core Values*—the belief and commitment that suicide can be eliminated in a population under care ... by improving service access and quality and through continuous improvement; *Systems Management*—taking systematic steps ... to create a culture that no longer finds suicide acceptable, [and] sets aggressive but achievable goals to eliminate suicide attempts and deaths among members; (and) *Evidence-Based Clinical Care Practice* delivered through ... standardized risk stratification, targeted evidence-based clinical interventions, accessibility, follow-up and engagement and education of patients, families and health care professionals ..." ([25], p. 4).

The comprehensive approach to suicide prevention recommended for healthcare organizations was named "Zero Suicide," representing both an aspirational goal and a specific set of practices. A care model and implementation toolkit for healthcare organizations was developed in 2012–2014 by the SAMHSA-funded Suicide Prevention Resource Center with the input of innovator sites in New York and Tennessee. By 2016, several hundred health and behavioral health organizations ranging from health plans to hospital systems to community mental health centers are implementing the Zero Suicide approach.

Elements of the Zero Suicide Model Provide an Evidence-Based Framework for Good Suicide Care

The Zero Suicide approach is both an amalgam of suicide care practices that have research support and an overall approach to care that also emphasizes supporting elements such as leadership, training, and quality improvement (see www.zerosuicide.com). For the purposes of this chapter and as a resource for health and behavioral health professionals, we will emphasize the clinical elements of the model. For each element, we will discuss recommended practices with a brief summary of the research evidence for the approach. Readers should be aware that many resources for each element (e.g., streaming video courses, archived webinars) are accessible via the www.zerosuicide.com website.

Screening and Assessment

The first key clinical principle is that healthcare organizations and practitioners should systematically screen for, identify, and assess suicide risk among people receiving care. As The Joint Commission notes in its recent alert, failure to assess suicide risk was the most common root cause of suicides qualifying as sentinel events [6]. Additionally, it appears clear (e.g., in the data on suicides following soon after primary care contacts) that the failure to screen for suicidality is the first and perhaps largest "crack" in healthcare that suicidal patients fall through. Whether universal screening of patients in good health is justified is not settled, given the very low baseline rate of suicide. The Joint Commission's alert recommends suicide screening of all patients likely to have elevated risk; the risk factors that should trigger screening for suicide include mental illness or substance use diagnoses, psychosocial trauma or conflict, recent loss (e.g., of a job or the death of a family member), family history of suicide, and personal history of suicide attempts [6].

The evidence for screening comes primarily from two areas. First, it is clear that the failure to screen/assess is a gap in care contributing to deaths. Second, it is clear that screening will identify people at elevated risk [12]. It is important to note that the research is not sufficient to suggest that screening tools and professional judgment can predict suicide risk with certainty or that the timing of self-harm can be accurately predicted. However, the Simon et al. research [12] and early experience with suicide care suggest that it is possible to predict when individuals face periods of elevated risk, during which better care can make a difference.

Credible screening and assessment tools should be incorporated in clinical practice and care protocols, as use of such tools coupled with clinical judgment has been found to be more accurate than clinician judgment alone [6, 26]. Concerns uncovered via screening should lead to assessment by a skilled clinician, and tools that specifically focus on suicide risk, such as the Columbia Suicide Severity Rating Scale [27], can provide more nuanced information than a single item that asks about thoughts of suicide. (For example, some individuals who live with persistent thoughts of suicide and thus might be thought of as "high risk" may have protective factors such as strong family relationships, faith, or learned skills to move past these thoughts which protect them.) Suicide risk assessment should be a comprehensive clinical evaluation to evaluate risk and protective factors, estimate the immediate danger to the patient, and consider treatment strategies that are relevant and acceptable to the patient.

Safety Planning Intervention with Means Reduction

The traditional approach to managing suicidal patients is inpatient hospitalization, often involuntary. While placement in such a controlled environment may meet short-term safety goals, there is no body of evidence that hospitalization for suicidality reduces risk in the long term. Hospitalization is also costly, both in economic terms and considering the fact that patients may find it unpleasant, perhaps to the point where they resolve to not disclose future suicidal thoughts to health professionals. Since inpatient care is usually brief and since treatment usually does not directly target suicidality, patients are often discharged at elevated risk; rates of completed suicide are very high in the period following discharge.

This is not to say that inpatient care must always be avoided; it may be the only way to keep some intensely suicidal patients alive. However, treatment outside the hospital may be preferable. The community care of patients with high suicide risk is like systematic approaches used for other health conditions, such as diabetes or high blood pressure. While specific treatment strategies are unique to each condition, a care protocol should systematically encourage use of evidence-based approaches for management of that condition. In the case of suicide, safety planning is one such approach. Safety planning is a brief, collaborative clinical intervention to strengthen an individual's ability to cope with suicidality and yielding a written personal plan of coping strategies and supports, developed by a clinician and patient [28]. The safety plan intervention should be completed in the same visit where elevated suicide risk is identified. The plan may include ways to manage thoughts of suicide in between provider visits, steps to reduce access to lethal means, and supports that the patient can access, collaboratively developed by a clinician and patient. This approach should replace use of "no-harm contracts," a practice now judged ineffective and perhaps harmful [29, 30]. A streaming video instructional course in the safety planning intervention may be accessed at http://zerosuicide.sprc.org/sites/zerosuicide.sprc.org/files/sp/course.htm.

An essential component of helping patients with suicide risk keep safe is restricting access to means of self-harm, especially those that they report having thought about using. This is an essential element of developing a safety plan, but it is emphasized here because of its crucial role. If suicidal patients are to be treated in community care, making their environment safe is critically important. Public health studies of reducing lethal means (e.g., firearms storage, bridge enclosures, replacing lethal cooking fuel with less toxic fuel) consistently show effectiveness.

(An excellent instructional course in reducing lethal means—CALM: Counseling on Access to Lethal Means—is at http://zerosuicide.sprc.org/resources/counseling-access-lethal-means-calm.) Additionally, leaders of the successful Henry Ford Health System initiative (perfect depression care) have reported that they believe intensive and personal efforts to reduce lethal means of self-harm are one of the most important contributors to their dramatically reduced suicide rates [31].

To summarize, developing a collaborative safety plan is the first clinical priority after suicide risk is assessed. Reviewing and updating the plan should be the first order of business at each clinical contact while the patient continues to report suicidal thoughts or feelings. Taking actions with the patient and family to reduce access to lethal means (and confirming that these steps have been taken) is a cornerstone of suicide care.

Evidence-Based, Direct Treatment of Suicidality

Treatment for suicidal patients has typically focused on the underlying mental health disorder in the hope that this will by itself reduce suicidal thoughts and feelings. The evidence now suggests that treatment should also directly target and treat suicidal thoughts and behaviors, preferably using evidence-based interventions. Controlled trials show that cognitive therapy for suicide prevention (CT-SP), dialectical behavior therapy (DBT), and collaborative assessment and management of suicidality (CAMS) are more effective than usual care in reducing suicidal thoughts and behaviors. These intervention approaches are summarized here:

Cognitive behavioral therapy (CBT) is based on the assumption that individuals with problems like depression lack skills for coping effectively with troubling thoughts or feelings; the therapy teaches patients to recognize these thoughts and provides alternative ways to cope. Many studies have demonstrated CBT's effectiveness with conditions such as depression and anxiety [32–34]; CT-SP is an adapted therapy focused on helping patients to directly manage suicidal thoughts and feelings. Research shows CT-SP results in reductions in suicide attempts and symptoms [35, 36].

Dialectical behavior therapy (DBT) is an adaptation of cognitive behavioral therapy, developed to help patients with chronic suicidality and other behavior problems. DBT has four components: a skills training group, individual treatment, phone coaching, and consultation team meetings. DBT is effective in reducing suicidal behavior. Linehan et al. [37] found that those receiving DBT were significantly less likely to drop out of treatment, attempt suicide, visit psychiatric EDs, or be hospitalized. Evidence suggests the skills training component of DBT is particularly significant for patients who are suicidal.

CAMS is an intensive psychological treatment that is suicide specific, helping patients develop other means of coping and problem-solving to replace or eliminate thoughts of suicide as a coping strategy. One of the core values of CAMS is that most suicidal patients can be treated effectively in outpatient settings. Studies of CAMS show reductions in suicidal ideation, depression, hopelessness, and visits to primary care and EDs [38].

A core practice principle shared by these treatment approaches is that all focus directly on thoughts and/or feelings of self-harm, as opposed to more traditional treatment approaches that generally target mental disorders in the hope that suicidality will abate. The implication for professionals working with suicidal patients is that the traditional approach can no longer be considered adequate. At a minimum, ongoing assessment and safety planning with means restriction are essential. Direct attention and assistance to the patient to help manage suicidal thoughts and feelings are also essential. Some resources on treating suicidality are available on the www.zerosuicide.com website (e.g., an archived webinar on this approach at http://zerosuicide.sprc.org/webinar/principles-effective-suicide-care-evidence-based-treatments).

As these therapies are further studied and as suicide care becomes more commonplace, we can expect access to training in these approaches will become easier.

Supportive Contacts During Care Transitions and High-Risk Periods

Isolation is a strong risk factor in suicide. Therefore, timely supportive contacts (which may include calls, texts, letters, visits) should be standard after acute care episodes or when ongoing services are interrupted (e.g., a scheduled visit is missed). Follow-up "caring contacts" with high-risk individuals have been demonstrated to be effective in reducing self-harm and suicide attempts [39]. These contacts can be completed by staff in any program that has provided acute care (e.g., ED or inpatient programs), by outpatient programs that provide ongoing care (during high-risk periods or when an appointment is missed), or by crisis centers that can conduct follow-up under contract with other services. The evidence supporting caring contacts finds various methods of supportive contacts can be effective [40].

Caring contacts are an especially important intervention during care transitions. The risk of a suicide attempt or death is high within the first month after discharge from inpatient or ED care, while up to 70% of patients who leave the ED after a suicide attempt never attend their first appointment [40]. Compounding the problem of follow-up care, the 2014 average performance on the Healthcare Effectiveness

Data and Information Set (HEDIS) measure—a national set of health plan quality measures—for one completed outpatient visit within 7 days of discharge from inpatient psychiatric hospitalization was only 51% [41]. Caring contacts are thus an additional tool—aside from successful linkages to follow-up treatment—that is both urgent and effective for suicidal patients. A streaming video course on conducting supporting follow-ups may be accessed at http://zerosuicide.sprc.org//sites/zerosuicide.actionallianceforsuicideprevention.org/files/monitor_suicidal_individuals/.

Summary and Conclusion

Attention to suicide prevention in healthcare settings is gaining momentum. Policy support is still needed to motivate adoption of suicide prevention by health systems. Attention to suicide prevention as a "core goal of health care services" in the updated national strategy [4] and The Joint Commission's recent alert will help stimulate change. SAMHSA has emphasized Zero Suicide approaches in its suicide prevention grant programs, and the National Institute of Mental Health recently released an announcement soliciting research proposals on Zero Suicide.

While policy change takes place, practitioners in all healthcare settings have the opportunity to learn and apply new actions and interventions to support their patients who are or might be suicidal. The key clinical activities presented in this chapter (with online resources to help practitioners learn the skills) are likely to become commonplace in healthcare settings, based on recommendations of major accrediting bodies and experts in suicide prevention. The essential clinical activities include:

- *Screening* all patients with suicide risk factors for suicidality. Risk factors include mental health and substance use disorders, recent loss, trauma history, and personal/family history of suicide. If screening reveals thoughts of suicide, a more complete *clinical assessment* should be completed immediately to guide treatment and suggest steps to keep patients safe.
- *Safety planning with means reduction.* Working with the patient to complete a collaborative safety plan, with steps they can take to ensure safety, is an essential step that should be carried out during the same visit where suicide risk is detected. An essential aspect of safety planning is identifying and carrying out *lethal means reduction* to remove means of self-harm, especially those the patient has identified. Reviewing suicide risk and updating the safety plan are the first order of business whenever the patient is seen, until risk is reduced.
- *Direct treatment of suicidality*, in addition to treatment for any mental disorder that the individual has, is suggested for any individual with high levels of suicide risk. Evidence-based approaches to managing and treating suicidality are preferable, and sessions at least once a week are suggested when patients remain at high risk. If individuals are able and willing to participate in safety activities and treatment, outpatient care is often preferable to hospitalization. If safety cannot reasonably be assured in the community, inpatient care may be necessary.

- *Supportive "caring contacts*" are perhaps the best-researched effective tool in caring for suicidal individuals. Caring contacts may be carried out by phone, text, email, letter, or visit, with the patient's preferences guiding the method of contact. Caring contacts are especially useful during care transitions or breaks in care (e.g., a missed therapy appointment).
- The ability of health professionals to implement these changes will vary considerably by the kind of settings they practice in. There are many challenges to improving screening, assessment, and basic management of suicidality in general medical settings including primary care. This is where most patients who subsequently die by suicide are seen, so improving detection in these settings, as The Joint Commission has urged, is important. Good suicide care including treatment of suicidality requires skilled mental health professionals, who are not yet present in many primary care and general medical settings. When suicidal patients are detected in these settings, care should include safety planning and an assured transition (including supportive contacts in the transition) to a mental health setting.

Much work to improve assessment and treatment of suicidality in the behavioral health sector is needed. This is essential because suicidal patients are generally referred to behavioral health providers, and as discussed earlier, professional training is not adequate [16]. Additionally, essential aspects of managing and treating suicidality (safety planning, lethal means reduction, direct treatment of suicidality, and persistent supportive contacts) are not yet standard in most behavioral health settings. As more states evaluate data on deaths and amend their suicide prevention plans, their attention will turn to improving suicide care in their behavioral health systems, and adoption of improved suicide care is likely to accelerate. The experience at Henry Ford and among early adopters demonstrates that implementing improved suicide care/Zero Suicide is feasible in ordinary care settings.

Change does not happen overnight, even in an area of obvious importance like suicide prevention. There is still much to do to turn the tide of suicide deaths but also much to be hopeful about. We hope that this discussion provides options for healthcare professionals that are seeking to improve the care they provide and stimulates action by health systems to reduce this preventable and tragic form of death.

References

1. Centers for Disease Control and Prevention. Web-based Injury Statistics Query and Reporting System (WISQARS): welcome to WISQARS. http://www.cdc.gov/injury/wisqars/index.html.
2. Centers for Disease Control and Prevention. WISQARS: fatal injury reports. http://www.cdc.gov/injury/wisqars/fatal_injury_reports.html.
3. Schmitz WM, Allen MH, Feldman BN, Gutin NJ, Jahn DR, Kleespies PM, et al. Preventing suicide through improved training in suicide risk assessment and care: an American Association of Suicidology Task Force report addressing serious gaps in U.S. mental health training. Suicide Life Threat Behav. 2012;42(3):292–304.
4. U.S. Department of Health and Human Services. National Strategy for Suicide Prevention: goals and objectives for action. http://www.sprc.org/library/nssp.pdf.

5. U.S. Surgeon General, National Action Alliance for Suicide Prevention. National Strategy for Suicide Prevention: goals and objectives for action, 2012. http://www.surgeongeneral.gov/library/reports/national-strategy-suicide-prevention/index.html.
6. The Joint Commission. Sentinel Event Alert, Issue 56: Detecting and treating suicide ideation in all settings. http://www.jointcommission.org/assets/1/18/SEA_56_Suicide.pdf.
7. Commission on Accreditation of Rehabilitation Facilities (CARF International). Quality practice notice—September 2016. Suicide prevention in CARF-accredited organizations: advancing clinical and workforce preparedness. http://www.carf.org/QPN_SuicidePrevention/.
8. Knox KL, Litts DA, Talcott GW, Feig JC, Caine ED. Risk of suicide and related adverse outcomes after exposure to a suicide prevention programme in the US Air Force: cohort study. BMJ. 2003;327(7428):1376–80. https://doi.org/10.1136/bmj.327.7428.1376.
9. Walrath C, Garraza L, Reid H, Goldston D, McKeon R. Impact of the Garrett Lee Smith Youth Suicide Prevention Program on suicide mortality. Am J Public Health. 2015;105(5):986–93.
10. Ahmedani B, Simon G, Stewart C, Beck A, Waitzfelder B, Rossom R, et al. Health care contacts in the year before suicide death. J Gen Intern Med. 2014;29(6):870–7.
11. Boschert S. New strategies target suicidality in EDs. Irving, TX: American College of Emergency Physicians; 2009. https://www.acep.org/Clinical---Practice-Management/New-Strategies-Target-Suicidality-in-EDs/.
12. Simon G, Rutter C, Peterson D, Oliver M, Whiteside U, Operskalski B, et al. Does response on the PHQ-9 Depression Questionnaire predict subsequent suicide attempt or suicide death? Psychiatr Serv. 2013;64(12):1195–202. http://www.ncbi.nlm.nih.gov/pmc/articles/PMC4086215/pdf/nihms598768.pdf.
13. Suicide Prevention Resource Center. Surveillance success stories: Kentucky. Waltham, MA: Education Development Center; 2015. http://www.sprc.org/library_resources/items/surveillance-success-stories-kentucky.
14. Suicide Prevention Resource Center. Surveillance success stories: Vermont. Waltham, MA: Education Development Center; 2015. http://www.sprc.org/sites/sprc.org/files/library/SPRC_Vermont_compliant.pdf.
15. Hiance-Steelesmith DL, Fontanella CA, Sweeney HA, Campo JV. Behavioral health service use among suicide decedents in the public behavioral health system. Poster session presented at: 48th Annual Conference of the American Association of Suicidology; 2015 Apr 15–18; Atlanta, GA.
16. Bertolote JM, Fleischmann A. Suicide and psychiatric diagnosis: a worldwide perspective. World Psychiatry. 2002;1(3):181–5.
17. Bickley H, Hunt I, Windfuhr K, Shaw J, Appleby L, Kapur N. Suicide within two weeks of discharge from psychiatric inpatient care: a case-control study. Psychiatr Serv. 2013;64(7):653–9.
18. Siegfried N, Bartlett M. Navigating suicide assessment: a roadmap for providers. Plenary presented at: The Joint Commission's 2014 Annual Behavioral Health Care Conference; 2014 Oct 15–16; Rosemont, IL.
19. Valenstein M, Kim HM, Ganoczy D, McCarthy JF, Zivin K, Austin KL, et al. Higher-risk periods for suicide among VA patients receiving depression treatment: prioritizing suicide prevention efforts. J Affect Disord. 2009;112(1):50–8.
20. Institute of Medicine. Crossing the quality chasm: a new health system for the 21st century. Washington, DC: National Academies Press; 2001.
21. Coffey CE. Building a system of perfect depression care in behavioral health. Jt Comm J Qual Patient Saf. 2007;33(4):193–9.
22. Stone D, Crosby A. Suicide prevention: state of the art review. Am J Lifestyle Med. 2014;8(6):404–20.
23. Coffey MJ, Coffey CE, Ahmedani BK. Suicide in a health maintenance organization population. JAMA Psychiatry. 2015;72(3):294–6.
24. Gould MS, Munfakh JL, Kleinman M, Lake AM. National suicide prevention lifeline: enhancing mental health care for suicidal individuals and other people in crisis. Suicide Life Threat Behav. 2012;42(1):22–35.

25. National Action Alliance for Suicide Prevention: Clinical Care & Intervention Task Force. Suicide care in systems framework. Washington, DC: The Alliance; 2012. http://actionallianceforsuicideprevention.org/sites/actionallianceforsuicideprevention.org/files/taskforces/ClinicalCareInterventionReport.pdf.
26. Assessment and Management of Risk for Suicide Working Group. VA/DoD clinical practice guideline for assessment and management of patients at risk for suicide. Washington, DC: Department of Veterans Affairs, Department of Defense; 2013. http://www.healthquality.va.gov/guidelines/MH/srb/VADODCP_SuicideRisk_Full.pdf.
27. Posner K, Brown G, Stanley B, Brent D, Yershova K, Oquendo M, et al. The Columbia-Suicide Severity Rating Scale: initial validity and internal consistency findings from three multisite studies with adolescents and adults. Am J Psychiatry. 2011;168(12):1266–77.
28. Stanley B, Brown G. Safety planning intervention: a brief intervention to mitigate suicide risk. Cogn Behav Pract. 2012;19(2):256–64.
29. Edwards SJ, Sachmann MD. No-suicide contracts, no-suicide agreements, and no-suicide assurances: a study of their nature, utilization, perceived effectiveness, and potential to cause harm. Crisis. 2010;31(6):290–302.
30. Jacobs DG, Baldessarini RJ, Conwell Y, Fawcett JA, Horton L, Meltzer H, et al. Assessment and treatment of patients with suicidal behaviors. APA Practice Guidelines. 2010. http://psychiatryonline.org/pb/assets/raw/sitewide/practice_guidelines/guidelines/suicide.pdf.
31. Coffey, E. Personal communication. 2013 Sept 16.
32. Gloaguen V, Cottraux J, Cucherat M, Blackburn IM. A meta-analysis of the effects of cognitive therapy in depressed patients. J Affect Disord. 1998;49(1):59–72.
33. Churchill R, Hunot V, Corney R, Knapp M, McGuire H, Tylee A, et al. A systematic review of controlled trials of the effectiveness and cost-effectiveness of brief psychological treatments for depression. Health Technol Assess. 2002;5(35):1–73.
34. Stewart RE, Chambless DL. Cognitive–behavioral therapy for adult anxiety disorders in clinical practice: a meta-analysis of effectiveness studies. J Consult Clin Psychol. 2009;77(4):595–606.
35. Brown G, Ten Have T, Henriques G, Xie S, Hollander J, Beck A. Cognitive therapy for the prevention of suicide attempts: a randomized controlled trial. JAMA. 2005;294(5):563–70.
36. Stanley B, Brown G, Brent D, Wells K, Poling K, Curry J, et al. Cognitive-Behavioral Therapy for Suicide Prevention (CBT-SP): treatment model, feasibility, and acceptability. J Am Acad Child Adolesc Psychiatry. 2009;48(10):1005–13.
37. Linehan M, Comtois K, Murray A, Brown M, Gallop R, Heard H, et al. Two-year randomized controlled trial and follow-up of dialectical behavior therapy vs therapy by experts for suicidal behaviors and borderline personality disorder. Arch Gen Psychiatry. 2006;63(7):757–66.
38. Comtois KA, Jobes DA, O'Connor SS, Atkins DC, Janis K, Chessen CE, et al. Collaborative assessment and management of suicidality (CAMS): feasibility trial for next-day appointment services. Depress Anxiety. 2011;28(11):963–72.
39. Knesper DJ, American Association of Suicidology, Suicide Prevention Resource Center. Continuity of care for suicide prevention and research: suicide attempts and suicide deaths subsequent to discharge from an emergency department or an inpatient psychiatry unit. Education Development Center: Newton, MA; 2010. http://www.sprc.org/library_resources/items/continuity-care-suicide-prevention-and-research.
40. Luxton D, June J, Comtois K. Can postdischarge follow-up contacts prevent suicide and suicidal behavior? Crisis. 2013;34(1):32–41.
41. Group Health. 2015 HEDIS and CAHPS measures and performance. Group Health Cooperative: Seattle; 2016. https://www1.ghc.org/static/pdf/public/about/hedis.pdf.

Preventing Suicide in Hospital-Based Care

12

Clare C. Mitchell and Jeanne M. Lackamp

Introduction

Healthcare providers typically equate preservation of life with clinical success. Loss of life, then, is often viewed as the "enemy" of modern medicine. Even more devastating than death from so-called natural causes is death at someone's hand—another person killing the patient or, worse still, the patient killing themselves. In cases of patients taking their own lives, one of the most upsetting and dramatic events is when patients take their own lives *while under direct medical care*. This chapter will address suicide management and prevention in hospital settings.

Several things should be noted as we begin this discussion. Firstly, according to the World Health Organization, suicide results in almost a million deaths worldwide each year, and the increasing rate of suicides in the USA has now made suicide the tenth leading cause of death nationally [1–4]. While it is unknown exactly how many of these occur in hospitalized patients, authors report that inpatient suicides constitute *one of the most common* sentinel events reported to the Joint Commission on Hospital Accreditation (JCAHO) [3, 5–7]. Concern over inpatient suicides led to the 2007 JCAHO National Patient Safety Goal (NPSG.15.01.01), mandating that "general hospitals treating patients with a primary diagnosis or a primary complaint of an emotional or behavioral disorder and psychiatric hospitals identify patients at risk for suicide" ([5], p. 472). Sadly, as of 2012, JCAHO reported that psychiatric hospitals were "the most frequent setting for a sentinel event" [8].

Secondly, healthcare providers, even highly trained mental health providers, cannot predict (let alone prevent) all patient suicides [9]. Many providers endeavor to establish rapport with patients via sensitive patient interviews and detailed suicide assessment scales, in order to identify suicide risk factors and current acute level of risk [10]. Unfortunately, providers do not meet with consistent success. As noted by

C. C. Mitchell, Ph.D. (✉) · J. M. Lackamp, M.D.
University Hospitals Cleveland Medical Center, Cleveland, OH, USA
e-mail: Clare.Mitchell@UHhospitals.org; Jeanne.Lackamp@UHhospitals.org

T. Falcone, J. Timmons-Mitchell (eds.), *Suicide Prevention*,
https://doi.org/10.1007/978-3-319-74391-2_12

one author, "Suicidal ideation does not accurately predict suicide, nor is the absence of suicidal ideation a guarantee that no suicide will occur" ([11], p. 267). As alarming as this realization may be, patients who die by suicide may or may not have cardinal features, and/or prodromal signs, predicting their behavior.

Another complicating factor in modern healthcare is an increasing push for cost-effective care provision. This can lead to pressures to reduce what are seen as extraneous inpatient staffing costs—which can include reduction or elimination of constant observation ("CO") of at-risk patients [7]. In addition, pressures toward reduced length of stay ("LOS") may prompt clinicians to discharge patients, leaving some of the most ill patients on the unit (thus stressing nursing staff and resources) [6] or creating a "revolving door" where a prematurely discharged patient's suicide risk remains elevated despite inpatient treatment ([8], p. 393). These issues, and countless others, can come together to create an environment where the threat of inpatient suicide persists despite caring and motivated clinicians.

Note that while many patients may have sentinel events while hospitalized—including those who attempt to *harm* themselves (i.e., not trying to kill themselves) and those who engage in other surreptitious behaviors which *may* result in harm (e.g., using drugs or alcohol in the hospital)—this chapter will focus on patients who are *purposely attempting to end their lives* while admitted to the hospital.

High-Risk Patients: What Are Common Risk Factors and How Should We Assess Them?

Though limited research exists to describe the characteristics of patients who attempt and complete suicide in both inpatient psychiatric and general medical hospital settings [12], it does appear that risk factors for suicidal behavior in the hospital differ from risk factors for suicide in the general population [13]. Furthermore, recent research has demonstrated risk factors for suicide in hospital settings are likely different for different groups, including those experiencing suicidal ideation versus those who go on to make attempts [14] and those hospitalized across different settings (i.e., medical-surgical units vs. psychiatric units vs. freestanding psychiatric hospitals). Additionally, different risk factors may exist for patients hospitalized on medical-surgical units following suicide attempts. For the purpose of this chapter, we will focus on risk factors for suicide in patients admitted to psychiatric and medical-surgical units.

For patients admitted to psychiatric units, those at high risk for inpatient suicide include those with serious psychiatric diagnoses (mood and psychotic disorders), substance use, past suicide attempts or psychiatric admissions, family histories of mental health problems, stressors such as financial or family tensions, acute anxiety and agitation while hospitalized, and severe anhedonia at the time of their attempt/completion [6, 15, 16]. Additionally, suicide on inpatient units appears to peak shortly after admission, with young males dying by suicide more often than older patients and females [17]. It should be noted, however, that reliance on the predictive power of these risk factors may have limited utility given the rarity of completed suicides [18]. Powell and colleagues suggest a focus instead on making changes to the environment aimed at promoting patient safety [12].

Suicide completion on medical-surgical units appears to be rarer than suicide completion on psychiatry units [19, 20]. Not surprisingly, much less is known about risk factors for suicide in the general hospital setting [21, 22]. A recent longitudinal, case-controlled study found those who completed suicide in a hospital had a history of psychiatric comorbidities, did not communicate any suicidal ideation to staff during admission, and died by suicide shortly after admission [3]. Other studies suggest acute anxiety and conditions leading to agitation and impulsivity may result in suicide on medical-surgical units [23, 24]. Finally, times of transition and changing health conditions likely constitute higher-risk times for medically hospitalized patients [1].

Despite identification of correlates associated with completed suicide on inpatient psychiatric and medical-surgical units, they cannot be used to predict suicide attempts or completion with accuracy. In fact, several authors suggest suicide risk assessment as it is usually performed, looking at the number of risk factors present and determining a "low," "moderate," or "high" level of risk, has little utility [25–28]. This method of risk stratification may produce too many false positives where patients falling into the "high-risk" group may never attempt suicide [12]. Conversely, patients deemed "low risk" may go on to attempt suicide, despite being given this reassuring label.

At present, few better alternatives exist to replace the standard psychiatric risk assessment in hospital practice, since risk assessment generally forms the cornerstone for treatment planning and disposition. Hawgood and De Leo [9] suggest not eliminating risk assessment entirely but rather shifting the focus away from determining categories of risk and toward assessment focused on collaboration with the patient. Lieberman and colleagues [28] suggest a focus on decreasing environmental risk factors as opposed to attempting to identify patients who may be at risk. Clearly, we cannot stop assessing our hospitalized patients; however, questions remain about the most useful ways to pursue the assessment process.

Common Methods: How Do Patients Attempt Suicide While Hospitalized?

It is interesting to note that hospitalized patients have different methods of suicide attempt/completion as compared to outpatients. Suicide researchers note that one of the most common methods of outpatient suicide is via the use of firearms [22]. However, methods of inpatient suicide appear to be different, largely based on access and location.

Both medical and psychiatric hospital settings can limit suicide methods simply by virtue of the patient being in a more controlled environment than if they were in the community. Steps that should be taken with *all* patients who pose a risk of harm to themselves include searching belongings, ensuring that patients do not have access to dangerous items, and ensuring that visitors do not bring (and/or leave) potentially dangerous items when they come to see their loved ones [4]. If these limitations are imposed, then access to some suicide methods (medications for overdose, items for cutting, and firearms) should be drastically reduced as compared to outpatients. Indeed, authors describe restriction of access to dangerous items as "one of the few interventions found to be effective" ([29], p. 486). In one thorough description of a suicide prevention program, failure to secure patient belongings was identified as a significant safety factor [8]. Further, attiring patients in hospital clothing can reduce elopement risk (or make elopement more evident if a patient attempts to leave hospital grounds).

Many authors have found that the most common methods of attempting/completing suicide while hospitalized were serious and violent, which include *hanging* and *jumping from a height* [6, 30–32]. (Some authors [22] even distinguish further that inpatient psychiatry patients tend to hang themselves, while inpatient medical patients tend to jump from heights.) Despite safety precautions, these two methods remain readily available to hospitalized patients because of linens and clothing, as well as building construction with multiple floors. Additionally, if patients are in close proximity to a potentially dangerous area, patients may utilize that proximity for attempting suicide—for instance, eloping from hospital units and running into traffic, toward train tracks, or toward a body of water [20, 33].

Hospital administration, medical providers, and legal teams often collaborate in the creation of safety policies, to ensure reasonable, consistent, and fair treatment of all patients. Citing the importance of adherence to safety restrictions, the rationale behind such restrictions, and the criteria for when restrictions can be lifted often help staff and patients feel reassured. Though implementation of safety policies may prove challenging, the importance of protocols including limiting access to potentially dangerous items and maintaining patients in hospital clothing cannot be overstated.

Inpatient Units: Risks and Strategies

Guidelines

In response to the painful reality of inpatient suicide, JCAHO implemented guidelines regarding care of suicidal patients. Unfortunately, as authors note, "[t]he Joint Commission emphasized the need for around-the-clock observation for inpatients assessed as being at high risk for suicide. It did not, however, define how adequate around-the-clock observation should be implemented" ([31], p. 17).

Personnel

Each hospital system has its own culture of caring, and its own sets of limitations, including financial, staffing, and motivational limitations which can impact patient safety [5]. Staff also naturally vary in their skills regarding patient assessment, communication, comfort level, and personal reactions when treating patients demonstrating psychiatric symptoms [34]. Nurses on both medical-surgical units and psychiatric units may feel overwhelmed, stressed, or burdened when faced with patients having acute mental health issues accompanied by the risk of self-injury or death. Lack of supervision, support, and training can lead to difficulty interacting with this patient population, thus impacting patient care. Other personnel (supervisors, nursing assistants, and sitters) can be similarly inclined. Combining training limitations with hospital culture can lead staff to undervalue the process of suicide prevention program creation, implementation, and adherence [5].

Patients at risk of inpatient suicide merit increased level of staff involvement and direct observation. Despite the edict to have staff observers for suicidal patients, specific guidelines and reasonable mechanisms for observation are lacking—which can lead to subpar patient safety. This will be further addressed in the sections on "sitters" below.

Unit-Specific Issues

Medical-Surgical Units

Inpatient medical and surgical units (including general units, OB units, and ICU settings) are fraught with challenges when attempting to keep patients safe. In some cases patients are admitted to medical units with suicidal ideation. Others may never make suicidal statements while in the hospital. It should be noted that patients on medical-surgical units who are at risk for suicide may present with medical conditions marked by impulsivity (i.e., alcohol withdrawal delirium and various neurological conditions). For this reason, the ability to recognize symptoms associated with these conditions, and communicate concerns to other staff, is essential [4, 21]. Dlugacz and colleagues also recommend increased nursing and medical education, as well as ensuring appropriate communication between staff at hand-off times, to improve identification of at-risk patients [11].

Importantly, staff must be attentive to the patient environment, because inpatient medical-surgical rooms often are equipped with items/objects which can be harmful for a patient intent on suicide. Items such as IV poles/tubing, oxygen tubing, sharps containers, and other medically necessary implements (e.g., suture kits, wound care kits, syringes, and flushes) can prove dangerous. Staff vigilance is crucial, especially for patients who are confused and distressed or who do reveal suicidal ideation. While hospitals vary in their policies, consideration should be given to removing unnecessary items from patient rooms, to reduce potential for harm.

Psychiatry Units

Providing appropriate observation and milieu activities on inpatient psychiatric units, while maintaining safety, can be challenging [35]. Inpatient psychiatric units may have unique obstacles to patient safety, including specific areas (e.g., physical therapy, occupational therapy, art therapy rooms) which may have implements or items contained within them which could be potentially dangerous [32]. Furthermore, in contrast to medical-surgical units where patients are restricted to their own room, patients on psychiatry units typically have more freedom for movement around the unit (unless they are in seclusion or in restraints). Thus, even on locked wards and even on wards where seclusion is an option, there can be more potential for exposure to dangerous elements in individual rooms, other patients' rooms, and the general unit as compared to medical-surgical units.

Over the years, structural changes have emerged—from breakaway elements in bathrooms to no-hang bars (with seamless attachments to walls), each step of safety evolution has led to additional challenges. Breakaway bars were initially deemed reasonable, so that bars could not provide anchor points for patients to hang themselves. However, adoption of breakaway bars quickly proved unsafe, as the jagged or sharp edges of the bars could be used as weapons against self or others [36]. No-hang bars were deemed safer but can pose infectious disease challenges when cleaning the small "trough" created by the attachment between the bar and the wall ([36], p. 9). Elimination or replacement of unnecessary doors (such as cupboard doors) and modification of other anchor points to prevent hanging can be effective [29], as are safety features on doors including pressure sensors, so that weight of a ligature and body triggers an alarm and release of the door [36]. Of course, one must remember that patients can attach ligatures lower down and then "slump" from a kneeling position, so lower level attachment points must be identified and modified [36], p. 9).

Previously, risk factors unique to inpatient psychiatric units included weekend leave and passes, as well as the chronic risk of elopement [33]. It should be noted that, in recent years, it is less common for inpatient psychiatric units to provide weekend leave and passes off the unit. Risks of suicide when patients are "off" inpatient units now largely relate to time of discharge, with authors noting that patients remain at elevated risk of suicide in the weeks/months immediately following their discharge home [30].

What About Sitters?

One of the most common (yet contentious) interventions for suicidal inpatients is direct observation. It is likely that every reader has had subpar experiences with staff observation of suicidal patients, from staff sleeping while observing to staff distracted by television or cellphones to staff getting into altercations with patients. Thus, we acknowledge that a staff observer is neither a perfect nor foolproof method of ensuring patient safety. Additionally, staff observers can be employed for various reasons unrelated to suicide risk; we will not address those scenarios here. [*Please note that in this section, we will use various terms such as "CO," "observer," and "sitter" interchangeably to denote a staff member assigned for direct, constant observation of a potentially suicidal patient.*]

Despite the frequency of their use, there is a relative dearth of evidence about observation interventions with regard to safety and harm reduction [35, 37, 38]. Many articles echo the theme that there is "little empirical evidence" ([37], p. 272) to support the use of direct observation. Numerous articles cite the high cost of constant observation, and some researchers even found that decisions about a patient's risk for suicide can be influenced by staffing elements more so than actual patient assessment [6]. Other articles note that implementation of constant observation does not always prevent bad outcomes. In one review of 76 suicides while inpatient (or immediately after discharge), 20% of those who died by suicide were on q30 min checks, or were observed within 30 minutes, of their suicide; another 42% were on q15 min checks, or were observed within 15 minutes, of their suicide—and a tragic 9% of these patients were on 1:1 observation at the time of their suicide [23]. Some authors suggest, provocatively, that constant observation may be associated with increased episodes of self-harm [35]. The reader is asked to consider this statement closely, understanding that the most acute patients are assigned to constant observation (thus, there exists a selection bias toward the potential for bad outcomes).

One problem identified in the literature is the variety of terms and strategies for direct observation of suicidal patients [7, 31]. Some patients are observed on "general" or "routine" observation, some are observed every 30 minutes ("q30"), some are observed every 15 minutes ("q15"), and some patients are assigned to constant observation ("CO"). This typically entails use of a nurse or other staff member assigned as a 1-to-1 (or "1:1") companion, sometimes called a "sitter." This level of observation had long been considered the gold standard for observation of suicidal patients [7]. [Another, even more intense, form of observation is sometimes called "intensive psychiatric observation" where a staff member is within arms' length of the patient at all times [31]. This is typically reserved for the most acute, highest-risk patients.] Throughout the literature, it is clear that protocols for constant observation are anything but consistent and often depend on individual hospital systems, staffing issues, and administrative pressures.

In addition to variability of procedures and terms, staff observers possess varying levels of training and experience. Staff members may be inconsistently or improperly trained in safety assessment and maintenance, may have limited understanding of the risks inherent in the patients they treat, and may have limited knowledge of how to communicate those risks [7, 8, 37, 39, 40]. While we will not address constant observation based on specific diagnoses, it also should be noted that staff observers may be less vigilant about a patient's risk of suicide depending on patient presentation (for instance, confused patients may be considered more likely to fall or pull out an IV line), and staff can thus have an inappropriately low estimation of suicide risk.

In addition to simple lack of training, staff may unwittingly put patients at higher risk if they take shortcuts, make protocol adjustments, fail to communicate appropriately with colleagues, or commit other errors which lead to less-than-optimal observation of a potentially dangerous patient [31]. Furthermore, staff may consider observation to be a low-level task that is not clinically useful; this attitude may contribute to lack of perceived efficacy because of lack of staff buy-in and implementation [31]. Communication failures were mentioned as particularly significant, especially during patient transfers and transitions of care [11, 31]. One comprehensive review of an inpatient psychiatry unit suicide prevention program identified "areas of failure" including failure in patient assessment (including failure to reassess each shift), lack of control/supervision/restraint of patients, and failure to monitor (and/or medicate) patients in a timely fashion, in addition to failure to secure the patient environment ([8], p. 395). Thus, perhaps it is not CO which is ineffective but rather the way in which CO is implemented. Each one of the potential pitfalls noted above should be kept in mind, as hospitals attempt to create and implement reasonable suicide prevention strategies of their own.

Other struggles include the stress associated with CO, on both patients and staff members providing the observation. Staff have described feeling challenged, frustrated, afraid, overwhelmed, and powerless when caring for patient with self-harming and suicidal behavior as inpatients [35]. To combat the stresses of CO, some literature suggests that CO staff and patient be of the same gender and that CO staff observe for very short amounts of time (e.g., an hour at a time) [7]. Some authors postulate that suicide observation may further stigmatize fragile patients by drawing attention to their symptomatic acuity [41] and that the restriction (and lack of privacy) associated with CO is a disadvantage for patients [37]. Finally, there is a question of secondary gain for patients who are getting direct staff attention by virtue of safety concerns [37].

While there seem to be many negatives related to the use of sitters for suicidal patients, it is important to acknowledge another side to this debate. Several recent articles highlight critical errors in the arguments against CO. Firstly, there is no way to objectively study the benefit of constant observation, since engaging in any intervention (e.g., stopping CO) which could potentially put patients at risk of suicide or self-harm would be unethical [7]. Additionally, what is meant by CO—and which patients are placed on CO—may directly impact staff's impression of the intervention's efficacy [7]. Rather than CO being a flawed idea at baseline, authors posit that a significant contributor to CO failure is *improper, inappropriate, or inadequate creation and implementation of CO policy* [7, 8]. One strong proponent of correct usage of CO states "I would suggest we acknowledge the face validity that CO, when performed correctly, prevents suicide in the short run. CO, like some medical procedures, may be unpleasant and unwanted but nevertheless life saving" ([7], p. 387).

Alternatives to Sitters?

Given the lack of evidence to support CO in reducing self-harm and suicide on psychiatric and medical-surgical units, many authors have proposed CO alternatives. Suggested alternatives have included cohorting patients with similar issues (e.g., placing two patients who require constant observation in the same room), having family members stay with patients, utilizing hospital volunteers to sit with patients, having patients located closer to nursing stations, utilizing as-needed medications, using standardized behavioral charting, and (strangely) utilizing physical restraints [38–40, 42–44]. It should be noted that one of the original reasons that direct patient observation was initiated was the desire to *reduce* the use of physical restraints. It is unfortunate, then, to have modern-day authors suggesting this backward step in patient care. Furthermore, one wonders what message the use of such "lesser" interventions sends to patients and families—if potentially at-risk patients are treated with more cost-effective (but not necessarily more safe) interventions.

With regard to using CO alternatives to reduce patient harm, the most notable research findings seem to be that there are no findings—or at least very limited ones. While many proposals seem to be well-intentioned, seem to reduce the use of sitters, and seem to increase staff satisfaction [45], research to date does not appear to support a relationship between the implementation of these alternatives and increase in patient safety. One reason for limited outcome data related to sitter alternative interventions may be the (relative) rarity of suicide in hospital settings. A multi-year study utilizing patient video monitoring on two medical-surgical units resulted in decreased use of sitters but no significant decreases in falls or self-harm behavior [46]. The authors of this study noted that self-harm events were so rare that they could not perform relevant inferential statistical analyses.

A few studies highlight various process improvement measures as alternatives to the use of sitters, as opposed to implementing and examining the effects of just one intervention. Process improvement measures reported in the literature include educating staff on how to identify patients at-risk for delirium; engaging in "lightening rounds" with an attending physician, nurse, and care coordinator to develop and communicate individualized care plans; improving communication about patient behaviors through charting in electronic medical records; using psychiatric nurse liaisons to educate nursing staff about appropriate sitter use; and using sitter evaluation tools and algorithms [38, 39, 43, 47]. While these measures are indeed likely to improve the quality of care patients receive, and may even work together to reduce patient harm, studies to date appear to be mostly descriptive in nature. Thus, we cannot draw conclusions about their effects on reduction in patient harm.

With little evidence to support the use of sitters and little evidence to support alternatives to sitters, what measures can we take to improve patient safety and decrease the risk of suicide on inpatient psychiatric and medical-surgical units? As mentioned above, better education and training of sitters could improve patient safety, as well as protect sitters from potentially violent patients [48]. Finally, a paradigm shift away from research examining the relationship between intervention and sitter reduction, and toward the relationship between intervention and patient harm reduction, would be useful.

Future Directions

Many authors cite environmental safety issues, patient assessment limitations, poor staff communication, and limited staff training as critical risk factors for patient suicide [1, 6–8]. Fortunately, many of these elements are dynamic risk factors which can be changed, with appropriate effort. Thus, while we cannot "control" or "predict" patient behavior, we *can* increase patient safety by improving the patient environment and by training our staff thoroughly in assessment, communication, and safety procedures.

As we move forward in the study of suicide assessment and prevention on inpatient hospital units, it is crucial to maximize effective interventions with patients. Elements of inpatient psychiatry suicide prevention programs described in the literature include patient assessment and management, staff education/training, episodic assessment of the patient care environment (with corrections as needed), and root cause analyses (RCA) of any untoward events ([8], p. 397). These strategies, in addition to the process improvement steps noted in the section above, demonstrate how challenging it is to identify inpatient safety opportunities and create a reasonable suicide prevention programs—yet how vitally important this is for the safety and wellbeing of our patients.

Remaining tenacious about the importance of reasonable safety interventions, in the face of hospital budget cuts, staffing shortages, and administrative stressors, is a vital step toward keeping our patients safe. Providers, administrators, and patient care advocates are encouraged to work together in the spirit of excellence, to attain and maintain the highest level of safety, and to prevent the ultimate tragedy of inpatient hospital suicides.

References

1. Pompili M, Lester D, Innamorati M, Del Casale A, Girardi P, Ferracuti S, et al. Preventing suicide in jails and prisons: suggestions from experience with psychiatric inpatients. J Forensic Sci. 2009;54(5):1155–62. https://doi.org/10.1111/j.1556-4029.2009.01122.x.
2. Nichols H. The top 10 leading causes of death in the United States. 2015. http://www.medicalnewstoday.com/articles/282929.php#top_10_leading_causes_of_death. Accessed Dec 2016.
3. Shekunov J, Geske JR, Bostwick JM. Inpatient medical–surgical suicidal behavior: a 12-year case–control study. Gen Hosp Psychiatry. 2013;35(4):423–6. https://doi.org/10.1016/j.genhosppsych.2013.03.005.
4. Mills PD, Watts BV, Hemphill RR. Suicide attempts and completions on medical-surgical and intensive care units. J Hosp Med. 2014;9(3):182–5. https://doi.org/10.1002/jhm.2141.
5. Cullen SW, Marcus SC. Suicide in inpatient settings: are our hospitals safe enough? Jt Comm J Qual Saf. 2008;34(8):472–3. https://doi.org/10.1016/s1553-7250(08)34059-8.
6. Tishler CL, Reiss NS. Inpatient suicide: preventing a common sentinel event. Gen Hosp Psychiatry. 2009;31(2):103–9. https://doi.org/10.1016/j.genhosppsych.2008.09.007.
7. Russ MJ. Constant observation of suicidal patients. J Psychiatr Pract. 2016;22(5):382–8. https://doi.org/10.1097/pra.0000000000000175.
8. Jayaram G. Inpatient suicide prevention. J Psychiatr Pract. 2014;20(5):392–404. https://doi.org/10.1097/01.pra.0000453369.71092.69.
9. Hawgood J, De Leo D. Suicide prediction—a shift in paradigm is needed. Crisis. 2016;37(4):251–5. https://doi.org/10.1027/0227-5910/a000440.
10. Bolton JM, Spiwak R, Sareen J. Predicting suicide attempts with the SAD PERSONS scale. J Clin Psychiatry. 2012;73(06):e735–41. https://doi.org/10.4088/jcp.11m07362.
11. Dlugacz YD, Restifo A, Scanlon KA, Nelson K, Fried AM, Hirsch B, et al. Safety strategies to prevent suicide in multiple health care environments. Jt Comm J Qual Saf. 2003;29(6):267–78. https://doi.org/10.1016/s1549-3741(03)29031-6.
12. Powell J, Geddes J, Hawton K, Deeks J, Goldacre M. Suicide in psychiatric hospital in-patients: risk factors and their predictive power. Br J Psychiatry. 2000;176(3):266–72. https://doi.org/10.1192/bjp.176.3.266.

13. Wint DP, Akil M. Suicidality in the general hospitalized patient. Hosp Physician. 2006;42(1):13.
14. May AM, Klonsky ED. What distinguishes suicide attempters from suicide ideators? A meta-analysis of potential factors. Clin Psychol. 2016;23(1):5–20. https://doi.org/10.1111/cpsp.12136.
15. Goh SE, Salmons PH, Whittington RM. Hospital suicides: are there preventable factors? Profile of the psychiatric hospital suicide. Br J Psychiatry. 1989;154(2):247–9. https://doi.org/10.1192/bjp.154.2.247.
16. Roy A, Draper R. Suicide among psychiatric hospital in-patients. Psychol Med. 1995;25(01):199. https://doi.org/10.1017/s0033291700028233.
17. Appleby L. Suicide in psychiatric patients: risk and prevention. Br J Psychiatry. 1992;161(6):749–58. https://doi.org/10.1192/bjp.161.6.749.
18. Cassells C, Paterson B, Dowding D, Morrison R. Long- and short-term risk factors in the prediction of inpatient suicide. Crisis. 2005;26(2):53–63. https://doi.org/10.1027/0227-5910.26.2.53.
19. Suominen K, Isometsä E, Heilä H, Lönnqvist J, Henriksson M. General hospital suicides: a psychological autopsy study in Finland. Gen Hosp Psychiatry. 2002;24(6):412–6. https://doi.org/10.1016/s0163-8343(02)00222-0.
20. Cheng IC, Hu FC, Tseng MC. Inpatient suicide in a general hospital. Gen Hosp Psychiatry. 2009;31(2):110–5. https://doi.org/10.1016/j.genhosppsych.2008.12.008.
21. Bostwick JM, Rackley SJ. Completed suicide in medical/surgical patients: who is at risk? Curr Psychiatry Rep. 2007;9(3):242–6. https://doi.org/10.1007/s11920-007-0026-6.
22. Ballard ED, Pao M, Henderson D, Lee LM, Bostwick JM, Rosenstein DL. Suicide in the medical setting. Jt Comm J Qual Saf. 2008;34(8):474–81. https://doi.org/10.1016/s1553-7250(08)34060-4.
23. Busch KA, Fawcett J, Jacobs DG. Clinical correlates of inpatient suicide. J Clin Psychiatry. 2003;64(1):14–9. https://doi.org/10.4088/jcp.v64n0105.
24. Rogers ML, Ringer FB, Joiner TE. A meta-analytic review of the association between agitation and suicide attempts. Clin Psychol Rev. 2016;48:1–6. https://doi.org/10.1016/j.cpr.2016.06.002.
25. Large MM, Ryan CJ. Disturbing findings about the risk of suicide and psychiatric hospitals. Soc Psychiatry Psychiatr Epidemiol. 2014;49(9):1353–5. https://doi.org/10.1007/s00127-014-0912-2.
26. Large M, Smith G, Sharma S, Nielssen O, Singh SP. Systematic review and meta-analysis of the clinical factors associated with the suicide of psychiatric in-patients. Acta Psychiatr Scand. 2011;124(1):18–9. https://doi.org/10.1111/j.1600-0447.2010.01672.x.
27. Ryan C, Nielssen O, Paton M, Large M. Clinical decisions in psychiatry should not be based on risk assessment. Australas Psychiatry. 2010;18(5):398–403. https://doi.org/10.3109/10398562.2010.507816.
28. Lieberman DZ, Resnik HLP, Holder-Perkins V. Environmental risk factors in hospital suicide. Suicide Life Threat Behav. 2004;34(4):448–53. https://doi.org/10.1521/suli.34.4.448.53740.
29. Mills PD, DeRosier JM, Ballot BA, Shepherd M, Bagian JP. Inpatient suicide and suicide attempts in Veterans Affairs hospitals. Jt Comm J Qual Saf. 2008;34(8):482–8.
30. Spießl H, Hübner-Liebermann B, Cording C. Suicidal behaviour of psychiatric in-patients. Eur Psychiatry. 2002;17:205. https://doi.org/10.1016/s0924-9338(02)80877-x.
31. Janofsky J. Reducing inpatient suicide risk: using human factor analysis to improve observation practices. J Am Acad Psychiatry Law. 2009;37(1):15–24.
32. Mills PD, Watts BV, Miller S, Kemp J, Knox K, DeRosier JM, et al. A checklist to identify inpatient suicide hazards in Veterans Affairs hospitals. Jt Comm J Qual Saf. 2010;36(2):87–93. https://doi.org/10.1016/s1553-7250(10)36015-6.
33. Deisenhammer EA, DeCol C, Honeder M, Hinterhuber H, Fleischhacker WW. In-patient suicide in psychiatric hospitals. Acta Psychiatr Scand. 2000;102(4):290–4. https://doi.org/10.1034/j.1600-0447.2000.102004290.x.
34. Colson DB, Allen JG, Coyne L, Dexter N, Jehl N, Mayer CA, et al. An anatomy of countertransference: staff reactions to difficult psychiatric hospital patients. Psychiatr Serv. 1986;37(9):923–8. https://doi.org/10.1176/ps.37.9.923.

35. James K, Stewart D, Bowers L. Self-harm and attempted suicide within inpatient psychiatric services: a review of the literature. Int J Ment Health Nurs. 2012;21(4):301–9. https://doi.org/10.1111/j.1447-0349.2011.00794.x.
36. Environment of Care News. Suicide prevention and the inpatient room: bricks and sticks and beyond. 2008;11(12):8–11. http://www.ingentaconnect.com/contentone/jcaho/ecn/2008/00000011/00000012/art00006.
37. Manna M. Effectiveness of formal observation in inpatient psychiatry in preventing adverse outcomes: the state of the science. J Psychiatr Ment Health Nurs. 2010;17(3):268–73. https://doi.org/10.1111/j.1365-2850.2009.01512.x.
38. Laws D, Crawford CL. Alternative strategies to constant patient observation and sitters. J Nurs Adm. 2013;43(10):497–501. https://doi.org/10.1097/nna.0b013e3182a3e83e.
39. Rausch DL, Bjorklund P. Decreasing the costs of constant observation. J Nurs Adm. 2010;40(2):75–81. https://doi.org/10.1097/nna.0b013e3181cb9f56.
40. Björkdahl A, Nyberg U, Runeson B, Omérov P. The development of the suicidal patient observation chart (SPOC): Delphi study. J Psychiatr Ment Health Nurs. 2011;18(6):558–61. https://doi.org/10.1111/j.1365-2850.2011.01758.x.
41. Large M. Risk of suicidal behavior in medical–surgical settings. Gen Hosp Psychiatry. 2013;35(6):676. https://doi.org/10.1016/j.genhosppsych.2013.07.008.
42. Worley LLM, Kunkel EJS, Gitlin DF, Menefee LA, Conway G. Constant observation practices in the general hospital setting: a national survey. Psychosomatics. 2000;41(4):301–10. https://doi.org/10.1176/appi.psy.41.4.301.
43. Salamon L, Lennon M. Decreasing companion usage without negatively affecting patient outcomes: a performance improvement project. Medsurg Nurs. 2003;12(4):230–6.
44. Nadler-Moodie M, Burnell L, Fries J, Agan DL. A S.A.F.E. alternative to sitters. Nurs Manage. 2009;40(8):43–50. https://doi.org/10.1097/01.numa.0000359209.42026.e9.
45. Rachh P, Wilkins G, Capodilupo TA, Kilroy S, Schnider M, Repper-Delisi J. Redesigning the patient observer model to achieve increased efficiency and staff engagement on a surgical trauma inpatient unit. Jt Comm J Qual Saf. 2016;42(2):77–85. https://doi.org/10.1016/s1553-7250(16)42009-x.
46. Davis J, Kutash M, Whyte J IV. A comparative study of patient sitters with video monitoring versus in-room sitters. J Nurs Educ Pract. 2016;7(3):137. https://doi.org/10.5430/jnep.v7n3p137.
47. Spiva L, Feiner T, Jones D, Hunter D, Petefish J, VanBrackle L. An evaluation of a sitter reduction program intervention. J Nurs Care Qual. 2012;27(4):341–5. https://doi.org/10.1097/ncq.0b013e31825f4a5f.
48. Schoenfisch AL, Pompeii LA, Lipscomb HJ, Smith CD, Upadhyaya M, Dement JM. An urgent need to understand and address the safety and well-being of hospital "sitters". Am J Ind Med. 2015;58(12):1278–87. https://doi.org/10.1002/ajim.22529.

Gatekeeper Training to Prevent Suicide in the Emergency Department and in Primary Care

13

Glenn Albright, Jane Timmons-Mitchell and Jeremiah McMillan

Introduction

The Centers for Disease Control and Prevention (CDC) reported in 2015 that suicide was the tenth leading cause of death for all age groups [1] and among 10–34 year-olds the second leading cause of death according to 2016 CDC data [2]. The cause of suicidal ideation and behavior is complex and multifaceted, but the goal of suicide prevention is simple: to reduce risk factors and promote protective factors. Gatekeeper training has been found to be an effective training model for suicide prevention by increasing awareness of suicide and suicidal behaviors and promoting protective factors within the community as a whole [2].

Although there are a number of suicide prevention and intervention programs available, suicide remains a significant public health issue in the USA. Suicide is one of the top three causes of death for adolescents, behind only homicides and unintentional injuries [3], and one of the top ten causes of death for citizens of all

G. Albright, Ph.D. (✉)
Department of Psychology, Baruch College, City University of New York, New York, NY, USA

Kognito, New York, NY, USA
e-mail: glenn.albright@baruch.cuny.edu

J. Timmons-Mitchell, Ph.D.
Begun Center for Violence Prevention Research and Education, Jack, Joseph, and Morton Mandel School of Applied Sciences, School of Medicine, Case Western Reserve University, Cleveland, OH, USA
e-mail: jct2@case.edu

J. McMillan, B.A.
University of Georgia, Athens, GA, USA
e-mail: jmcmillan@uga.edu

T. Falcone, J. Timmons-Mitchell (eds.), *Suicide Prevention*,
https://doi.org/10.1007/978-3-319-74391-2_13

ages [1]. In recent years, interventions have included universal training of gatekeepers in various high risk settings, including middle schools and high schools, universities, and the military. The general purpose of gatekeeper programs is to train key individuals in techniques for the early identification of suicidal ideation and behavior and make appropriate follow-up service referrals [4]. Gatekeeper training is listed as a promising intervention by the Suicide Prevention Resource Center [5]. A 2005 panel report published in the *Journal of the American Medical Association (JAMA)* examined evidence for the effectiveness of suicide-preventive interventions, including gatekeeper training [6]. They concluded that in systematic evaluations of impact, decreased suicide rates could be tied to the presence of gatekeeper training.

The Gatekeeper

Kurt Lewin was the first to use the term gatekeeper [7]; at its most general, a gatekeeper is someone who controls access, to information, for example. Shoemaker and Riccio provide a modern-day description [8]. Gatekeepers reduce a large amount of potentially available information to the smaller amount of information that is readily available. Gates are decision points at which the movement of information past one gate and toward the next gate can be facilitated or hindered.

Applied to suicide prevention, a gatekeeper is an individual who can recognize when a person is manifesting signs of psychological distress including depression and suicidal ideation, approach and talk with that person about concerns, and if necessary, make an effective referral to mental health support services. The need for individuals to learn gatekeeper skills to reduce suicide is recognized internationally for the United Nations has recommended that gatekeeper training be considered an important part in implementing an effective strategy to prevent suicide worldwide [9].

Unfortunately, most gatekeeper programs are less effective than planned for they do not employ active learning strategies such as role rehearsal, in which learners practice gatekeeper skills by role-playing with an individual who is portraying himself or herself as being a distressed or suicidal person, to aid skill development in the learner [10]. Although some gatekeeper programs have demonstrated increases in knowledge and self-efficacy, relatively few studies examined changes in gatekeeper behaviors [4, 6, 11–15]. Thus, legacy gatekeeper training programs that employ traditional didactic models where knowledge is presented and learners passively accept it, such as suicide prevention placards and listening to lectures/PowerPoint presentations or webinars, should be augmented with opportunities to engage in active learning strategies where users can practice gatekeeper skills.

There has been widespread agreement based on extensive research that conversation skills such as those used by gatekeepers are best learned when knowledge is actively constructed. Active learning, or situated learning, involves learning by doing and provides agency that allows the brain to make meaningful connections through physical, embodied experiences that are as authentic as possible to the context where the learning will be applied. There are hundreds of journal articles including meta-analytic studies that examine the impact of active learning strategies as applied to multiple disciplines, and for our purpose, we will address how newly developed virtual role-play simulations that integrate situated learning strategies are being used to teach gatekeeping skills to primary care professionals (PCP) and emergency department personnel (EDP).

Innovative Virtual Human Gatekeeper Simulation Technology

Recent developments in simulation and gaming technology and research into the efficacy of gatekeeper simulations have demonstrated effective use of virtual humans as an alternative to the traditional, live role-play methodology. These developments eliminate many of the barriers seen in face-to-face training. An example is Kognito's *At-Risk in Primary Care* and *At-Risk in the ED*: two simulations that were designed using a proprietary game-based Kognito Conversation Platform™, a new and innovative group of development, delivery, API, data collection, and analytic technologies integrated with components of neuroscience, social cognition, adult learning, applied game mechanics, and storytelling. These simulations are built around a series of game-based mini-conversation role-plays where users interact with emotionally responsive, fully animated virtual patients that have memory and personality and will react like real patients experiencing mental health disorders, including depression and thoughts of suicide.

Advantages of Virtual Humans

Virtual humans are defined as automated, three-dimensional agents that converse, understand, reason, and exhibit emotions (see Illustration 13.1). Their use has many educational and economic advantages allowing users to practice how to leverage conversations and drive meaningful change in behaviors and attitudes. Role-playing with virtual humans decreases the likelihood of negative transference reactions or the user feeling embarrassed or judged which often happens in live role-plays especially in the presence of peers [16, 17]. Both negative emotions in general and social evaluative threat in particular are known to impede cognitive performance, learning, and retention [18–24].

Learning through role-play with trained instructors has been widely used in health and behavioral health education. However, the cost and logistics of organizing live role-plays with trained actors (or standardized patients) to assess and teach communication skills is often prohibited. Other barriers facing live role-plays include addressing the challenge of standardizing the learning experience, and the discomfort participants often experience when role-playing in a workshop setting. Recent development and research into the efficacy of virtual humans as an alternative to the traditional, live role-play methodology provides an opportunity to eliminate these barriers. This alternative also has been shown to provide a highly effective learning experience (described later) building and assessing communication and conversation competencies in a digital, standardized, and risk-free medium that is available 24/7.

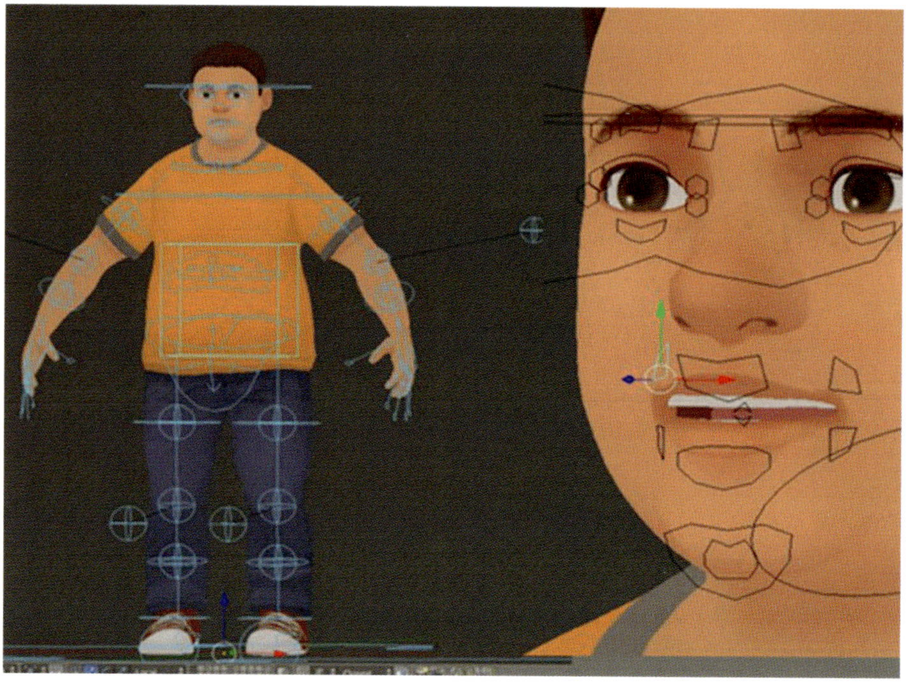

Illustration 13.1 Virtual humans are defined as automated, three-dimensional agents that converse, understand, reason, and exhibit emotions. Character from the simulation "Change Talk: Childhood Obesity." An initiative of the American Academy of Pediatrics Institute for Healthy Childhood and Kognito

Another advantage is that virtual humans are coded to support high fidelity of the learning experience. Fidelity refers to the quality of delivery across all trainers so there is a high standardization of the learning experience each time, including accurate knowledge dissemination, realistic and engaging role-plays, and appropriate feedback. This in part is due to the simulation being computer-delivered and not possible to modify the content and its delivery. Also, complex algorithms that drive multiple decision trees are incorporated such that selecting a particular conversation tactic to discuss with the virtual patient will result in an appropriate follow-up Thus, content available is uniform across participants and administrations. As data presented later in this chapter will indicate, the fidelity of the PCP and EDP simulations is very high due to the consistent delivery of accurate knowledge, realistic and engaging role-plays, and appropriate feedback. Adding to the fidelity is that virtual humans do not fatigue, have a neutral appearance, are not subject to trainer bias, and will continually respond in the most efficacious way to promote skill development. The high standardization and replicability is also due in part to the comprehensive and iterative development process involving nationally recognized subject matter experts and a variety of end users, whereas face-to-face training depends on the skill and experience of each individual trainer and his/her knowledge of the population and culture being trained. Not surprisingly, such skills and experience can vary from

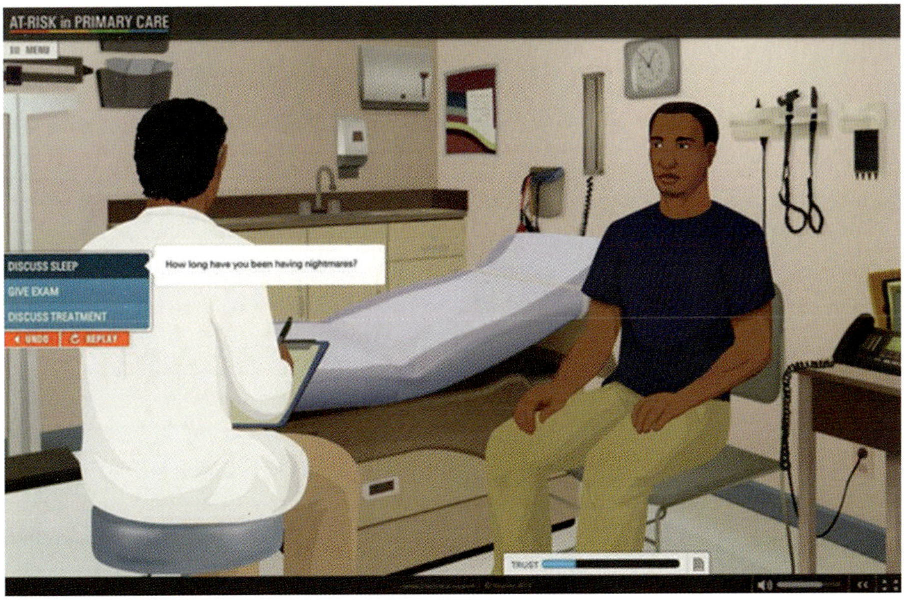

Illustration 13.2 Screenshot of a virtual role-play conversation with Antoine, a patient in *At-Risk in Primary Care*

person to person which can compromise the learning experience. Users also find it easier to talk to, develop a rapport with, feel safer and less judged when interacting with virtual humans [25, 26]. Since there is little fear of making mistakes, especially when practicing in the privacy of one's home or office, the learning experience is reinforced. In fact, it is not unusual for curious learners to retake the simulation and on purpose, choose the wrong communication tactics to observe patient responses, which further reinforces the learning experience. Lastly, the appearance and voice/language of the virtual human can be customized to each user and conversation setting to provide a high level of personalization, localization, and cultural appropriateness. These factors make digital simulations appropriate alternatives or supplements to traditional workshops and other non-interactive learning experiences.

How the Simulation Works

In the simulations, learners assume the role of a virtual PCP or EDP and must use motivational interviewing (MI) conversation skills (i.e., open-ended questions and reflective listening), empathy, and mindfulness in order to gain patient trust so that they will open up and provide more information (learning model described later). Learners communicate by selecting from a dynamic menu of dialogue options that represent a variety of effective, neutral, and ineffective conversation tactics (see Illustration 13.2). In some cases, a tactic that is ineffective at one point in the conversation may be effective elsewhere. Once learners choose a dialogue option, they see their virtual patient "perform" the dialogue and then observe the verbal and nonverbal responses of the virtual patient. A new set of dialogue options then appears, based on tactic selected. In some cases, a patient trust meter provides continual feedback based on the choices made by the learner as he or she progresses through the simulation. If the learner selects choices that include being judgmental or labeling, the trust meter will decrease, and learners will find it harder to complete the simulation within an allotted time frame.

Throughout the simulation, learners can occasionally view the patient's inner thoughts, which are designed to provide greater insight, understanding, and opportunities to practice empathic communication skills. Additionally, a virtual coach provides personalized feedback and gives users an opportunity to revise or undo their conversation tactic choice. Lastly, the relationship between the user's dialogue decision and the response of the emotionally responsive virtual humans are controlled by a set of mathematical behavioral models and algorithms specifically designed to simulate real interactions with patient types that represent particular personality traits or conditions. These algorithms ensure that users are repeatedly exposed to target conversation and behavior patterns as a way to develop skills and knowledge. To successfully complete the conversation, users must apply effective conversation tactics and adapt their decisions based on the virtual human's behavior.

Lastly, the simulation provides learners with opportunities to engage in sustained and deliberate practice in an environment that is visually and mechanically congruous with the setting in which learners will apply their skills in real settings (situated learning). Deliberate practice intends to improve real-world performance [26] by offering a challenge to learners' existing skills, a simulated environment that allows users to experiment with various techniques with no fear of the consequences real humans might experience, a protected environment with no fear of judgment from observers or patients (as opposed to live role-play with peers or standardized patients), time for users to reflect on their skills and adjust their strategies, and continuous analysis of performance through simulation features (e.g., a meter representing patient's current level of trust) and through individualized and immediate feedback from a virtual coach throughout the simulation. Evidence shows that practitioners' communication skills improve and endure when training incorporates deliberate practice, ongoing tailored feedback, and role-plays and establishes a connection between new skills learned such as those used in motivational interviewing and their application in live settings [27]. To the author's knowledge, there are no other conversation simulations within the field of medical education that integrate virtual human role-plays, game mechanics, and MI strategies to teach communication skills. Additionally, the increased functionality of the simulation including having access to a patient's inner thoughts, the trust meter and being able to undo conversation tactics to try new ones has yet to be duplicated.

Both the PCP and EDP simulations are listed in Section III of the SPRC/AFSP Best Practices Registry for Suicide Prevention and approved for 1.50 *CME AMA PRA Category 1 Credits*™ and 1.50 ANCC CNE contact hour. PCP is also listed in the Substance Abuse and Mental Health Services Administration's National Registry of Evidence-Based Programs and Practices (NREPP). The simulations take between 1

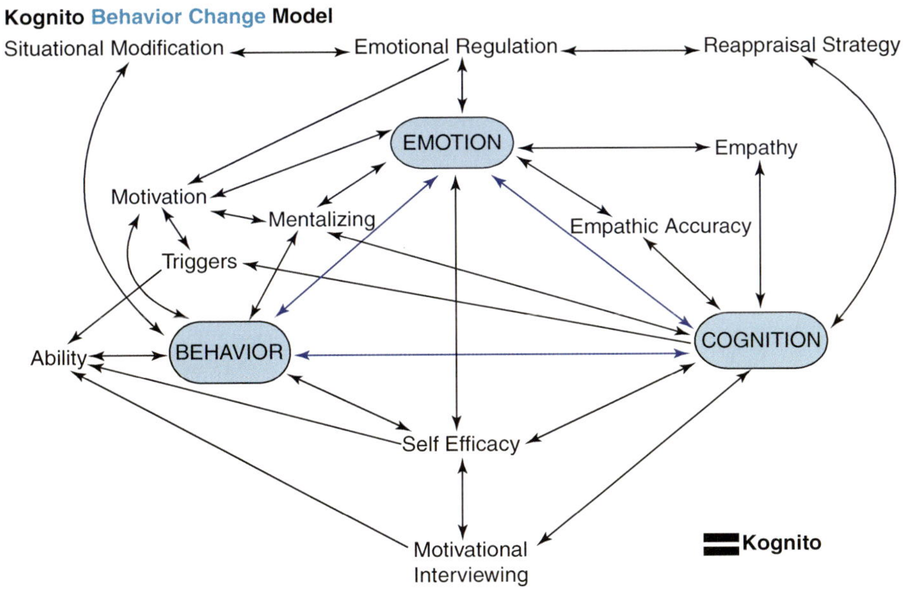

Illustration 13.3 Conversation components of the Kognito Behavior Change Model

and 1.5 h to complete and are self-paced (users can complete the simulation in multiple sittings) and available to each user online 24/7.

Kognito Behavior Change Model

To be effective, gatekeeper simulations need to employ instructional design components that motivate the learner to use evidence-based communication strategies to manage what can be difficult patient conversations about suicide. Thus, in teaching individuals to manage collaborative conversations with patients, a behavior change model was integrated into the Kognito Conversation Platform™ that drives the PCP and EDP simulations (see Illustration 13.3). This model involves several constructs to maximize skill acquisition and includes the following components:

Cognitive Load: According to cognitive load theory, the processing capabilities of the brain's short-term or working memory are limited, and in order for patients and healthcare providers to effectively engage in conversations about suicide risk, you want to minimize extraneous thoughts and concerns in working memory to increase processing capability [28]. The gatekeeper conversation and associated information that accompanies such a conversation must be presented in such a way as to reduce unnecessary cognitive load which on the patient's end means recognizing that their working memory is being inundated with competing information ranging from presenting physical complaint(s), anxious thoughts, predisposed beliefs/attitudes/stigma about mental health, cultural concerns, and other pertinent historical experiences. This competing information can compromise their ability to attend, comprehend, and ultimately adhere to treatment recommendations. Additionally, the working memory of the PCP or EDP is being loaded by their perceptions, beliefs, awareness of time being spent, patient backlog, etc., all of which can interfere with one's ability to implement effective gatekeeper conversation tactics. The simulations discussed in this chapter are designed to give the healthcare professional the practice and ultimately the skill to prevent cognitive overload or to observe when it is happening and correct for it by meeting the patient at their level of knowledge, understanding, and functioning. The evidence-based conversation strategies that facilitate this process are described below which are integrated into the simulation's Conversation Platform™ and include:

Motivational Interviewing (MI): MI is a set of communication strategies originally designed by clinical psychologists for use in counseling sessions with problem drinkers [29]. MI is a goal-oriented, person-centered counseling approach designed to help people resolve their ambivalence about behavior change. By strategically evoking the patient's own thoughts and feelings, the healthcare professional facilitates the safe exploration in managing a conversation about suicide risk [30]. MI skills are quite intuitive yet take practice to use them in an effective and time-conscious manner. The four core MI communication skills are:

(a) *Ask open-ended questions* to invite the patient to share their thoughts while focusing the conversation in a particular direction.
(b) *Affirm* the patient's strengths, values, or efforts. This builds trust and instills the power to change.
(c) Listen closely and *reflect* the patient's statements to selectively emphasize them and confirm understanding.
(d) *Summarize* what the patient has told you to show that you're listening, link to related information, or transition to a new topic.

Mentalizing: Mentalizing, also known as "theory of mind," is the ability to attribute intentions and other mental states to other beings [31]. Neuroimaging research has identified a network of brain regions involved in mentalizing. This network includes portions of the medial prefrontal cortex and the temporal lobes [32]. While all healthy adults understand that other beings have independent minds, both the inclination to attend to the minds of others and the ability to accurately assess what others think or know vary among individuals. Thus, mentalizing is the ability to recognize and accept nonjudgmentally or non-critically that patients have their own thoughts, beliefs, intentions, and emotions which may differ from one's own and is crucial for effective interactions. Practicing mindfulness has been shown to lead to better mental health outcomes [33–35].

Empathy: Empathy is the capacity to feel the emotions of another person [36, 37]. In most cases, an empathic response is incumbent on mentalizing, in that one is unlikely to experience the emotions of another if one fails to consider that other as an autonomous agent capable of independent thoughts and feelings [32]. In fact, neuroimaging research has shown that mentalizing and empathy rely on overlapping yet distinct brain networks [38]. While both showed activity in many of the typical mentalizing areas, including prefrontal and temporal regions, empathy uniquely showed increases in areas of the brain associated with emotional experience and assessment, including the anterior cingulate and the amygdala. An intact empathic response is important for healthy social and emotional functioning. There are numerous studies on the impact of empathy in medical practice including increases in patient satisfaction, reduced stress, adherence to treatment recommendations, and improved health outcomes [39, 40]. High-empathic individuals have been found to be more altruistic, less aggressive [41], more likely to engage in prosocial behavior, and more socially competent [42], all of which can build patient trust. Lastly, research has shown that empathic responsiveness can be enhanced through training [43–45].

Empathic Accuracy (EA): EA also sometimes described as "cognitive empathy" is the ability to correctly assess or identify the emotions of another and in this case, patients [46]. This skill may be thought of as the ability to "read people." EA and empathy are conceptually distinct for empathy does not necessarily imply the ability to accurately identify a shared emotion and EA does not necessarily require that one feel the emotions of another. However, research has shown a bidirectional relationship between empathy and EA, as long as there is sufficient expression [47]. EA also varies across individuals, and high EA is predictive of healthy interpersonal relationships [48, 49] thus relating to building patient trust. Neuroimaging research has found that EA relies not only on the medial prefrontal and temporal regions associated with mentalizing but also on structures within the human mirror neuron system thought to be involved in shared sensorimotor representations [50]. Lastly, EA has shown that it can be improved with training [37].

Situation Modification (SM): SM is when either the patient or healthcare professional attempts to avoid, leave, or modify conversations that are likely to elicit unwanted emotions and to enter into a conversation that is likely to elicit desired emotions [51]. Although situational modification is an understandable response in conversations involving suicide risk, it is best to recognize when it is happening and not let it sidetrack the purpose of the discussion.

Reappraisal Strategy (RS): RS is when one changes the way they interpret the meaning of a stimulus [52, 53]. For example, rather than view a patient who discloses thoughts of suicide as weak, it can be seen as a strength and an appropriate call for help. Reappraisal is an especially important strategy, as it has been shown to have lasting effects on the way in which one responds to an emotional stimulus. The tendency to reappraise is correlated with improved mental health, social functioning, and well-being [54, 55].

Outcome Studies

There have been many outcome studies that examine the impact of gatekeeper simulations that are based on the behavior change model described above. Below we summarize the results of two studies, one on *At-Risk in Primary Care* [56] and the other on *At-Risk in the ED* [57].

At-Risk in Primary Care Study

In this study, 614 participants were placed in either the treatment or control group. As would be expected from the random assignment design, the control group and treatment group did not differ significantly on gender, race, work role, years of experience, or previous training for mental health screening (all χ^2 test significance values were greater than $p = 0.05$), nor did they differ on initial knowledge and skills or likelihood (both *t*-test significance values were greater than $p = 0.05$). Participants in the treatment group first took a pre-training survey, completed the training simulation, and then completed a post-training survey. Participants in the control group completed the pre-training survey for comparison purposes.

Measures

All measures were included in the pre-training and post-training surveys, with the exception of means efficacy which was only included in the post-training survey.

Knowledge and skills were assessed using a Likert scale designed for this study pertaining to general abilities and preparedness to deal with mental health issues within the patient population (Cronbach's $\alpha = 0.96$). A composite score was created by averaging the six items in this scale.

Likelihood to screen and manage mental health issues was also assessed using the single item: "How likely are you to screen and manage the treatment of patients that exhibit signs and symptoms of trauma-related mental health disorders when visiting your primary care practice?"

Means efficacy is a measure of an individual's belief in the utility of the tools available for performing a job and has been correlated with changes in behavior [58]. It was measured by seven Likert scale items administered in the posttest.

Gatekeeper behavior was measured 3 months after completing the simulation and was comprised of self-reported impact of the simulation on relevant behaviors.

Evaluation of *At-Risk in Primary Care*

The main set of statistical analyses consisted of evaluating knowledge and skills as well as likelihood to screen and manage mental health issues that were defined within the survey as mental health disorders such as alcohol and substance abuse, depression, generalized anxiety disorder, and post-traumatic stress disorder. Knowledge and skills of the treatment group measured in the post-training survey were significantly higher than the control group ($p < 0.001$). Note that there was no significant difference when comparing the treatment group pre-training to the control group ($p = 0.55$). The results of this quasi-experimental design study were analyzed using either an independent sample *t*-test or a two-way ANOVA and are summarized in Table 13.1.

Table 13.1 Summary of results from *At-Risk in Primary Care*: A professional development simulation for primary care professionals on how to conduct screening, brief interventions, and referral to treatment with patients suffering from substance use, depression, anxiety, and PTSD [56]

Simulation goals	Sample size and demographics	Results
1. Recognize risk factors and warning signs of alcohol and substance use, depression, and suicidal thoughts	$N = 614$ Gender 79%—Female 11%—Male Race/ethnicity White—73.6% Black—7.3% Hispanic—10.4% American Indian/ Alaska Native—0.9% Asian—5.2% Multiple ethnicities—2.6%	Satisfaction data: 94% said they would recommend to colleague; 99% said they would recommend to fellow nursing or medical students; 97% stated the simulation enhanced their skill as a healthcare professional; 86% rated the simulation as "excellent" to "very good" Statistically significant ($p < 0.001$) changes in knowledge and skill to (1) identify risk factors and warning signs of behavioral health disorders, (2) recognize when a patient is exhibiting signs and symptoms, (3) screen patients for behavioral health disorders, (4) discuss treatment options, (5) engage in collaborative decision-making about treatment plans, and (6) build intrinsic motivation in patients to adhere to the suggested treatment plan
2. Conduct brief interventions using motivational interviewing to build patients' motivation and increase protective behaviors	Participants recruited from six different states in the Midwest, Southwest, and Northeast regions of the USA	Behavior change: 3-month self-reported follow-up data revealed that participants either agreed or strongly agreed that as a result of the simulation, there was an increase in the number of at-risk patients they: • Identified—51% • Screened—60% • Discussed treatment options with—58% • Engaged in collaborative decision-making about treatment plans—53%
3. Engage in collaborative treatment planning with patients	Work role 35%—Nurse 11%—Doctor 17%—Nursing or medical student 21%—Mental health or social worker	
4. Refer patients to treatment services and follow-up on referrals	Industry experience Mean = 7.4 years (9.87) Received prior training for screening mental health disorders—55.3%	

Table 13.2 Means efficacy items for at-risk in primary care—percentage of participants who endorsed each option

	Not at all/ very little	A little	Some	Greatly	Very greatly
Please indicate to what extent you think that the course is:					
A useful tool	0.5%	0.9%	15.3%	54.1%	29.3%
Well constructed	0.0%	0.9%	7.7%	55.9%	35.6%
Easy to use	0.0%	0.5%	8.6%	51.4%	39.6%
Relevant to your patient population	1.4%	3.2%	15.3%	50.9%	29.3%
Helpful in learning how to identify and manage the care of patients with trauma-related mental health disorders	0.5%	1.8%	18.9%	52.7%	26.1%
Helpful in learning effective conversation tactics to increase patient engagement, trust, and adherence to treatment plans	0.5%	2.3%	14.9%	52.7%	29.7%
Realistic representations of conversations you have or may have with your patients	0.9%	1.8%	21.6%	48.2%	27.5%

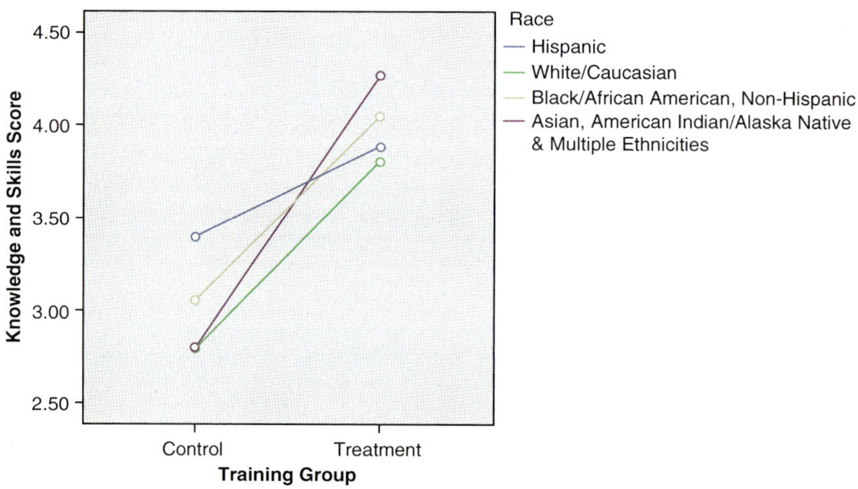

Fig. 13.1 Knowledge and skills by race and training group

Means Efficacy

All measures of means efficacy were high for the trainings were rated as being a useful tool, well constructed, easy to use, and helpful in learning how to identify and manage the care of patients with mental health disorders and in using effective conversation tactics to increase patient engagement, trust, and adherence to treatment plans (see Table 13.2).

A second set of analyses was conducted to determine if participant ethnicity/race moderated the relationship between condition and outcomes. A two-way ANOVA determined that participant race did not interact significantly with treatment group for likelihood of helping behaviors. However, there was a significant interaction between participant race and treatment group for the knowledge and skills composite score ($p < 0.05$). See Fig. 13.1 for a graphical representation of the interaction effect. Post hoc pairwise comparisons revealed that, within each racial/ethnic group, the control and treatment means were significantly different (Bonferroni-corrected $p < 0.05$ in all four cases). The source of the interaction seems to be a significant difference between Hispanics and Whites in the control group but no significant difference in the treatment group, resulting in differential amounts of improvement but ultimately similar outcomes on average. Additionally, Whites and "Other" (i.e., Asian, American Indian/Alaska Native, or multiple ethnicities) are not different in the control condition but Other is significantly higher than Whites in the treatment condition. These results suggest that training was effective for all four groups but is most efficacious for those in the Other category. An important caveat in interpreting these results is the difference in sample sizes. The total sample sizes for the control group for Whites, Hispanics, Blacks, and Other are as follows: 160, 18, 18, and 16. The total sample sizes for the treatment group for Whites, Hispanics, Blacks, and Other are as follows: 153, 26, 13, and 21.

Student Status as a Moderator

Because many of the participants in this study were students, we were interested in determining if student status would moderate the impact of the training simulation. Thus, we ran two two-way ANOVAs with the likelihood and the knowledge and

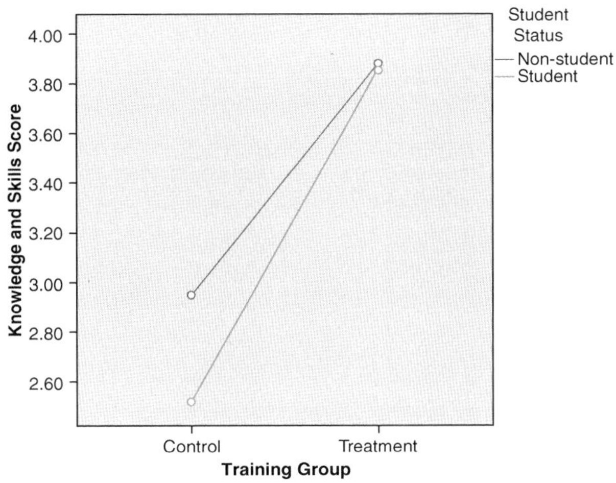

Fig. 13.2 Knowledge and skills by student status and training group

skills composite score as dependent variables. While there was no significant interaction between student status and treatment condition ($p > 0.05$) on likelihood, there was a significant interaction between student status and treatment group on knowledge and skills ($p < 0.05$). An illustration of this interaction (Fig. 13.2) suggests that the source of the effect is from differences between students in the control group, whereby non-students score higher on knowledge and skills, but these differences are minimized after training.

The Role of Completion Time and Fidelity

Completion time from beginning of the pretest to end of the posttest differed widely among participants. Median completion time was 166 min, while mean completion time was 4370 min; many participants took several days to complete the entire process, indicating that they did not complete it in a single sitting. Thus, it was important to evaluate if this variable might be associated with the impact of the training simulation. Treatment group participants were grouped into two categories: (1) those who completed the entire study in less than 4 h—considered to be the upper limit of a reasonable completion time—"short completers" ($n = 123$) and (2) those who completed it in greater than 4 h, "long completers" ($n = 99$). Independent sample t-tests for both likelihood of helping behaviors and knowledge and skills (composite score and all individual items) indicated no significant differences between short completers and long completers (all $ps > 0.6$). Thus, evidence suggests that the training simulation is equally effective regardless of time to complete the pretest—training simulation—posttest process. This also suggests that the fidelity of the simulation was maintained in light of the different completion times.

Discussion

Regarding the effectiveness of the *At-Risk in Primary Care* intervention, when compared to the control group, participants in the training group improved significantly on all knowledge and skills and likelihood-dependent measures. This included (1) identifying risk factors and warning signs of mental health disorders, (2) recognizing when a patient is exhibiting signs and symptoms of mental health disorders, (3) screening patients for mental health disorders, (4) discussing treatment options with patients exhibiting signs and symptoms of mental health disorders, (5) engaging in collaborative decision-making about treatment plans with patients exhibiting signs and symptoms of mental health disorders, (6) building intrinsic motivation in patients with mental health disorders to adhere to your suggested treatment plan, and (7) likelihood to screen and manage the treatment of patients that exhibit signs and symptoms of mental health disorders. Furthermore, even though students started out lower in their knowledge and skills when compared to non-students, they also benefited more, which suggests the simulation might be particularly useful for this population.

The results also showed that participants endorsed a high level of means efficacy with relation to the intervention. Most participants find the training to be useful, realistic, and helpful in learning new valuable skills. Lastly, at a 3-month follow-up, a large number of the training group participants reported that as a result of the intervention, there were increases in the number of at-risk patients identified, screened, discussed treatment options with, and engaged in collaborative decision-making about treatment plans.

At-Risk in the ED Study

In this study, 1707 participants completed the *At-Risk in the ED* simulation. Of those, 89 matched samples from five states completed all three surveys, the pre-, post-, and follow-up. All participants were recruited by email from a hospital or medical school administrator. Participants completed a pre-simulation survey, followed by the *At-Risk in the ED* simulation, then the post-simulation survey, and 3 months later, the follow-up survey.

Measures

All the surveys included the 11-item Gatekeeper Behavior Scale (GBS), a validated tool that has been used to assess the impact of online virtual human gatekeeper training simulations [59]. The GBS's items measure attitudes and intentions drawn from major theories of motivation that have been shown to predict changes in behavior [60]. This includes assessing three dimensions or subscales: learner preparedness, likelihood, and self-efficacy to engage in gatekeeper behaviors. The GBS's construct and content validity was assessed via confirmatory factor analysis (CFA). Criterion validity was examined via correlations with behavioral measures, and convergent validity was assessed via correlations with similar but distinct constructs. The three factor CFA model showed all subscale items correlated highly with theoretical constructs ($r \geq 0.84$, $p < 0.001$). The full 11-item GBS was found to have high internal consistency ($\alpha = 0.93$). Criterion-related validity for likelihood to discuss concerns significantly related to actually approaching people that they believe are in psychological distress ($r = 0.219$, $p < 0.001$). Likelihood to refer someone to psychological services significantly correlated with the actual number of people referred ($r = 0.235$, $p < 0.001$). Convergent validity was established via a robust correlation between self-efficacy in motivating someone to seek help and general self- efficacy ($r = 0.519$, $p < 0.001$). For this study, the GBS was slightly modified by changing the items to focus on suicide risk and substance abuse as opposed to more general psychological distress. We also added preparedness and self-efficacy items to assess non-gatekeeper learning objectives.

The preparedness survey items were based on Likert scale prefaced by the phrase "A patient is admitted into the ED with a non-mental health complaint (such as a bone fracture). How would your preparedness to recognize when a patient's:" (1)

behavior is a sign of suicide risk/substance abuse, (2) physical appearance is a sign of suicide risk/substance abuse, and (3) emotional state is a sign of suicide risk/substance abuse. Other items included how prepared are you to (4) screen patients for suicide risk/substance abuse, (5) discuss with a patient your concern about signs of suicide risk/substance abuse, (6) decide on next steps for patients who screen positive for suicide risk/substance abuse, (7) conduct a brief intervention with a patient who screens positive for suicide risk/substance abuse, (8) make an appropriate referral to treatment for a patient who screens positive for suicide risk/substance abuse, and (9) adequately document your screening and referral of patients for suicide risk/substance abuse.

The likelihood or behavioral intent items were also based on a Likert scale and included (1) how likely are you to discuss with a patient your concern about signs of suicide risk/substance abuse and (2) how likely are you to conduct a brief intervention and referral with a patient who screens positive for suicide risk/substance abuse.

The self-efficacy Likert scale items included statements beginning with "I feel confident in my ability to" (1) discuss my concerns with an ED patient exhibiting signs of suicide risk/substance abuse, (2) screen ED patients for suicide risk/substance abuse, (3) make an appropriate referral of an ED patient exhibiting signs of suicide risk/substance abuse, and (4) conduct a brief intervention with a patient who screens positive for suicide risk/substance abuse.

To determine impact on ED behavior, participants responded to a follow-up survey where they were asked to respond via a 4-point Likert scale ranging from strongly disagree to strongly agree to the following items prefaced by the statement "As a result of taking the *At-Risk in the ED* simulation, there has been an increase in the number of patients that I have:" (1) recognized as exhibiting signs of substance abuse, (2) discussed my concerns with about substance abuse, (3) screened for substance abuse, (4) referred for substance abuse treatment, (5) recognized as exhibiting signs of suicide risk, (6) discussed my concerns with about suicide risk, (7) screened for suicide risk, and (8) referred for suicide risk treatment.

Evaluation of *At-Risk in the ED*

In this study, three composite variables were formed that included the attitudinal measures of preparedness, likelihood, and self-efficacy for both suicide risk and substance abuse. Summary ANOVA results from a within-group longitudinal study design (pre- and post-simulation surveys and 1-month follow-up survey) are summarized in Table 13.3.

Means Efficacy

All measures of means efficacy were high for the trainings and were rated as being a useful tool, well constructed, easy to use, likely to help you help ED patients exhibiting signs of substance abuse, likely to help you help ED patients exhibiting

Table 13.3 Summary of results from *At-Risk in the ED*: A professional development simulation to prepare emergency department personnel on how to screen for risk of suicide and substance use and conduct brief interventions [57]

Simulation goals	Sample size and demographics	Results
Recognize and screen patients at risk for suicide substance use	*N* = 1707 *N* = 89 matched samples (completed all three surveys) Gender Female—84% Male—16% Race/ethnicity White—89% Black—4.9% Hispanic—10.8% American Indian/ Alaska Native—3.3% Asian—5.0%	Satisfaction data: Participants gave the learning experience highly positive ratings—97% said they would recommend it to a colleague, and all participants rated the course as good (9.5%), very good (45.9%), or excellent (43.2%) Longitudinal data showed statistically significant ($p < 0.001$) and sustained increases from pre-survey to 3-month follow-up measures in participant's preparedness and self-efficacy composite scores to (1) recognize, (2) screen, (3) discuss concerns and next steps with patients who screen positive, (4) conduct a brief intervention, (5) make an appropriate referral, and (6) adequately document screening and referral for patients at risk for substance use and suicide. Participants also reported statistically significant ($p < 0.001$) increases in the likelihood that they will discuss concerns and conduct brief interventions and referrals with a patient that screens positive for suicide risk and substance use
1. Conduct brief interventions using motivational interviewing to build patients' trust and motivation and to increase compliance to treatment plans	Participants recruited by email from hospital or medical school administrators from five sites	Behavior change: 3-month self-reported follow-up data revealed that participants either agreed or strongly agreed that as a result of the simulation, there was an increase in the number of patients they: • Recognized as exhibiting signs of substance abuse—80%. • Discussed concerns with about substance abuse—75% • Screened for substance abuse—74% • Referred for substance abuse treatment—70% • Recognized as exhibiting signs of suicide risk—76% • Discussed my concerns about suicide risk—78% • Screened for suicide risk—79% • Referred for suicide risk treatment—72%

(continued)

Table 13.3 (continued)

Simulation goals	Sample size and demographics	Results
2. Engage in collaborative treatment planning with patients	Work role	
	46.5%—Nurse	
	2.1%—Doctor	
	45.0%—Nursing student	
	0.9%—Medical student	
	3.4%—Social worker	
	1.6%—Nurse practitioner	
3. Refer patients to treatment services and document screening and referral	Received prior training in:	
	43%—Suicide risk screening	
	34%—Substance abuse training	

Table 13.4 Means efficacy items for *At-Risk in the ED*—percentage of participants who endorsed each option

	Not at all/very little	A little	Some	Greatly	Very greatly
Please indicate to what extent you think that the course is:					
A useful tool	0.0%	1.9%	11.3%	56.6%	30.2%
Well constructed	0.0%	3.8%	11.3%	50.9%	34.0%
Easy to use	0.0%	5.7%	9.4%	43.4%	41.5%
Likely to help you help ED patients exhibiting signs of substance abuse	0.0%	3.8%	13.2%	52.8%	30.2%
Likely to help you help ED patients exhibiting signs of suicide risk	0.0%	3.8%	11.3%	52.8%	32.1%
Based on scenarios that are relevant to you and your patients	0.0%	3.8%	7.7%	55.8%	32.7%

signs of suicide risk, and based on scenarios that are relevant to you and your patients (see Table 13.4).

Discussion

Regarding the effectiveness of the *At-Risk in ED* interventions, participants showed significant and sustained increases in preparedness and self-efficacy to (1) recognize, (2) screen, and (3) discuss concerns and next steps with patients who are at risk for suicide or substance use. Additionally, there were significant increases in (4) conducting brief interventions, making an appropriate referral, and adequately documenting screening and referral for patients at risk for suicide risk and substance use. Participants also reported significant increases in likelihood or behavioral intent to discuss concern and conduct a brief intervention and referral with a patient that screens positive for suicide risk and substance use. Lastly, a large number of participants reported at the 3-month follow-up that as a result of the simulation, there were increases in the number of patients (1) recognized as exhibiting signs of suicide risk or substance abuse, (2) discussed concerns with about suicide risk or substance abuse, (3) screened for suicide risk or substance abuse, and (4) referred for suicide risk or substance abuse treatment.

Conclusion

The simulations described above show great promise in augmenting suicide prevention efforts into primary care and the emergency department. There are numerous advantages in implementing these types of simulations that go well beyond detecting and referring those at risk. In a broader sense, digital learning experiences such as *At-Risk in Primary Care and the ED* demonstrate a capability to address major health and public health concerns where effectively managing conversations are necessary to bring about changes in attitudes and behaviors. Whether online or mobile, innovative use of simulation technology increases participant engagement so learners not only enjoy the experience but also find themselves transformed from passive receivers to active constructors of the learning experience. In conclusion, the authors are truly excited about the possibilities of reaching large numbers of geographically dispersed PCPs and EDs that often serve vulnerable populations to bring about positive changes in people's lives.

Additional research is needed involving randomized controlled trials that examine the actual number of patients identified, screened, and referred as well as the impact on health outcomes of these patients. Lastly, research is needed to compare the efficacy of simulated role-plays with face-to-face and other methods used to teach gatekeeper skills.

References

1. Centers for Disease Control and Prevention. Web-based Self Injury Statistics Query and Reporting System https://www.cdc.gov/nchs/data/nvsr/nvsr66/nvsr66_06.pdf/.
2. Chagnon F, Houle J, Marcoux I, Renaud J. Control-group study of an intervention training program for youth suicide prevention. Suicide Life Threat Behav. 2007;37(2):135–44. https://doi.org/10.1521/suli.2007.37.2.135.
3. US Surgeon General, National Action Alliance for Suicide Prevention. National strategy for suicide prevention: goals and objectives for action, 212. Washington, DC: HHS; 2012. http://www.surgeongeneral.gov/library/reports/national-strategy-suicide-prevention/index.html.
4. Wyman PA, Brown CH, Inman J, Cross W, Schmeelk-Cone K, Guo J, et al. Randomized trial of a gatekeeper program for suicide prevention: 1-year impact on secondary school staff. J Consult Clin Psychol. 2008 Feb;76(1):104. https://doi.org/10.1037/0022- 006X.76.1.104.
5. Suicide Prevention Resource Center. Best practices registry section III adherence to standard QPR (Question Persuade Refer). Waltham, MA: Suicide Prevention Resource Center; 2013.

6. Mann JJ, Apter A, Bertolote J, Beautrais A, Currier D, Haas A, et al. Suicide prevention strategies: a systematic review. JAMA. 2005;294(16):2064–74. https://doi.org/10.1001/jama.294.16.2064.
7. Lewin K. Forces behind food habits and methods of change. Bull Natl Res Council. 1943;108(1043):35–65.
8. Shoemaker PJ, Riccio JR. Gatekeepeing. New York: John Wiley & Sons; 1991. https://doi.org/10.1002/9781118541555.wbiepc202.
9. United Nations Department for Policy Coordination and Sustainable Development. Prevention of suicide: guidelines for the formulation and implementation of national strategies. New York: United Nations; 1996.
10. Cross WF, Seaburn D, Gibbs D, Schmeelk-Cone K, White AM, Caine ED. Does practice make perfect? A randomized control trial of behavioral rehearsal on suicide prevention gatekeeper skills. J Prim Prev. 2011;32(3–4):195. https://doi.org/10.1007/s10935011- 0250-z.
11. Aseltine RH Jr, DeMartino R. An outcome evaluation of the SOS suicide prevention program. Am J Public Health. 2004;94(3):446–51. https://doi.org/10.2105/AJPH.94.3.446.
12. Cross W, Matthieu MM, Lezine D, Knox KL. Does a brief suicide prevention gatekeeper training program enhance observed skills? Crisis. 2010;31:149–59. https://doi.org/10.1027/0227-5910/a000014.
13. Isaac M, Elias B, Katz LY, Belik SL, Deane FP, Enns MW, et al. Gatekeeper training as a preventative intervention for suicide: a systematic review. Can J Psychiatr. 2009;54(4):260–8.
14. Kalafat J, Gagliano C. The use of simulations to assess the impact of an adolescent suicide response curriculum. Suicide Life Threat Behav. 1996;26(4):359–64. https://doi.org/10.1111/j.1943- 278X.
15. Schurtz DR, Cerel J, Rodgers P. Myths and facts about suicide from individuals involved in suicide prevention. Suicide Life Threat Behav. 2010;40(4):346–52. https://doi.org/10.1521/suli.2010.40.4.346.
16. Nestel D, Tierney T. Role-play for medical students learning about communication: guidelines for maximising benefits. BMC Med Educ. 2007;7(1):3. https://doi.org/10.1186/1472-6920-7-3.
17. Stevenson K, Sander P. Medical students are from Mars-business and psychology students are from Venus-university teachers are from Pluto? Med Teach. 2002;24(1):27–31.
18. Baumeister RF, Twenge JM, Nuss CK. Effects of social exclusion on cognitive processes: anticipated aloneness reduces intelligent thought. J Pers Soc Psychol. 2002;83(4):817–27. https://doi.org/10.1037/0022-3514.83.4.817.
19. Bolte A, Goschke T, Kuhl J. Emotion and intuition effects of positive and negative mood on implicit judgments of semantic coherence. Psychol Sci. 2003;14(5):416–21.
20. Kuhlmann S, Piel M, Wolf OT. Impaired memory retrieval after psychosocial stress in healthy young men. J Neurosci. 2005;25(11):2977–82.
21. Lupien SJ, Gaudreau S, Tchiteya BM, Maheu F, Sharma S, Nair NP, et al. Stress-induced declarative memory impairment in healthy elderly subjects: relationship to cortisol reactivity 1. J Clin Endocrinol Metab. 1997;82(7):2070–5.
22. Payne J, Jackson E, Ryan L, Hoscheidt S, Jacobs J, Nadel L. The impact of stress on neutral and emotional aspects of episodic memory. Memory. 2006;14(1):1–6.
23. Payne JD, Jackson ED, Hoscheidt S, Ryan L, Jacobs WJ, Nadel L. Stress administered prior to encoding impairs neutral but enhances emotional long-term episodic memories. Learn Mem. 2007;14(12):861–8.
24. Smallwood J, Fitzgerald A, Miles LK, Phillips LH. Shifting moods, wandering minds: negative moods lead the mind to wander. Emotion. 2009;9(2):271–6. https://doi.org/10.1037/a0014855.
25. McGaghie WC, Siddall VJ, Mazmanian PE, Myers J. Lessons for continuing medical education from simulation research in undergraduate and graduate medical education: effectiveness of continuing medical education: American College of Chest Physicians Evidence-Based Educational Guidelines. Chest. 2009;135(3 Suppl):62S–8S.
26. Lucas GM, Rizzo A, Gratch J, Scherer S, Stratou G, Boberg J, Morency LP. Reporting Mental Health Symptoms: Breaking Down Barriers to Care with Virtual Human Interviewers. Frontiers in Robotics and AI. 2017 Oct 12;4:51. doi.org/10.3389/frobt.2017.0005126.

27. Ericsson KA, Prietula MJ, Cokely ET. The making of an expert. Harv Bus Rev. 2007;85(7–8):114–21.
28. Van de Wiel MW, Van den Bossche P, Janssen S, Jossberger H. Exploring deliberate practice in medicine: how do physicians learn in the workplace? Adv Health Sci Educ. 2011;16(1):81–95.
29. Van Merrienboer JJ, Sweller J. Cognitive load theory and complex learning: recent developments and future directions. Educ Psychol Rev. 2005;17(2):147–77.
30. Miller WR. Motivational interviewing with problem drinkers. Behav Psychother. 1983;11(2):147–72.
31. Miller WR, Rollnick S. Applying motivational interviewing. In: Miller WR, Rollnick S, editors. Motivational interviewing: helping people change. 3rd ed. New York: Guilford Press; 2012. p. 335–51.
32. Frith CD, Frith U. Interacting minds—a biological basis. Science. 1999;286(5445):1692–5.
33. Gallagher HL, Frith CD. Functional imaging of 'theory of mind'. Trends Cogn Sci. 2003;7(2):77–83.
34. Bateman AW, Fonagy P. Mentalization-based treatment of BPD. J Personal Disord. 2004;18(1):36–51.
35. Bateman A, Fonagy P. Mentalization based treatment for borderline personality disorder. World Psychiatry. 2010;9(1):11–5.
36. Allen JG, Fonagy P, editors. The handbook of mentalization-based treatment. Chichester, UK: John Wiley & Sons; 2006.
37. Decety J, Jackson PL. The functional architecture of human empathy. Behav Cogn Neurosci Rev. 2004;3(2):71–100.
38. Stotland E. Exploratory investigations of empathy. Adv Exp Soc Psychol. 1969;4:271–314.
39. Völlm BA, Taylor AN, Richardson P, Corcoran R, Stirling J, McKie S, et al. Neuronal correlates of theory of mind and empathy: a functional magnetic resonance imaging study in a nonverbal task. NeuroImage. 2006;29(1):90–8.
40. Mercer SW, Reynolds WJ. Empathy and quality of care. Br J Gen Pract. 2002;52(Suppl):S9–12.
41. Neumann M, Edelhäuser F, Tauschel D, Fischer MR, Wirtz M, Woopen C, et al. Empathy decline and its reasons: a systematic review of studies with medical students and residents. Acad Med. 2011;86(8):996–1009.
42. Mehrabian A, Young AL, Sato S. Emotional empathy and associated individual differences. Curr Psychol. 1988;7(3):221–40.
43. Eisenberg N, Miller PA. The relation of empathy to prosocial and related behaviors. Psychol Bull. 1987;101:91–119.
44. Şahin M. An investigation into the efficiency of empathy training program on preventing bullying in primary schools. Child Youth Serv Rev. 2012;34(7):1325–30.
45. Pecukonis EV. A cognitive/affective empathy training program as a function of ego development in aggressive adolescent females. Adolescence. 1990;25(97):59.
46. Riess H, Kelley JM, Bailey R, Konowitz PM, Gray ST. Improving empathy and relational skills in otolaryngology residents: a pilot study. Otolaryngol Head Neck Surg. 2011;144(1):120–2.
47. Ickes W. Empathic accuracy. J Pers. 1993;61(4):587–610. https://doi.org/10.1111/j.1467-6494.1993.tb00783.x.
48. Zaki J, Bolger N, Ochsner K. It takes two: the interpersonal nature of empathic accuracy. Psychol Sci. 2008;19(4):399–404.
49. Noller P, Ruzzene M. Communication in marrage: the influence of affect and cognition. In: Fletcher GJO, Fincham FD, editors. Cognition in close relationshpis. Hillsdale, NJ: Erlbaum; 1991. p. 203–33.
50. Noller P, Venardos C. Communication awareness in married couples. J Soc Pers Relat. 1986;3(1):31–42.
51. Zaki J, Weber J, Bolger N, Ochsner K. The neural bases of empathic accuracy. Proc Natl Acad Sci U S A. 2009;106(27):11382–7.
52. Gross JJ. Emotion regulation in adulthood: timing is everything. Curr Dir Psychol Sci. 2001;10(6):214–9.
53. Gross JJ. The emerging field of emotion regulation: an integrative review. Rev Gen Psychol. 1998;2(3):271–99. https://doi.org/10.1037/1089-2680.2.3.271.

54. Ochsner KN, Silvers JA, Buhle JT. Functional imaging studies of emotion regulation: a synthetic review and evolving model of the cognitive control of emotion. Ann N Y Acad Sci. 2012;1251(1):E1–24.
55. Ehring T, Tuschen-Caffier B, Schnülle J, Fischer S, Gross JJ. Emotion regulation and vulnerability to depression: spontaneous versus instructed use of emotion suppression and reappraisal. Emotion. 2010;10(4):563–72. https://doi.org/10.1037/a0019010.
56. John OP, Gross JJ. Healthy and unhealthy emotion regulation: personality processes, individual differences, and life span development. J Pers. 2004;72(6):1301–34.
57. Albright G, Bryan C, Adam M, McMillan J, Shockley K. Utilizing virtual patient simulations to prepare health professionals to conduct substance use and mental health screening and brief intervention. 2016. (Accepted for Review, NREPP: SAMHSA's national registry of evidence-based programs and practices).
58. Adams M, Albright G. Utilizing a simulation with virtual humans to prepare emergency department personnel to conduct substance use and mental health screening and brief interventions. 2015. https://resources.kognito.com//downloads/AtRisk_in_ED_Kognito_Research.pdf.
59. Eden D, Ganzach Y, Flumin-Granat R, Zigman T. Augmenting means efficacy to boost performance: two field experiments. J Manag. 2010;36(3):687–713.
60. Albright GL, Davidson J, Goldman R, Shockley KM, Timmons-Mitchell J. Development and validation of the Gatekeeper Behavior Scale. Crisis. 2016;37:271–80. https://doi.org/10.1027/0227-5910/a000382.
61. Bandura A. Self-efficacy: toward a unifying theory of behavioral change. Psychol Rev. 1977;84(2):191–215. https://doi.org/10.1037/0033-295X.84.2.191.
62. Centers for Disease Control and Prevention. Web-based Self Injury Statistics Query and Reporting System. https://doi.org/10.1037/0033-295X.84.2.191.

Medical Student Suicide: An Assessment of Risk Factors and Prevention Strategies

14

Carol Swetlik and Kathleen N. Franco

Worldwide, medical students experience high rates of burnout, depression, and suicidal ideation that may lead to suicide completion. The death of a caregiver has a dramatic impact on that person's family, peers, and the surrounding medical community [1]. Understanding the circumstances surrounding these emerging mental health issues in medical students is paramount for medical schools to identify at-risk students and serve the entire student body.

Suicide Completion Prevalence and Surrounding Circumstances

From 1947 to 1967, nearly one in five medical student deaths with known causes was attributable to suicide, second only to accidental deaths [2]. This number has decreased to 5.9 deaths per 100,000 that occurred from 1989 to 1994 [3]. Subsequent studies have largely relied on survey-based elicitation from medical schools. Most recently, a 2014 survey revealed six medical student suicides occurred across 90 responding US medical schools from 2006 to 2011, at a rate of 2.3 per 100,000 [4]. While physicians are known to be at increased risk for suicide completion relative to their peers, suicide rates for medical students are most recently reported to be

C. Swetlik, B.A. (✉)
Cleveland Clinic Lerner College of Medicine of Case Western Reserve University, Cleveland, OH, USA
e-mail: swetlic@ccf.org

K. N. Franco, M.D. (✉)
Cleveland Clinic Lerner College of Medicine of Case Western Reserve University, Cleveland, OH, USA

Department of Psychiatry and Psychology, Cleveland Clinic, Cleveland, OH, USA
e-mail: francok@ccf.org

T. Falcone, J. Timmons-Mitchell (eds.), *Suicide Prevention*,
https://doi.org/10.1007/978-3-319-74391-2_14

lower than the national average rate of 13.6 deaths per 100,000 for adults ages 25–34 [5, 6].

Due to low numbers, changing demographics of medical students, and possible reporting bias from schools, it is difficult to provide a generalizable statement about medical students who are most at-risk for suicide completion. However, demographics and particular circumstances are known about individual cases. In the most recent survey by Cheng, four of the six students identified were men, with equal distribution across the first 3 years of school [4]. Of the five with known methods, two were by hanging, two by gunshot, and one by overdose. Half were in the presence of a known psychiatric morbidity, with two having major depression. No students were married, and none were suspected to have substance or alcohol use involved in their deaths. This careful analysis of previously identified risk factors for depression and suicidal ideation can assist in identifying those who need rapid attention.

Suicidal Ideation

Suicidal ideation has been shown to increase risk of suicide completion [7, 8]. Studies have shown suicidal ideation rates range from 3 to 6% at smaller, single-medical school studies to 10–20% in longitudinal multicenter and older unicenter studies [9–11]. Recent analysis of 24 longitudinal studies reveals the median rate of suicidal ideation to be 11.1% (range 7.4–24.2%) [12]. Possible risk factors for suicidal ideation include depression, anxiety, life events, gender, marital status, and race. The literature exploring these will be addressed in this chapter. Importantly, rates of depression and suicidal ideation in medical students have been shown to be at least on par with that of residents and in some studies nearly double that of residents, emphasizing the importance of screening and detection early in training [12, 13].

Assessment of ideation, as well as depression and burnout, can be completed with a variety of instruments. While rates detected will depend on the instrument used and population surveyed, the persistent findings of depression, suicidal ideation, and plans among medical students are areas of concern that schools can be primed to address. As medical school is an opportunity to build required medical knowledge, it is also a time for students to build required coping skills, resilience, and an understanding of their own vulnerabilities and strengths before beginning practice as a licensed physician.

Depression

Rates of depression and depressive symptoms among medical students have varied widely across studies and periods of time. An analysis of 183 studies on mood problems in medical students concluded that rates of depression of first-year medical students range from 1.4% to 73%, with some studies showing higher rates of depression relative to nonstudent young adult controls and others showing the same or lower [12]. Overall, the prevalence in medical students was found to be 27.2%, higher than the estimated prevalence of 9.3% in the general population of 18- to 25-year-olds. While the mental health profile of first-year medical students is not shown to differ from other types of entering students, changes in mental health status that emerge after starting medical school are less clear [14]. In longitudinal studies, students in their later years of training were found to have nearly double the rates of depression compared to students with fewer years, suggesting that the stresses of medical school may directly contribute to depressive symptoms [11, 16]. Spikes in depressive symptoms during medical school have been reported, particularly at the end of second year, coinciding with the time when many students take their first USMLE examination, Step 1. Of note, a recently documented suicide took place in the context of receipt of a board score [4].

Severity of depression is a risk factor for suicidal ideation. In a recent study, almost 70% of students and physician residents who screened positive for major depression endorsed suicidal ideation [13]. In contrast, a much smaller proportion of those with minor or moderate depression (20.4%) endorsed suicidal ideation. Those with a personal history of depression and family history of depression were 3.7 times and 2.3 times, respectively, more likely to report suicidal ideation themselves. Only 15.7% of students who have endorsed symptoms of depression have sought treatment [12].

Anxiety

There is less literature describing the role of medical student anxiety leading to suicidal ideation than depression. A recent cross-sectional investigation revealed that 44% of medical students are anxious, with more female students than male reporting symptoms [17]. Anxiety levels have shown to increase during the first few years of medical school, particularly between years 1 and 2, but may drop in later years [17–21]. Additionally, anxiety levels have been shown to climb faster in medical students than in other types of students [18]. Regardless of trends, prevalence of anxiety in medical students across all 4 years has been shown to be higher than age-matched controls, with mental distress linked to increased risk of suicidal ideation [22, 23].

Anxiety and most specifically panic disorder are associated with a significantly greater risk for suicide, particularly with coexisting depression and substance abuse [24]. When looking at the connection between these mental states to suicidal ideation and attempts, overall anxiety symptoms, level of anticipatory anxiety, avoidance of bodily sensations, vigilance of bodily disturbances, and fear of cognitive incapacitation are highly predictive [25].

Additionally, other comorbid conditions may contribute to anxiety. Undergraduate college students with ADHD are more likely to develop anxiety than those without ADHD [26]. There has been an increase in medical students using medications to treat ADHD, but whether all of the students have been properly diagnosed remains a question [27]. In younger students, anxiety is associated with lower levels of academic attainment and increased risk to leave school early [28, 29]. Whether this is true of medical students is yet to be determined, but it would be worthwhile to assess students at the time of dropout or earlier, should they begin to show a pattern of academic underachievement that may indicate a change in mental health.

Sex

In the general population, male sex is a known risk factor for suicide completion, particularly in populations with major depression [30]. Across all 25- to 34-year-olds, the CDC reports the rate of male suicides to be 21.8 per 100,000 [6]. In contrast, the rate of female suicides is calculated to be 5.2 per 100,000. These numbers are lower in African-American and Asian populations and higher in the Caucasian population. In medical students, a recent survey by Cheng et al. reveals a suicide completion rate that is more equal across sexes than that previously seen [4]. From the early 1990s to 2011, the risk of male medical student suicide has fallen from 8.80 to 2.96 [3, 4]. The rate of female suicide, however, has increased from 1.03 to 1.63 per 100,000 [3, 4]. As the proportion of female medical students has risen dramatically, it is possible that increased or additional representation of this group has contributed to the decrease in rate in student suicide to 2.3 per 100,000, along with improved wellness programs and postulated increases in cohort resiliency [4]. However, historically, female and male medical student suicide rates have not differed significantly, and significant differences between male and female physicians are also not detected [31]. Therefore, normal fluctuations and small sampling may explain the recent gender discrepancy detected in the 1990s and its recent resolution, rather than sociological or psychological phenomena.

While a clear difference between rates of depression exists in the general population, this trend is not as clear in medical students. Longitudinal studies and systematic reviews have not found clear differences in rates of depression or suicidal ideation between male and female students throughout medical school [11, 32–34]. However, some have found that temporary discrepancies emerge at peak periods of stress, with midyear depressive and anxiety score discrepancies greater than end-of-year scores between male and female students [32, 33, 35]. The same trend between the general population and the medical student community is not consistently reproducible and possibly implies that male students may be at particular increased risk for depression and suicidal ideation compared to their male nonmedical student peers at baseline. One study has reported higher rates of depression in females, but this did not translate to discrepancies in suicidal ideation [13]. Additionally, males and females are generally reported to have similar scores of global psychological state in their first year, but female students showed higher global psychological distress than their male counterparts at the end of medical school [22, 35]. In a cross-sectional study of four classes of medical students, females had higher anxiety than their male peers [22]. Therefore, the stress of medical school may create differential mental health outcomes in males and females, but these may not necssarily tranlate into differential rates of suicidal ideation.

Personal, Familial, and Curricular Factors

Environmental factors, including personal events, familial attitudes, and stressors from training, have also been evaluated in assessing risk of suicidal ideation. A 2006 study by Dyrbye et al. evaluated the effect of major positive and negative personal life events, including illness, divorce, and death of a loved one, that often occur during medical training [15]. Personally experiencing a major illness in the previous 12 months was strongly associated with symptoms of depression. Adverse personal life events increased the risk of depression and alcohol use and have been linked to burnout. Familial behaviors can also directly impact risk of suicide; lifetime prevalence of suicidal behavior, including ideation, plan, and attempt, increased in medical students exposed to continuous parental emotional abuse, compared to those who experienced physical, sexual abuse, or general trauma [36]. In a similar vein, increased social support has been suggested to decrease likelihood of depression, particularly in at-risk groups, such as African-American females [37]. Low socioeconomic status has also been associated with increased risk of suicidal ideation [38].

Curricular events may also put students at risk for depression. Students who were not as academically successful reported higher levels of depression [20]. Difficult events on the wards, including high workloads and death of patients, also occur and may contribute to levels of stress [39]. As Haglund describes, in the third year of medical school, non-traumatic stressful events, such as poor role modeling and mistreatment by superiors, were associated with increased anxiety scores at the end of the year and were suggested to decrease personal well-being [39]. Interestingly, the number of direct trauma exposures, such as stressful patient-student interactions, was not significantly associated with personal distress at the end of the year. This suggests that while students may become accustomed to working in a medical environment, the attitudes and behaviors of those supervising them may be more important in medical student well-being.

Burnout

Burnout, comprised of emotional exhaustion, depersonalization, and a low sense of personal accomplishment, is postulated to begin during medical school. Using an inventory developed by Meehan and colleagues, medical students from five schools were surveyed longitudinally in a study by Dyrbye and colleagues [10]. In the 12 months preceding survey completion, prevalence of ideation among medical students from these schools was reported to be 10%. The majority of students with suicidal ideation endorsed lower quality of life, depressive symptoms, and burnout with depersonalization. However, the severity of burnout was predictive of the prevalence of suicidal ideation, independent of depression, supporting a dose-response association. Burnout was estimated to occur in approximately 50% of all students, with high depersonalization and high emotional exhaustion commonly occurring. Of the students experiencing burnout, longitudinal follow-up revealed approximately one-quarter recovered from burnout over the following year. Recovery was associated with a decreased risk of having reported suicidal ideation in the previous year and a rate of ideation similar to those who had never experienced burnout. This supports the notion that burnout severity, suicidal ideation, and suicide attempts exist along a continuum of personal distress. Programs that promote screening and support at any point along the continuum may be beneficial, but by far burnout was shown to be the most common experience among students.

Race

In a recent study of students who completed suicide, four students were Caucasian and one was Asian [4]. However, a nationwide prospective cohort study drawing from 49 schools recently reported baseline data showing significantly increased rates of depression and anxiety in entering African-American medical students, possibly due to lower social support [37]. Interestingly, the authors found that African-American female medical students have a less-than-expected risk of depression than either their African-American or female status alone would predict. Multiple smaller studies have previously found no difference between minority and nonminority students in rates of depression, emphasizing the importance of sampling in studying these phenomena [41, 42]. In one study, rates of depression did not differ, but rates of suicidal ideation have been shown to increase in the African-American medical students and residents compared to Caucasian students (13.5% vs. 4.5%) [13]. While 11.3% of minority medical students reported that their minority status had negatively affected their medical student experience, minority students were found to have decreased rates of burnout compared to nonminority students [42]. In the progression toward suicide, it may be that minority students do not present with depressive symptoms or burnout symptoms as the first indication as frequently as nonminority students. Further investigation of protective factors minority students may possess, including increased resilience or coping mechanisms, should be done.

Marital Status

Marriage prevalence in medical students has been demonstrated to be lower than in the general population [15]. However, marriage is believed to serve as a protective factor against depression, particularly under high-stress circumstances [43]. High levels of quality support within the marriage, not marriage itself, modulate the experience of distress. An inverse relationship between the Beck Depression Inventory and the Perceived Stress Scale was found in married medical students reporting higher emotional support but not those indicating lower spousal support [43–45]. Others found that married students had higher baseline depression scores and did not provide buffer over the next 2 years [16]. Female medical students with children have greater rises in depression scores between the first and second years than women without children. The same was not true for men [16].

Substance Abuse

Studies have shown that medical students, on average, report decreased use of tobacco and alcohol compared to age-matched peers [46]. In a survey of medical students across Minnesota, medical students' binge drinking rates of 15% were much lower than those of the states and national average of 27.8% and 24.1%, respectively [15]. A recent study by Jackson et al. assessed nearly 3000 medical students across the United States for alcohol abuse with the AUDIT-C screening tool [47]. 32.4% of those surveyed met criteria for alcohol abuse/dependence, and nearly 80% surveyed met criteria for burnout, depression, or alcohol abuse. 4.9% of students endorsed all three. Of note, burnout, higher levels of debt, and being younger were independently associated with increased risk of alcohol abuse/dependence. While alcohol abuse/dependence did not independently associate with suicidal ideation, the authors emphasize the link between alcohol abuse and risk of completed suicide, which was not assessed in their study.

Other studies have evaluated the abuse of other substances in the medical student population. Studies have consistently shown that 10–15% of medical students have used stimulants non-medically to help them study in school [27, 48]. Multiple studies have shown that approximately one-third of medical students have used cocaine [46, 49, 50]. Studies have revealed that both personality factors and environmental factors may contribute to these patterns of behavior. One study has shown that students with higher degrees of aggressive-hostility personality as measured by the Zuckerman-Kuhlman Personality Questionnaire have a higher likelihood of abusing stimulants [50]. Binge drinking episodes correlated with white race, intention to enter a subspecialty, and being unmarried [51]. Experiences of belittlement and harassment in school were significantly associated with alcohol and drug abuse [52].

A review of medical school handbooks revealed that most studied medical schools had formal policies regarding substance abuse. Most revealed direct referrals to formal health services, a dean, or a student-faculty committee. A subset of schools also stated that students struggling with substance abuse who self-referred would not face disciplinary action and would be offered the greatest degree of confidentiality legally permitted throughout and after treatment [53].

Assessment of Suicide Risk and Others in Medical Students

Authors have used a variety of assessment methods and tools to determine the level of medical student stress. A review of various programs by Shiralkar et al. demonstrates the great variety of questionnaires requested of students. Some are well known, such as the Profile of Moods States, the Beck Depression Inventory, the Brief Symptom Inventory, the Hopkins Symptom Checklist, the Perceived Stress Scale, and the UCLA Loneliness Scale [54]. In the Healer Education Assessment and Referral (HEAR) program, the nine-item Patient Health Questionnaire (PHQ-9) was selected as a rapid and familiar instrument known to many services. Assessment of suicidal ideation can be completed via an inventory developed by Meehan and colleagues [40]. This instrument evaluates suicidal ideation, attempts, and subsequent medical care needed for attempts. Alternatively, other studies have evaluated suicidal ideation over the past 2 weeks using PRIME-MD [13, 55]. In a review by Dyrbye et al., in 2006, the Beck Depression Inventory was frequently used in studies to evaluate depression [34].

Some student surveys are done in order to evaluate the effects of student wellness programs [56]. An interesting study by Ito and colleagues tested new interns just before starting internship and then again 3 months later. They compared the Sense of Coherence (SOC) Scale to new-onset depression identified by the Center for Epidemiologic Studies Depression (CES-D) Scale. They believed that those with lower SOC scores might benefit from additional support, as they were at higher risk for depression. At Vanderbilt, students take the Eating Disorder Examination Questionnaire (EDE-Q), the Beck Depression Inventory II (BDI-II), the State-Trait Anxiety Inventory for Adults (STAIA), the Michigan Alcoholism Screening Test (MAST), and the Drug Abuse Screening Test (DAST) [57].

Because all of the instruments given require confidentiality and anonymity, it is understandably hard to get all students who might benefit into therapy. Moutier and colleagues wrote about similarities between medical personnel and the military: "They do not complain, do not show pain, do not shrink work and above all do not ever show signs or symptoms of mental illness, especially depression" [58]. Because the medical culture has not permitted or encouraged physicians, residents, and medical students to be human or have personal needs, it remains challenging to achieve full participation in any of the screening programs.

At UCSD, the HEAR protocol has been used for years to ultimately bolster use of mental health of the student body [59]. Although statistical significance was not achieved, the trend over the 4 years was increased mental health usage by the students and reduced suicide risk. Downs and colleagues provide extensive face-to-face educational programs to physicians at all levels of training and practice. These are followed by waves of emails inviting participants to a screening website. They request chairs, program directors, deans, and other leaders to invite both medical trainees and physicians to complete surveys. If the web-based screening denotes concern for depression, anxiety, or suicide risk, a personalized report is sent back to the anonymous individual. They are invited for an interview and offered treatment if appropriate. It is impressive that some students reported they would not have availed themselves of treatment and were only identified by participating in this screening. This anonymous web-based suicide prevention program has been adopted by over 60 colleges and 8 medical schools [59].

Prevention

There are some curricular changes that have been noted to alter stress. Two studies noted that switching from grades to a pass-fail system reduced stress and students' licensing exam scores and residency placement were unchanged [60, 61].

Out of 90 surveyed medical schools, 92% have a formal stress reduction program in place [4]. Multiple schools promote a healthy lifestyle with physical exercise, adequate sleep, and healthy foods [62, 63]. Mindfulness plays a central role at SUNY Downstate. Erogul and colleagues offered an 8-week course to first-year students: a 75-minute session weekly and 20 minutes of meditation daily [64]. Initially the homework was completed using a 20-minute video that could include body scan, breath meditation, or yoga. They found improvements in the PSS and Self-Compassion Scale (SCS) but not in the Resilience Scale (RS). In a similar approach, Hassed and colleagues combined eight lectures with six tutorials [63]. One hour of the tutorial was spent reviewing the stress release program or mindfulness skills, and the other hour was dedicated to essence lifestyle and fostering conscious choice behavior strategies from pre-contemplative to the contemplative stage. They demonstrated improved student well-being in a pre-exam period but had no control group to which the students could be compared. Of the half of participants who responded to the survey at the end of the course, slightly over 90% reported using mindfulness practices.

Vanderbilt's Medical Student Wellness Program has five major components: mentoring, community, body, mind, and social [57]. Although the Office of Student Affairs has a coordinating role, the program is trifold with faculty advisors teaming with student advisers, as well as the VMS LIVE curriculum and a formidable student wellness committee with five programming subcommittees. There is also an offsite wellness retreat for the students and faculty. It is well worth reviewing the Drolet and Rodgers' paper which describes the project in great detail and the positive feedback from participating students. Another paper from the same university indicates that depression and anxiety continue to be more prevalent in medical students than nonmedical peers, but exercising one to three times per week provided some protection from depression and anxiety [61].

The model described by Laura Dunn and colleagues on promotion of resilience and prevention of burnout is very worthwhile reading for both faculty and students [65]. The authors describe a coping reservoir with both negative and positive input as well as outcomes of burnout or resilience. On the negative input side, stress and internal conflict, along with time and energy demands, are the clear detractors from student success. For positive input, psychosocial support, social and healthy activities, mentorship, and intellectual stimulation will fill the coping reserve. Quite influential are the personality and temperamental factors that mix with both the negative and positive inputs.

The same authors also present typical student difficulties, levels of distress, and the importance of tailoring interventions to each student. For example, if the student has no history of academic problems and no history of depression or anxiety, their intervention would differ from the student with higher academic risks and a history of depression or anxiety. There are two intermediate levels: one with higher academic risk but no history of mental illness and a second with a history of mental illness but no prior concern with academic risk. For each of these four scenarios, the authors describe a typical method for assessing the student, be that investigation or analysis of the situation, along with the provision of reassurance and resources. Some may need help with time management and organizational skills to improve the quality of their study time or may require a tutor. Others may need coaching about healthy attitudes and choices, while a smaller number need referrals for psychological services with close follow-up. Drawing the coping reservoir, with its negative and positive inputs and looking at the outcomes, allows the student and faculty member to match the correct strategies with the problems observed or felt. Another benefit of this model is its ability to normalize what has happened with the individual student in distress and destigmatize asking for help and accepting the resources the medical school has to offer.

Another interesting article by Austenfeld and colleagues describes writing activities that impact psychological and physical well-being of third-year medical students [66]. This randomized controlled trial gave students assignments of writing about a traumatic situation and expressing deep emotion (EMO). At other times, students were required to write about a disturbing circumstance from the position of their best possible self (BPS) and how they saw themselves handling this type of situation in the future. Students who began the study with greater hostility benefited more from writing about EMO, resulting in less hostility 3 months later. Some students tended to have more emotional processing (EP) and thinking about the circumstances, while others were more inclined to outwardly express emotional (EE) to others. Students with higher EP/EE demonstrated fewer symptoms of depression when they wrote about the EMO they had experienced, while students with lower EP/EE had less depression when they wrote from the best personal self condition. However, the authors also reported that the lower EP individuals who wrote from the best personal self had fewer healthcare visits at 3 months compared to the control group or the lower EP students who wrote about their raw emotions. This study needs replication but is certainly an interesting one, reminding us that one size does not fit all or every student in this case. Depending on the student's style of expression or processing and the symptoms she or he is experiencing, it might be possible to match an exercise with an individual student.

Conclusion

In conclusion, it is clear that a significant number of medical students experience depression, anxiety, or substance abuse as they handle increased stress or mistreatment. The stress from high stakes exams and feeling competition from brilliant peers around the country for selective residency programs are among the burdens they carry. Assessment or screening can help identify those needing support or therapy. Their confidentiality must be protected including knowledge that their treatment will not be shared with others. Building in a healthy multifaceted wellness program can help them strengthen positive lifestyle changes, which if continued can increase their resilience in the years ahead.

References

1. Schernhammer E. Taking their own lives: the high rate of physician suicide. N Engl J Med. 2005;352(24):2473–6.
2. Simon HJ. Mortality among medical students, 1947–1967. J Med Educ. 1968;43(11):1175–82.

3. Hays LR, Cheever T, Patel P. Medical student suicide, 1989–1994. Am J Psychiatry. 1996;153(4):553–5.
4. Cheng J, Kumar S, Nelson E, Harris T, Coverdale J. A national survey of medical student suicides. Acad Psychiatry. 2014;38(5):542–6.
5. Hawton K. Suicide in doctors while under fitness to practise investigation. BMJ. 2015;350:h813.
6. Centers for Disease Control and Prevention, National Center for Health Statistics: underlying cause of death 1999–2015 on CDC WONDER online database. 2017. http://wonder.cdc.gov/ucd-icd10.html. Accessed 3 Mar 2017.
7. Baca-Garcia E, Perez-Rodriguez MM, Oquendo MA, Keyes KM, Hasin DS, Grant BF, et al. Estimating risk for suicide attempt: are we asking the right questions? Passive suicidal ideation as a marker for suicidal behavior. J Affect Disord. 2011;134(1):327–32.
8. Beck AT, Kovacs M, Weissman A. Assessment of suicidal intention: the Scale for Suicide Ideation. J Consult Clin Psychol. 1979;47(2):343–52.
9. Dahlin M, Joneborg N, Runeson B. Stress and depression among medical students: a cross-sectional study. Med Educ. 2005;39(6):594–604.
10. Dyrbye LN, Thomas MR, Massie FS, Power DV, Eacker A, Harper W, et al. Burnout and suicidal ideation among U.S. medical students. Ann Intern Med. 2008;149(5):334–41.
11. Clark DC, Zeldow PB. Vicissitudes of depressed mood during four years of medical school. JAMA. 1988;260(17):2521–8.
12. Rotenstein LS, Ramos MA, Torre M, Segal JB, Peluso MJ, Guille C, et al. Prevalence of depression, depressive symptoms, and suicidal ideation among medical students: a systematic review and meta-analysis. JAMA. 2016;316(21):2214–36.
13. Goebert D, Thompson D, Takeshita J, Beach C, Bryson P, Ephgrave K, et al. Depressive symptoms in medical students and residents: a multischool study. Acad Med. 2009;84(2):236–41.
14. Carson AJ, Dias S, Johnston A, McLoughlin MA, O'connor M, Robinson BL, et al. Mental health in medical students: a case control study using the 60 item General Health Questionnaire. Scott Med J. 2000;45(4):115–6.
15. Dyrbye LN, Thomas MR, Huntington JL, Lawson KL, Novotny PJ, Sloan JA, et al. Personal life events and medical student burnout: a multicenter study. Acad Med. 2006;81(4):374–84.
16. Rosal MC, Ockene IS, Ockene JK, Barrett SV, Ma Y, Hebert JR. A longitudinal study of students' depression at one medical school. Acad Med. 1997;72(6):542–6.
17. Saravanan C, Wilks R. Medical students' experience of and reaction to stress: the role of depression and anxiety. Sci World J. 2014. https://doi.org/10.1155/2014/737382.
18. Aktekin M, Karaman T, Senol YY, Erdem S, Erengin H, Akaydin M. Anxiety, depression and stressful life events among medical students: a prospective study in Antalya, Turkey. Med Educ. 2001;35(1):12–7.
19. Inam SB. Anxiety and depression among students of a medical college in Saudi Arabia. Int J Health Sci (Qassim). 2007;1(2):295–300.
20. Stewart SM, Betson C, Marshall I, Wong CM, Lee PW, Lam TH. Stress and vulnerability in medical students. Med Educ. 1995;29(2):119–27.
21. Bassols AM, Okabayashi LS, Silva AB, Carneiro BB, Feijó F, Guimarães GC, et al. First- and last-year medical students: is there a difference in the prevalence and intensity of anxiety and depressive symptoms? Rev Bras Psiquiatr. 2014;36(3):233–40.
22. Lloyd C, Gartrell NK. Psychiatric symptoms in medical students. Compr Psychiatry. 1984;25(6):552–65.
23. Tyssen R, Vaglum P, Grønvold NT, Ekeberg O. Suicidal ideation among medical students and young physicians: a nationwide and prospective study of prevalence and predictors. J Affect Disord. 2001;64(1):69–79.
24. Noyes R. Suicide and panic disorder: a review. J Affect Disord. 1991;22(i):1–11.
25. Schmidt N, Woolaway-Bickel K, Bates M. Evaluating panic specific factors in the relationship between suicide and panic disorders. Behav Res Ther. 2001;39(6):635–49.
26. O'Rourke SR, Bray AC, Anastopoulos AD. Anxiety symptoms and disorders in college students with ADHD. J Atten Disord. 2017. https://doi.org/10.1177/1087054716685837.

27. Tuttle J, Schuerich N, Ranseen J. Prevalence of ADHD diagnosis and nonmedical prescription stimulant use in medical students. Acad Psychiatry. 2010;34(3):220–3.
28. Mazzone L, Ducci F, Scoto MC, Passaniti E, D'arrigo VG, Vitiello B. The role of anxiety symptoms in school performance in a community sample of children and adolescents. BMC Public Health. 2007;7(1):347.
29. Esch P, Bocquet V, Pull C, Couffignal S, Lehnert T, Graas M, et al. The downward spiral of mental disorders and educational attainment: a systematic review on early school leaving. BMC Psychiatry. 2014;14(1):237.
30. Blair-West GW, Cantor CH, Mellsop GW, Eyeson-annan ML. Lifetime suicide risk in major depression: sex and age determinants. J Affect Disord. 1999;55(2–3):171–8.
31. Pepitone-Arreola-Rockwell F, Rockwell D, Core N. Fifty-two medical student suicides. Am J Psychiatry. 1981;138(2):198–201.
32. Vitaliano PP, Maiuro RD, Russo J, Mitchell ES. Medical student distress: a longitudinal study. J Nerv Ment Dis. 1989;177(2):70–6.
33. Richman JA, Flaherty JA. Gender differences in medical student distress: contributions of prior socialization and current role-related stress. Soc Sci Med. 1990;30(7):777–87.
34. Dyrbye LN, Thomas MR, Shanafelt TD. Systematic review of depression, anxiety, and other indicators of psychological distress among U.S. and Canadian medical students. Acad Med. 2006;81(4):354–73.
35. Lloyd C, Gartrell NK. Sex differences in medical student mental health. Am J Psychiatry. 1981;138(10):1346–51.
36. Jeon HJ, Roh MS, Kim KH, Lee JR, Lee D, Yoon SC, et al. Early trauma and lifetime suicidal behavior in a nationwide sample of Korean medical students. J Affect Disord. 2009;119(1):210–4.
37. Hardeman RR, Przedworski JM, Burke SE, Burgess DJ, Phelan SM, Dovidio JF, et al. Mental well-being in first year medical students: a comparison by race and gender. J Racial Ethn Health Disparities. 2015;2(3):403–13.
38. Fan AP, Kosik RO, Mandell GA, Tran DT, Cheng HM, Chen CH, et al. Suicidal ideation in medical students: who is at risk? Ann Acad Med Singap. 2012;41(9):377–82.
39. Haglund ME, aan het Rot M, Cooper NS, Nestadt PS, Muller D, Southwick SM, et al. Resilience in the third year of medical school: a prospective study of the associations between stressful events occurring during clinical rotations and student well-being. Acad Med. 2009;84(2):258–68.
40. Meehan PJ, Lamb JA, Saltzman LE, O'carroll PW. Attempted suicide among young adults: progress toward a meaningful estimate of prevalence. Am J Psychiatry. 1992;149(1):41–4.
41. Pyskoty CE, Richman JA, Flaherty JA. Psychosocial assets and mental health of minority medical students. Acad Med. 1990;65(9):581–5.
42. Dyrbye LN, Thomas MR, Huschka MM, Lawson KL, Novotny PJ, Sloan JA, et al. A multicenter study of burnout, depression, and quality of life in minority and nonminority US medical students. Mayo Clin Proc. 2006;81(11):1435–42.
43. Katz J, Monnier J, Libet J, Shaw D, Beach SR. Individual and crossover effects of stress on adjustment in medical student marriages. J Marital Fam Ther. 2000;26(3):341–51.
44. Coombs RH, Fawzy FI. The effect of marital status on stress in medical school. Am J Psychiatry. 1982;139(11):1490–3.
45. Cohen S, Kamarck T, Mermelstein R. A global measure of perceived stress. J Health Soc Behav. 1983;24(4):385–96.
46. Baldwin DC, Hughes PH, Conard SE, Storr CL, Sheehan DV. Substance use among senior medical students: a survey of 23 medical schools. JAMA. 1991;265(16):2074–8.
47. Jackson ER, Shanafelt TD, Hasan O, Satele DV, Dyrbye LN. Burnout and alcohol abuse/dependence among U.S. medical students. Acad Med. 2016;91(9):1251–6.
48. Wasserman JA, Fitzgerald JE, Sunny MA, Cole M, Suminski RR, Dougherty JJ. Nonmedical use of stimulants among medical students. J Am Osteopath Assoc. 2014;114(8):643–53.
49. Conard S, Hughes P, Baldwin DC, Achenbach KE, Sheehan DV. Substance use by fourth-year students at 13 U.S. medical schools. J Med Educ. 1988;63(10):747–58.

50. Bucher JT, Vu DM, Hojat M. Psychostimulant drug abuse and personality factors in medical students. Med Teach. 2013;35(1):53–7.
51. Frank E, Elon L, Naimi T, Brewer R. Alcohol consumption and alcohol counselling behaviour among US medical students: cohort study. BMJ. 2008;337:a2155.
52. Shoukat S, Anis M, Kella DK, Qazi F, Samad F, Mir F, et al. Prevalence of mistreatment or belittlement among medical students: a cross sectional survey at a private medical school in Karachi, Pakistan. PLoS One. 2010;5(10):e13429.
53. Dumitrascu CI, Mannes PZ, Gamble LJ, Selzer JA. Substance use among physicians and medical students. Med Student Res J. 2014;3:26–35.
54. Shiralkar MT, Harris TB, Eddins-Folensbee FF, Coverdale JH. A systematic review of stress-management programs for medical students. Acad Psychiatry. 2013;37(3):158–64.
55. Thompson D, Goebert D, Takeshita J. A program for reducing depressive symptoms and suicidal ideation in medical students. Acad Med. 2010;85(10):1635–9.
56. Kiessling C, Schubert B, Scheffner D, Burger W. First year medical students' perceptions of stress and support: a comparison between reformed and traditional track curricula. Med Educ. 2004;38(5):504–9.
57. Drolet BC, Rodgers S. A comprehensive medical student wellness program: design and implementation at Vanderbilt School of Medicine. Acad Med. 2010;85(1):103–10.
58. Moutier C, Norcross W, Jong P, Norman M, Kirby B, McGuire T, et al. The suicide prevention and depression awareness program at the University of California, San Diego School of Medicine. Acad Med. 2012;87(3):320–6.
59. Downs N, Feng W, Kirby B, McGuire T, Moutier C, Norcross W, et al. Listening to depression and suicide risk in medical students: the Healer Education Assessment and Referral (HEAR) Program. Acad Psychiatry. 2014;38(5):547–53.
60. Rohe DE, Barrier PA, Clark MM, Cook DA, Vickers KS, Decker PA. The benefits of pass-fail grading on stress, mood, and group cohesion in medical students. Mayo Clin Proc. 2006;81(11):1443–8.
61. Bloodgood RA, Short JG, Jackson JM, Martindale JR. A change to pass/fail grading in the first two years at one medical school results in improved psychological well-being. Acad Med. 2009;84(5):655–62.
62. Ghodasara SL, Davidson MA, Reich MS, Savoie CV, Rodgers SM. Assessing student mental health at the Vanderbilt University School of Medicine. Acad Med. 2011;86(1):116–21.
63. Hassed C, De lisle S, Sullivan G, Pier C. Enhancing the health of medical students: outcomes of an integrated mindfulness and lifestyle program. Adv Health Sci Educ Theory Pract. 2009;14(3):387–98.
64. Erogul M, Singer G, Mcintyre T, Stefanov DG. Abridged mindfulness intervention to support wellness in first-year medical students. Teach Learn Med. 2014;26(4):350–6.
65. Dunn LB, Iglewicz A, Moutier C. A conceptual model of medical student well-being: promoting resilience and preventing burnout. Acad Psychiatry. 2008;32(1):44–53.
66. Austenfeld JL, Paolo AM, Stanton AL. Effects of writing about emotions versus goals on psychological and physical health among third-year medical students. J Pers. 2006;74(1):267–86.

15 Teaching Psychiatry Residents About Suicide Prevention and Postvention

Farah Munir, Sarah Nagle-Yang, and Cathleen Cerny

> *"My job is to determine who has a true and acute mental illness and who is an imminent danger to themselves or others. Admit those. Determine who is malingering, who has a chronic mental illness with no acuity, who is low risk for actually attempting or completing suicide; Discharge those."*—Trisha M. Danz [1]

Introduction

From day 1 as interns and then as residents, psychiatry trainees learn the practical arts involved in rapid suicide assessment and formulation, as they spend much of the first 2 years of training covering the emergency department and working with acutely ill inpatients. As seen in the resident quote above, sometimes the work of residency can seem as if it is distilled to this one topic area alone. This is also the period of time where most adverse events are experienced by residents [2]. Such events may include violence and aggression from patients and even the dreaded event of completed suicide. As will become clear in this chapter, residents often feel pressured to make split-second decisions which can have far-reaching consequences. They may buckle under the pressure of an angry emergency room attending or go along with the disposition formulated by a supervising attending despite personal misgivings. When an adverse event, such as the suicide of a patient, occurs under their "watch," they are especially vulnerable, particularly when they receive little anticipatory guidance or support from their residency program and hospital administration. This chapter incorporates recent literature from the field of academic psychiatry to illustrate some of the current practices and consensus within the field and also highlights some of the aspects of residency curriculum, which are

F. Munir (✉) · S. Nagle-Yang · C. Cerny
University Hospitals Cleveland Medical Center, Case Western Reserve University School of Medicine, Cleveland, OH, USA
e-mail: farah.munir@uhhospitals.org

T. Falcone, J. Timmons-Mitchell (eds.), *Suicide Prevention*,
https://doi.org/10.1007/978-3-319-74391-2_15

currently under question and likely will continue to evolve in the near future, to meet the needs of our current psychiatric workforce.

This chapter is divided into four sections: section I reflects on the various components of education and training needed to prepare psychiatric residents to perform suicide risk assessment and formulation; section II discusses suicide prevention education; section III highlights the importance of proactive education to residents about the likelihood of encountering patient suicide during training and supportive interventions to be implemented to survivors and caregivers in the aftermath of a patient suicide; and finally, section IV describes an individual patient cared for in multiple clinical settings (outpatient, ED, etc.) to illustrate the clinical roles of psychiatry residents in suicide risk assessment and management, linking the requisite ACGME core competencies required in each scenario. The chapter section titles are summarized below:

I. Suicide Risk Assessment and Formulation
II. Suicide Prevention Strategies
III. Suicide Postvention Approaches
IV. ACGME Core Competencies: Patient Vignette Through Care Path

Suicide Risk Assessment and Formulation

Suicide risk assessment and management are essential skills for every psychiatrist. While these are tasks that psychiatrists complete on a daily basis, they are anything but simple. To adequately assess and manage a patient's suicidal risk, one must not only have knowledge of the large body of literature pertaining to known risk and protective factors for suicide but must also conduct the clinical interview in such a way that a patient feels comfortable disclosing his suicidal thoughts and behaviors. Concomitantly, a skillful clinician must be mindful of her own countertransference and outside pressures that may potentially influence the interview. Academic training offered to psychiatry residents must recognize this competency as a complex skill set that should be taught, nurtured, and evaluated in an ongoing and purposeful manner throughout the duration of a psychiatric residency. Training in this area must include not only classic lecture-style pedagogical methods but must incorporate active learning that allows the trainee opportunities for continuing practice and coaching.

Silverman describes a two-part risk assessment process: the identification of risk factors for suicide, followed by the more complex task of suicide risk assessment and formulation [3]. Accordingly, this chapter on academic training for psychiatric residents will comment only briefly on the use of clinical practice guidelines and the use of known risk and protective factors for suicide, which have been described thoroughly in professional organization guidelines [4] and elsewhere in this textbook. The focus of this chapter will be more on the interviewing methods helpful to elicit suicidal risk, models of suicide risk formulation, and pedagogical methods for effectively teaching these foundational skills to future psychiatrists, and the next sections will review suicide prevention and postventions.

Psychiatric Interviewing and Suicide Risk Assessment

It is safe to assume that all practicing psychiatrists encounter suicidal patients. However, there are many reasons that a patient may not choose to share this information. Feelings of shame or concerns about hospitalization may make it difficult for the patient to disclose suicidal thoughts or behaviors. In that regard, asking the "right questions" is sometimes insufficient unless a trainee has also developed rapport with a patient and illustrated to her that he is comfortable and familiar with the topic. Thus, a suicide risk assessment calls upon the trainee to utilize all of his available interviewing skills in order to obtain the most truthful information from the patient. The topic of suicide risk assessment is therefore an essential component of any academic psychiatric interviewing course and conversely can be a useful avenue to illustrate multiple fundamental interviewing skills. Many of the concepts presented in this section are discussed in more detail in the 2nd edition of Shea's *Psychiatric Interviewing: The Art of Understanding* textbook [5].

Introducing the Suicide Assessment in a Psychiatric Interview

It is advisable that any discussion with trainees centered on suicide assessment first include instruction on how to introduce the topic of suicide into a psychiatric interview. When well-timed and sensitively introduced, an inquiry into suicidality might allow the patient to feel better understood and engaged in the interview. When such questions are "thrown into" an interview, there is a risk that the patient could experience this as an intrusion or a doctor who is "just checking off boxes." It should be emphasized to trainees that part of a skillful interview is to be "on the lookout" for natural openings in the interview that lead to a suicide assessment. Shea recommends three primary "gates" that might signal an opportunity to shift into a suicide assessment: (1) exploration of psychotic content, (2) discussion of depressive symptoms, or (3) examination of a life crisis [5]. When such natural lead-ins do not present themselves, the trainee may consider preempting the inquiry with a normalizing statement (i.e., "Many people who struggle with severe anxiety sometimes have the feeling that life isn't worth living. Is that ever something that runs through your mind?").

The CASE Approach

Suicide assessment often occurs in busy work environments (such as a booked clinic or emergency room) with various background pressures (i.e., a patient who may be fearful about inpatient admission or a doctor with liability concerns). Recognizing this, Shea argues that a trainee must develop an approach that can become instinctual in that it is available to the trainee even when he is stressed or fatigued [5]. Shea's proposed approach, the Chronological Assessment of Suicide Events (CASE), is a convenient tool for trainees to utilize when making specific queries about a patient's suicidal thoughts and behaviors. This four-step approach to gathering information specifically about suicidal thoughts and behaviors can be helpful for a psychiatric trainee in developing a flexible yet consistent approach to this section of the interview.

The first step in the CASE approach is to explore the presenting suicidal event, when applicable. This exploration should occur using the interviewing technique "the behavioral incident." This technique, originally described by Pascal in the 1980s, focuses on the facts and sequence of the event [6]. The interviewer avoids asking the patient subjective questions about this emotionally charged topic and instead sticks to objective facts. The goal is to create a "verbal videotape" where the interviewer can describe the facts of the event with as much precision as possible. Examples of questions include "How many pills did you take? What happened next?" or "What were you thinking at that moment?" The interviewer can then analyze the facts to assess the severity of the attempt, the degree of planning that took place prior to the attempt, and the intention of the patient during the attempt.

The second step in the CASE approach is to explore the patient's recent suicidal events, specifically in the preceding 6–8 weeks. This region should again be explored concretely using objective information with the goal of determining what other plans the patient has considered, how close did the patient come in carrying out those plans, and a view of how much time the patient has been preoccupied with thoughts of suicide.

An exploration of more remote past suicide attempts follows as "step 3" in the CASE approach. Shea's recommendation is to limit time on this section to focus on key points, as an interviewer can easily get diverted into extraneous information with a patient who has a lengthy suicide history. The focus here should be on understanding (1) the most serious past attempt, (2) the approximate numbers of past attempts, and (3) the most recent past attempt.

The final section of the CASE approach circles back to the present. The goal here is to elicit the patient's immediate level of suicidality. This section of the interview should include an assessment of the patient's level of hopelessness or future orientation, plans for ongoing mental health support, and the patient's ideas about coping with current stressors.

Complementary Interviewing Skills Needed for a Suicide Assessment

Taken together, the four steps of the CASE approach provide trainees with an easy-to-remember guide for covering the important points of a suicide assessment. However, as has been mentioned, simply asking the right questions is sometimes not sufficient. Specific interviewing techniques, described by Shea [7], aimed at uncovering "taboo" information should be incorporated into any interviewing or suicide assessment course. Some of these techniques include:

1. The use of exact language ("kill yourself") reduces the possibility of miscommunications and signals to the patient that this is a subject that the interviewer is comfortable discussing.
2. Normalizing statements, as exemplified above, notify the patient that she is not the only person who has experienced suicidal thoughts or behaviors.
3. The use of gentle assumptions is a way to signal that suicidal thoughts or behaviors are something that the clinician has encountered before. (i.e., "How many times have you tried this before?" instead of "Have you ever tried this before?").

4. Finally, trainees should be coached to avoid asking questions in the negative (i.e., "You would never go through with an overdose, right?"). Questions asked in this way likely signal to the patient that the clinician is expecting or hoping for a negative answer and reduce the likelihood of the patient disclosing their true experience [5, 7].

Attunement to nonverbal language is a necessary component of a suicide risk assessment and a skillful psychiatric interview. Patients may indicate emotionally meaningful content in nuanced ways, which require the doctor's attention to appreciate. A patient who starts fidgeting in his chair or diverts his gaze when the topic of suicidality is approached may be signaling to the interviewer that this is a topic that calls for increased attention and sensitivity. Learning to be attuned to these subtle messages can be difficult for the trainee who may feel anxious about collecting a sufficient and accurate factual database on each patient. Furthermore, time-pressures and electronic charting often necessitate that doctors practice concurrent charting during patient visits. For these reasons it is crucial that psychiatric trainees are coached to balance these pressures in a way that allows them to remain attuned to the nonverbal language of the patient. At minimum, excessive note writing or typing should be avoided during crucial parts of the interview, including during the suicide assessment.

Collateral history taking is another essential skill in a suicide risk assessment. Even the most practiced interviewer will encounter patients who are not able or willing to fully disclose their suicidal thoughts, behaviors, or other risk factors. Furthermore, talking with friends or family members provides crucial information about a patient's history of suicidality as well as her support system, psychosocial stressors, and environmental risks (such as guns in the home). If a patient does have an elevated risk but does not meet criteria for involuntary hospitalization, then the collateral interview may allow for necessary treatment planning in order to address specific risk factors. Instruction on collateral history taking should encourage trainees to take an organized approach to the collateral interview and to incorporate questions on each of these topics.

Countertransference

Training on suicide risk assessment must also incorporate countertransference. The topic of suicide is often emotionally laden, especially for trainees who have been affected by suicide in their personal lives or who may have been exposed to strong beliefs about suicide through their religious or cultural background. For these trainees, the nonjudgmental and open demeanor that is a necessary component of a suicide risk assessment may be difficult to create. In these instances, a trainee may himself provide nonverbal communication to the patient that the interview is not a safe place to explore this topic. The trainee may unknowingly cope with his anxiety by not asking about suicidality or by asking about it in a rushed or close-ended manner. Instruction about suicide risk assessment must alert trainees to this possibility, encourage self-reflection, and provide practical resource support.

Model for Formulating Suicide Risk

The ultimate goal of the suicide risk assessment is to translate clinical information into an estimate of risk and to develop an appropriate treatment plan. The estimation of suicide risk represents the culmination of the suicide assessment and requires the trainee to incorporate all information that has been gathered into a succinct summary statement and risk category. Central to this task is clinical judgment, as no specific risk factors or set of risk factors has found to be absolutely predictive of suicide. Unfortunately experience alone does not equate to increased clinical judgment [2], and thus it is recommended that instruction about suicide risk estimation should include a standardized model with opportunities for trainees to practice and receive corrective feedback.

One such model has been developed by the American Association of Suicidology's Recognizing and Responding to Suicide Risk (RRSR) clinical training program. This model asserts that the presence of chronic risk factors for suicide establishes the patient's baseline risk, while the presence of acute risk factors establishes the basis for short-term risk. The interplay between acute and chronic risk factors and known protective factors is utilized to assign each patient to a suicide risk category: low, medium, or high [2].

The APA practice guidelines [3] for suicide assessment further emphasize the following points:

1. Risk factors are typically additive; however, they may interact in a synergistic manner (i.e., patient with depression and medical illness has a higher risk than when each is considered separately).
2. Certain risk factors (i.e., presence of a suicide note) are serious alone, even when not in combination of other risks.
3. The effect of life events or psychological strengths will vary on an individual basis.
4. Because of the low rate of suicide in the general population, only a small fraction of individuals with any particular risk factor will die from suicide.

Pedagogical Methods for Teaching Suicide Assessment

Considering the importance and complexity of assessing and managing suicidality, it is essential that psychiatry residency training programs develop a comprehensive curriculum on this topic, including opportunities for trainees to build their skills in an active manner. While a didactic session or assigned reading may be necessary for trainees to build a knowledge base, it is useful to think about these experiences as preparation for more active learning, rather than the sole methodology. Active learning methods allow the trainee to more fully interact with the material by putting it into practice, noticing challenges, and encountering unexpected events and problem-solving difficulties. The following section will outline some common and innovative teaching methods that employ active learning in the academic teaching of suicide assessment.

Clinical Vignettes

Clinical vignettes are an accessible and widely used active teaching methodology. Typically utilized in conjunction with appropriate pre-reading, they can be employed during a group learning session without the need for direct patient interaction. When vignettes are provided in written form, they require no additional technology, although some do chose to use video vignettes for engagement purposes. As clinical vignettes do not provide real or simulated patient interactions, they cannot offer practice in the subtleties of the psychiatric interview. They can, however, be useful in engaging trainees in the process of identifying an individual patient's risk factors, estimating that patient's level of risk (low, medium, or high), developing a treatment plan in accordance to the patient's risk, and documenting thoroughly all of the above [7].

Popular Film

Film can be a powerful learning tool for a variety of topics in psychiatry, including suicide assessment. The high production values of popular films can create an emotionally intense experience for the viewer and can illustrate psychopathology in a prototypic manner not commonly found in a live patient. Furthermore, film has the ability to tell the story of the patient as it unfolds, rather than the retrospective account that is collected in clinical encounters [8]. Similar to clinical vignettes, the film clips shown are prerecorded and thus not amenable to the practice of the psychiatric interview. They can be especially helpful in illustrating the larger spiritual or cultural aspects of suicide for the psychiatric trainee or for illustrating the impact of suicide on surviving families. Some examples of films that have been utilized to teach trainees about suicide are *Scent of a Woman* (1992), to illustrate a serious suicide plan [8], or *The Bridge* (2007), which emotionally portrays the impact of suicide on family members [9]. It is recommended that film clips be used in conjunction with a forum for discussion or reflective writing.

Video-Recorded Patient Interviews

Video-recorded patient interviews can be an engaging tool for teaching psychiatric interviewing around suicide. Using an actual patient interview allows a seasoned clinician to model a suicide assessment in a "real-life" scenario and can also help to illustrate how the clinician flexibly adapted to the patient's individual personality and challenges. While watching a video, the facilitator may consider pausing at key parts of the interview to allow for discussion on the patient's presentation or "where to go next" in the interview. One might also consider using the video as an "entry-way" into a workshop on risk formulation or documentation. At our institution (University Hospitals Cleveland Medical Center), trainees are shown a video of a patient interview recorded by a senior faculty member and then are asked to determine the patient's individual risk and protective factors for suicide.

Role-Playing and Standardized Patient

Role-playing is a valuable tool in skills training that requires the trainee to put her knowledge into active practice. Used in a multitude of medical training settings, it has shown to be a highly adaptable and effective strategy for teaching complex skill sets. Role-playing can be modified to illustrate a variety of patient presentations with the aim of increasing the flexibility of the interviewer. In addition, the trainer and trainee can at times "switch places" to allow the trainee the experience of both being the interviewer and the interviewee. The experience of being the interviewee can allow a trainee insight into what certain techniques "feel like" to the patient as well as allowing the trainer to model interviewing techniques [6]. Use of standardized patients (role-played by actors) can also be employed as a way to provide a more consistent experience between trainees during a role-play. This can be especially helpful when utilizing the role-play for assessment or formal feedback.

Virtual Patient

Virtual patient (VP) technology is one of the newer and more technologically advanced active learning methodologies in academic medicine. While VP technology has been increasingly adopted by emergency medicine, surgery, and internal medicine programs, academic psychiatry has been slower to embrace this approach. The unique strengths of VPs include its ease of access: VPs can be stored online and are accessible from a trainee's home or in a remote location. Furthermore, this methodology may have particular appeal to millennial students, who have a high comfort with technology. An example of the use of VP for teaching suicide risk assessment was described by Foster et al. [10], at Medical College of Georgia. In this example, the authors created a VP "Denise" using a web-based VP system. While participating in the experience, students visualized a static image of Denise and interacted with her by typing questions that she would answer in text. Denise was able to answer thousands of questions with hundreds of answers, allowing for some flexibility and perceived spontaneity. After their interview with Denise, trainees were given feedback regarding their ability to elicit specific elements of the suicide risk assessment [10].

II. Suicide Prevention Strategies

Information about recent advances in the field of suicide prevention may be found elsewhere in this textbook. Here, we primarily focus on the approaches to education about suicide prevention in psychiatry residency training.

In Search of Consensus Guidelines for Suicide Prevention Education

As mentioned in the previous section, the use of direct questioning, no matter how skilled the interviewer, is an insufficient method to accurately predict suicide [1]. Psychiatry residents often feel unprepared to assess and manage suicidal patients [11]. Information elicited from patients, taken together with other case-specific clinical information to arrive at a formulation of a given patient's level of risk, is considered to be a core competency for psychiatry residents [2]. However, there does not appear to be clear consensus in the literature about the most valid approach to teach suicide risk formulation and prevention to psychiatric trainees [4, 12].

Bernert and colleagues [4] conducted a systematic review of clinical practice guidelines in suicide risk prevention in 2015 with the goal of informing emerging standards for clinical practice, research, and training in suicide prevention. They found that all of the guidelines and resource documents addressed assessment of risk factors but that there was "insufficient inclusion of recommendations for training and education, safety planning measures and standardized risk level or decision-tree rules" [4]. Thus clinical educators and supervisors may not have a clear set of guidelines at hand for how and what to teach psychiatry trainees or may be using outdated sets of clinical guidelines as mentioned previously.

Several publications describe the need for improvement in resident education about suicide risk prevention [2, 4, 9, 12–14] as well as anticipatory education about how to cope if/when residents lose patients to suicide and postventions [1, 7] which will be discussed in a later section of this chapter. Here we describe some approaches to education in suicide prevention and recent efforts to reconceptualize the process of risk assessment and formulation to more seamlessly result in risk reduction and prevention efforts.

The Public Health Approach to Suicide Prevention Education

Cornette and colleagues [14] advocate for the use of a public health approach to suicide prevention education in psychiatric training programs. Their article emphasized the need for interdisciplinary and interinstitutional collaboration to develop policies for restricting access/means to firearms and to enact other public safety measures. Other strategies included several empirically supported public health approaches to reduce suicide including pharmacological interventions, means restriction interventions, follow-up contact interventions, media-based interventions, emergency room interventions, and community-based interventions. The authors also recommend that supervisors and training faculty be prepared to take an active role in emphasizing the public health approach to suicide prevention and use approaches such as group problem-solving to identify systems issues and implement effective postventions [14].

Zisook et al. describe the prevention of suicide on college campuses as "an understudied public health problem training residents about prevention of suicide on college campuses" ([15], p. 3). The authors point out that the role of the academic psychiatrist is to educate the college community, including not only the residents but also the other members of the health-care staff and college community at large.

Citing statistics that indicate that firearm suicides account for a significant percentage of all suicides in the USA alone, the authors of the next article sought to review efforts to train residents in gun safety and patient access to firearms at home. To determine whether or not psychiatric residency programs provided firearm anticipatory guidance training, a survey in 2010 by Price et al. found that only 13% of respondents had been training residents in firearm injury prevention. Furthermore, the majority of training directors through the American Psychiatric Association (APA) should provide curriculum guidelines regarding firearm injury prevention training [16, 17].

In 2005, in response to a growing recognition that veteran suicides were on the rise, the Department of Veterans Affairs (VA) published the VA Mental Health Strategic Plan and invested funding to develop a comprehensive suicide research, education/training, and prevention program to address this serious public health concern. As part of the program, suicide prevention counselors (SPCs) are located at each VA. There is a flagging system to identify high-risk veterans throughout the system nationwide, and a focus on safety planning and means restriction was implemented, as well as a national crisis hotline, mandated staff education programs, and funding for research on the biological and clinical aspects of suicide prevention [18, 19].

The VA has been noted to be a potential resource for psychiatry training programs who are affiliated with the VA system to take advantage of the substantial training and research opportunities, as the psychiatry residency program affiliated with the University of Rochester has done. Furthermore, the VISN 2 Center of Excellence for Suicide Prevention is home to the VA Advanced Fellowship Program in Veteran Mental Health and Suicide Prevention, which is part of the fellowship program in Mental Illness Research and Treatment, sponsored by the VA Office of Academic Affairs. This 2-year postdoctoral fellowship is designed "to prepare psychologists, physicians and associated health professionals with the depth and breadth of knowledge and experience necessary to become leaders and innovators in suicide prevention research and education, as well as experts in Veteran mental health care." [17, 18, 20].

Education About Suicide in Primary Care Residency and Fellowship Training Programs

Note that while the scope of this chapter and textbook is to specifically address training in psychiatric residency programs, a growing body of literature is emerging with recommendations for suicide training in primary care in the USA [21–25] and in other countries where access to psychiatry is not as prevalent and/or where medical trainees receive less exposure to psychiatry during medical school [26, 27]. Some, like the Western Interstate Commission for Higher Education in partnership with the Suicide Prevention Resource Center [25], have developed a prevention toolkit and associated curriculum for use in primary care postgraduate medical training programs.

Moving from Prediction to Prevention

Pisani and colleagues, in a recent article in *Academic Psychiatry* [12], argue that the practice of assigning simple risk categories (low, moderate, high) to suicide risk is inherently outdated and that greater precision in describing risk should be undertaken. Formulation should provide enough information to directly lead to the determination of the proper method or risk reduction or prevention. They introduce a definition of risk formulation as "a concise synthesis of empirically based suicide risk information regarding a patient's immediate distress and resources at a specific time and place" ([12], p. 625).

Despite the recognition that assessing suicide risk is a complex, dynamic process that is dependent on numerous variables [12, 15], the assignment of risk categories and risk formulation which essentially requires them to make a probability judgment, often with limited or flawed information, are tasks that residents face early in their training and often. The stress associated with performing these assessments can be high for trainees, who are at an early stage of their careers.

The model for teaching and formulating suicide risk put forth by Pisani and colleagues [12] incorporates advances made in the area of suicide risk assessment and goes one step further to incorporate violence risk assessment concepts. Their model comprises a fluid assessment beginning with risk status, moving to risk state, and takes into account available resources and foreseeable changes. The latter two concepts are noteworthy for they do not rely on notions of "protective factors" which refer to epidemiological variables associated with lower risk across populations and take into account events or stressors which could be expected to either increase or decrease risk for suicide. This individualized approach to considering risk formulation is also more likely to directly lead to the development and communication of contingency plans with patients and families in a collaborative manner between practitioner and patient/family [12].

Thus, as shown in Fig. 15.1 below ([12], p. 626), the movement from risk formulation to the development of safety plans flows logically as it "redirects clinicians'

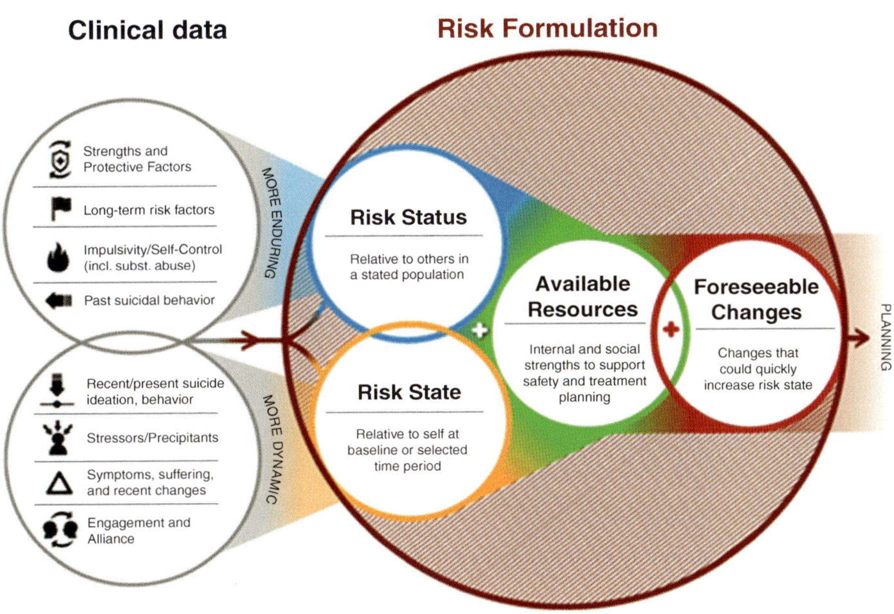

Fig. 15.1 Prevention-oriented risk formula ([12], p. 626)

attention away from prediction-oriented, categorical labeling and focuses on contextually anchored, prevention-oriented judgments. These judgments then directly inform person-specific plans and interventions ([12], p. 628)."

National surveys conducted on psychiatry residency programs have found that the majority of residency programs reported they received suicide management education through formal didactic lectures, seminars/courses, grand rounds, or journal clubs [11, 28]. All three surveys described here [11, 28, 29] noted a deficiency with respect to trainee education about the possibility of encountering suicide or postvention policies/procedures, which will be the focus of the next section of this chapter.

III. Suicide Postvention Approaches

Prevalence: Psychiatry Resident Experience of Patient Suicide

Psychiatry residents commonly experience the death of a patient by suicide, according to estimates from a systematic review by Puttagunta et al.; in 2014 [30], the prevalence of psychiatry residents experiencing the suicide of a patient ranged from 31 to 69%, across several studies. Of a survey of chief residents, only 19% felt prepared for the possibility of having to manage the aftermath of a patient suicide [11]. Ellis et al. [28] found that 18% of programs had postvention procedures specified in residency program policies and procedures and less than half overall reported that training activities instruct residents what to do should a patient die by suicide.

In a survey conducted by Tsai et al. [31], the authors noted that there had not been any progression in terms of findings of postvention across residency training programs, comparing their findings to that of Ellis et al. [28]. During the intervening 14 years, the authors reported that there may even have been a decline in the percentage of requirements and recommendations for certain activities following a patient suicide. In 2012 the authors speculate that this may be due to the lack of consensus about how to teach and implement postvention services. Of particular note was the finding that supervision and counseling to address the emotional impact of patient suicide were reported at a much higher rate in the earlier survey [31].

Emotional and Psychological Response: Resident Experience of Patient Suicide

The suicide of a patient is one of the most traumatic experiences that can overwhelm even the most seasoned clinician. So it follows that residents, who are at an early stage of their profession, would be uniquely vulnerable to emotional distress or self-doubt following the death of a patient by suicide. Sacks et al. [32] described the resident reaction as one of shock and disbelief, followed by a period of self-appraisal. A variety of emotional responses are possible, including severe stress responses, particularly when the individual does not receive adequate emotional support following the experience [32]. Ruskin et al. found that more than two-thirds of residents reported being unable to seek help after the suicide of a patient [33]. Yet, despite the fact that the death by suicide of a patient is hardly a rare occurrence for residents nor for their supervisors, anticipatory guidance early in training and resident debriefing or postvention strategies are not consistently included as part of residency curriculum [28, 31].

Fang and colleagues note in their review article that the reason for their decision to research the subject was that one-half of them had experienced at least one suicide by their 3rd year of training. Their review largely matched their discovery of their own program's lack of clear support both pre- and postexperience of a patient suicide. They note that the dilemmas of whether or not to communicate with the deceased patient's family and quality of supervisor relationship are of particular importance when considering how to prepare and support residents to deal with the suicide of a patient [34].

Another group of residents wrote a case study and review in 2009 [35] after each of them had experienced the suicide of a patient during their residencies and felt they needed to address the lack of institutional support following these distressing experiences. They reflected that after taking steps to implement a postvention program at their training program, and in the context of writing their journal article, the ability to implement a constructive response to their stressful experience helped them "to heal and grow a little more from this difficult experience," and the authors hoped their efforts would result in increased support for trainees at other programs [35].

Interventions with Trainees Following Patient Suicide: Postventions

As indicated by the shared experiences of trainees who have struggled with either their own reaction or dissatisfaction with their institution's response following the death of a patient by suicide described above, postvention responses have been called for by researchers and trainees alike. Yet, despite this fact, postvention is not a requirement in residency. A national survey of chief residents and program directors about patient suicides and postventions found that one in five residencies maintains a postvention protocol [31].

Like many of the residents who took matters into their own hands and helped to develop postventions at their programs described above, in 2012, Medical College of Wisconsin chief residents recognized the need for improvement in their residency program in helping residents talk about patient suicide and learn about the associated emotional and professional effects on clinicians. To this end, they initiated collaboration with the VA's suicide prevention team. They found that the development of a workshop focusing on the emotional and professional aspects of patient suicide helped those who had not had this experience as well as those who had experienced the suicide of a patient [18].

Jefee-Bahloul et al. reported on the impact of an educational program involving a panel presentation of suicide loss survivors from the American Foundation for

Suicide Prevention for the UT Southwestern Psychiatry Residency. Following the program, the majority of trainee participants reported they would be more likely to involve families in the care of suicidal patients and to call families after a patient suicide [36].

Prabhakar and colleagues developed an interactive curriculum for suicide postvention, called *Collateral Damages*. Their curriculum involved a video program with several clinical vignettes from psychiatrists and trainees who had personally experienced the suicide of one of their patients. It also included an instructive panel discussion and was followed by a fact-based presentation, a patient-based case learning exercise to reinforce the ACGME competencies involved, and both pre- and post-questions. The findings included the utility of pairing fact-based instruction with opportunity for personal reflection in a small group discussion format. It also emphasized appropriate responsiveness to the deceased patient's family [37, 38].

IV. Suicide Prevention and Management Core Competencies: An Examination of the Relevant ACGME Milestones and Clinical Case Correlation

Since July 2012 all ACGME-accredited graduate medical training programs have been responsible for training requirements related to six general core competencies: patient care (PC), medical knowledge (MK), practice-based learning (PBL), interpersonal and communication skills (IPC), professionalism (P), and systems-based practice (SBP).

Of these six core competencies, suicidality is most directly addressed in the ACGME milestones for patient care and medical knowledge (see Table 15.1). There is a patient care thread devoted to safety assessment with two milestones. Medical knowledge-2 has five milestones in the "knowledge to assess risk and determine level of care thread," whereas medical knowledge-6 has two milestones under "regulatory compliance" which speak to knowledge of involuntary treatment laws both regionally and internationally.

Core Competencies Viewed in Context: The Case of Angela

The following patient vignette illustrates the core competencies demonstrated by clinical activities performed by residents at different levels of training as the fictitious patient moves through the care path to different clinical settings and level of care, corresponding to the presentation of suicide risk at each point in time.

Setting: Outpatient College Mental Health Center

Angela is a 21-year-old woman who recently relocated from another state in order to attend college at the university after obtaining several credit hours at her local community college. She reports a history of treatment for depression and is seeking

Table 15.1 ACGME general psychiatry milestones related to assessment and treatment of suicidal risk

Competency domain	Sub-competency	Thread name	Milestone	Level
PC1	Psychiatric evaluation	C. Safety assessment	1.3/C screens for patient safety, including suicidal and homicidal ideation	1
PC1	Psychiatric evaluation	C. Safety assessment	2.4/C assesses patient safety, including suicidal and homicidal ideation	2
MK2	Psychopathology	B. Knowledge to assess risk and determine level of care	1.2/B lists major risk and protective factors for danger to self and others	1
MK2	Psychopathology	B. Knowledge to assess risk and determine level of care	2.2/B demonstrates knowledge of, and ability to weigh, risks and protective factors for danger to self and/or others in emergency and inpatient settings	2
MK2	Psychopathology	B. Knowledge to assess risk and determine level of care	3.2/B displays knowledge of, and the ability to weigh, risks and protective factors for danger to self and/or others across the life cycle, as well as the ability to determine the need for acute psychiatric hospitalization	3
MK2	Psychopathology	B. Knowledge to assess risk and determine level of care	4.2/B displays knowledge sufficient to determine the appropriate level of care for patients expressing, or who may represent, danger to self and/or others, across the life cycle and in a full range of treatment settings	4
MK2	Psychopathology	B. Knowledge to assess risk and determine level of care	5.1/B displays knowledge sufficient to teach assessment of risks and the appropriate level of care for patients who may represent a danger to self and/or others	5
MK6	Practice of psychiatry	B. Regulatory compliance	4.1/B describes the existence of state and regional variations regarding practice, involuntary treatment, health regulations, and psychiatric forensic evaluation	4
MK6	Practice of psychiatry	B. Regulatory compliance	5.1/B describes international variations regarding practice, involuntary treatment, and health regulations	5

Table 15.2 lists the didactic and clinical challenges of each training year as they relate to the suicidal patient and connect them to specific milestones

Table 15.2 Suicide risk assessment and management by training year—general psychiatry

Training year	Didactic learning	Experiential learning	Competency domain
PGY1	Suicide risk factors, protective factors, suicide risk tools, interviewing tips, how to document a risk assessment, regional statues about involuntary treatment, and civil commitment	Inpatient psychiatry, emergency psychiatry	PC1 1.3/C and 2.4/C; MK2 1.2/B, 2.2/B, 3.2/B; MK6 4.1/B
PGY2	Suicide risk assessment and management on the consultation liaison service	Inpatient psychiatry, psychosomatic medicine, emergency psychiatry	PC1 2.4/C; MK2 4.2/C; MK6 4.1/B
PGY3	Management of the suicidal patient in the outpatient setting	Outpatient psychiatry inclusive of community clinics, VA clinics, college mental health	PC1 2.4/C; MK2 4.2/B; MK6 4.1/B
PGY4	Management of the suicidal patient in the outpatient setting, teaching to teach suicide risk assessment and management to medical students and junior peers	Outpatient psychiatry, IOP/PHP, leadership positions (chief, integrated care, acting attending), forensic psychiatry elective	PC1 2.4/C; MK2 5.1/C; MK6 5.1/B

to establish care at campus mental health services. A 3rd year psychiatry resident is seeing her for an initial evaluation. Angela presents as a thin, anxious-appearing young woman with poor eye contact and a soft speaking voice. The resident also notes faint horizontal scarring on her left wrist. Angela tells the resident she is very depressed and homesick. She is not sleeping or eating well. She does not know anyone in the small college town and is feeling very lonely. She's had a hard time focusing on her classwork and has failed a few quizzes. She is also missing or arriving late to classes due to difficulty getting out of bed and completing her ADLs. Angela thinks she may have made a mistake going to school so far from home but fears that if she returns home, her parents will think she is a failure. Angela tells the resident she has been out of her antidepressant for 2 weeks. She is having daily suicidal thoughts and last night started writing a good-bye letter to her family. Angela reports a past history of suicide attempts and at least two psychiatric hospitalizations.

Core Competencies: PC1 1.3/C, MK2 1.2/B

Setting: Emergency Room

In the emergency room, a 1st year psychiatry resident is called to evaluate Angela for possible psychiatric admission. In addition to the information Angela provided to the outpatient resident, Angela also reports difficulty concentrating, ruminative worries, and frequent tearfulness. She does not see how things could possibly get any better for her. Angela reveals she has been thinking about overdosing on over-the-counter medications. She indicates that she has these thoughts daily and distracts herself with television or by calling her family. Angela has not told her parents about these thoughts or about how much she is struggling in school. When the resident tells Angela that she believes Angela requires psychiatric hospitalization for her safety, Angela tries to retract the suicidal thoughts she previously reported. The PGY1 involuntarily hospitalizes Angela.

Core Competencies: PC1 2.4/C, MK2 2.2/B, MD2 3.2/B

Setting: Inpatient Psychiatry Unit

On the psychiatric unit, Angela is assigned to a PGY2 resident. Also on the treatment are a PGY4 acting attending and two medical students. Under the supervision of her attending, the PGY2 resident restarts Angela on the antidepressant that had previously been helpful for her. The resident also suggests Angela participate in the on-unit occupational therapy groups. Initially, Angela is seclusive to her room and needs encouragement to even come out for meals. She often requests as needed medications for sleep and anxiety. She continues to report daily suicidal thoughts. At the suggestion of the PGY4 acting attending, the PGY2 resident obtains records from Angela's past psychiatrist and past hospitalizations. It is discovered that Angela has been significantly depressed since her teens and often has suicidal thoughts. She has made at least three serious suicide attempts and has a history of cutting.

The team decides to seek a court order for civil commitment as they believe Angela's risk for self-harm remains high at the end of her "pink slip" emergency hospitalization. The court order is granted. The PGY4 teaches the medical students about suicide risk factors and involuntary hospitalization in their state.

After 3–4 days, Angela seems mildly brighter. She comes out of her room for meals without being told to do so. She attends her first group and even sits in the common room with peers to watch television for short periods. An additional medicine to help manage anxiety is added, and Angela reports mild improvement in her mood. The team begins to talk about discharge planning.

Core Competencies: PC1 2.4/C, MK2 2.2/B, MK6 4.1/B

Setting: Partial Hospitalization Program

Angela is discharged to a partial hospitalization dialectical behavioral therapy (DBT) program after nearly 2 weeks in the hospital. Although her thoughts of death have not fully resolved, she indicates she has no plan or intent to die by suicide. A PGY4 resident is part of the PHP team and works with Angela both in groups and in individual therapy. They focus a lot on helping Angela develop coping skills. The resident therapist also makes suggestions for building a support network in the area. They talk about a safety plan for when Angela gets overwhelmed.

Core Competencies: PC1 2.4/C, MK2 4.2/B

Setting: College Mental Health Center

After PHP ends, Angela returns to campus mental health services to work with the PGY3 resident who did her initial outpatient psychiatric evaluation. In addition, she sees a psychologist for weekly therapy. The resident meets weekly with his psychiatrist supervisor and with Angela's psychologist at least twice a month to collaborate on Angela's care. The PGY3 resident also has Angela's permission to release treatment information to her out-of-state parents. In order to be successful at school, Angela reduced her credit hours. She obtained a tutor for the class that she has the most difficulty in. When she gets new assignments, Angela talks to her therapist about how to best complete the tasks without getting overwhelmed. Although she still occasionally has suicidal thoughts, Angela reports that they are fleeting and the coping strategies she learned in her DBT group help her manage her emotions.

Core Competencies: PC1 2.4/C, MK2 4.2/B

References

1. Danz TM. The gatekeeper. Acad Psychiatry. 2017;41(3):434–5. https://doi.org/10.1007/s40596-016-0645-5.
2. Silverman MM, Berman AL. Training for suicide risk assessment and suicide risk formulation. Acad Psychiatry. 2014;38(5):526–37.
3. Jacobs D, Brewer M. APA practice guideline provides recommendations for assessing and treating patients with suicidal behaviors. Psychiatr Ann. 2004;34(5):373–80.
4. Bernert RA, Hom MA, Roberts LW. A review of multidisciplinary clinical practice guidelines in suicide prevention: toward an emerging standard in suicide risk assessment and management, training and practice. Acad Psychiatry. 2014;38(5):585–92.
5. Shea SC. Psychiatric interviewing: the art of understanding. 2nd ed. Philadelphia: Elsevier Health Sciences; 1998.
6. Barney C, Shea SC. The art of effectively teaching clinical interviewing skills using role-playing: a primer. Psychiatr Clin North Am. 2007;30(2):e31–50.
7. Shea SC. My favorite tips for uncovering sensitive and taboo information from antisocial behavior to suicidal ideation. Psychiatr Clin North Am. 2007;30(2):253–9.
8. Hyler SE, Moore J. Teaching psychiatry? Let Hollywood help! Acad Psychiatry. 1996;20(4):212–9.
9. Retamero C, Walsh L, Otero-Perez G. Use of the film the bridge to augment the suicide curriculum in undergraduate medical education. Acad Psychiatry. 2014;38(5):605–10.
10. Foster A, Chaudhary N, Murphy J, Lok B, Waller J, Buckley PF. The use of simulation to teach suicide risk assessment to health profession trainees: rationale, methodology, and a proof of concept demonstration with a virtual patient. Acad Psychiatry. 2014;39(6):620–9.
11. Melton BB, Coverdale JH. What do we teach psychiatric residents about suicide? A national survey of chief residents. Acad Psychiatry. 2009;33(1):47–50.
12. Pisani AR, Murrie DC, Silverman MM. Reformulating suicide risk formulation: from prediction to prevention. Acad Psychiatry. 2015;40(4):623–9. https://doi.org/10.1007/s40596-015-0434-6.
13. Lomax JW. A proposed curriculum on suicide care for psychiatry residency. Suicide Life Threat Behav. 1986;16(1):56–64.
14. Cornette MM, Schlotthauer AE, Berlin JS, Clark DC, French LM, Miller ML, et al. The public health approach to reducing suicide: opportunities for curriculum development in psychiatry residency training programs. Acad Psychiatry. 2014;38(5):575–84.
15. Zisook S, Downs N, Moutier C, Clayton P. College students and suicide risk: prevention and the role of academic psychiatry. Acad Psychiatry. 2012;36(1):1–6.

16. Price JH, Thompson AJ, Khubchandani J, Mrdjenovich AJ. Firearm anticipatory guidance training in psychiatric residency programs. Acad Psychiatry. 2010;34(6):417–23.
17. Coverdale JH, Roberts LW, Balon R. The public health priority to address the accessibility and safety of firearms: recommendations for training. Acad Psychiatry. 2010;34(6):405–8.
18. Pheister M, Kangas G, Thompson C, Lehrmann J, Berger B, Kemp J. Suicide prevention and postvention resources: what psychiatry residencies can learn from the veteran's administration experience. Acad Psychiatry. 2014;38(5):600–4.
19. Coverdale JH, Roberts LW, Louie AK. Encountering patient suicide: emotional responses, ethics, and implications for training programs. Acad Psychiatry. 2007;31(5):329–32.
20. US Department of Veterans Affairs. VISN 2 Center of Excellence for suicide prevention. 2016. http://www.mirecc.va.gov/suicideprevention/fellowship.asp. Accessed 24 Jan 2017.
21. Sudak D, Roy A, Sudak H, Lipschitz A, Maltsberger J, Hendin H. Deficiencies in suicide training in primary care specialties: a survey of training directors. Acad Psychiatry. 2007;31(5):345–9.
22. Fallucco EM, Hanson MD, Glowinski AL. Teaching pediatric residents to assess adolescent suicide risk with a standardized patient module. Pediatrics. 2010;125(5):953–9.
23. Fallucco EM, Conlon MK, Gale G, Constantino JN, Glowinski AL. Use of a standardized patient paradigm to enhance proficiency in risk assessment for adolescent depression and suicide. J Adolesc Health. 2012;51(1):66–72.
24. Boris NW, Fritz GK. Pediatric residents' experiences with suicidal patients. Acad Psychiatry. 1998;22(1):21–8.
25. DeHay T, Ross S, McFaul M. Training medical providers in evidence-based approaches to suicide prevention. Int J Psychiatry Med. 2015;50(1):73–80.
26. Kato TA, Suzuki Y, Sato R, Fujisawa D, Uehara K, Hashimoto N, et al. Development of 2-hour suicide intervention program among medical residents: first pilot trial. Psychiatry Clin Neurosci. 2010;64(5):531–40.
27. Fujisawa D, Suzuki Y, Kato TA, Hashimoto N, Sato R, Aoyama-Uehara K, et al. Suicide intervention skills among Japanese medical residents. Acad Psychiatry. 2013;37(6):402–7.
28. Ellis TE, Dickey TO, Jones EC. Patient suicide in psychiatry residency programs. Acad Psychiatry. 1998;22(3):181–9.
29. Pilkinton P. Encountering suicide: the experience of psychiatric residents. Acad Psychiatry. 2003;27(2):93–9.
30. Puttagunta R, Lomax ME, McGuinness JE, Coverdale J. What is the prevalence of the experience of death of a patient by suicide among medical students and residents? A systematic review. Acad Psychiatry. 2014;38(5):538–41.
31. Tsai A, Moran S, Shoemaker R, Bradley J. Patient suicides in psychiatric residencies and postvention responses: a national survey of psychiatry chief residents and program directors. Acad Psychiatry. 2012;36(1):34–8.
32. Sacks M, Cohen A, Keats M, Turnquist K. Residency response to patient suicide. J Psychiatr Educ. 1987;11(4):217–26.
33. Ruskin R. Impact of patient suicide on psychiatrists and psychiatric trainees. Acad Psychiatry. 2004;28(2):104–10.
34. Fang F, Kemp J, Jawandha A, Juros J, Long L, Nanayakkara S, et al. Encountering patient suicide: a resident's experience. Acad Psychiatry. 2007;31(5):340–4.
35. Mangurian C, Harre E, Reliford A, Booty A, Cournos F. Improving support of residents after a patient suicide: a residency case study. Acad Psychiatry. 2009;33(4):278–81.
36. Jefee-Bahloul H, Hanna RC, Brenner AM. Teaching psychiatry residents about suicide loss: impact of an educational program. Acad Psychiatry. 2014;38(6):768–70.
37. Prabhakar D, Anzia JM, Balon R, Gabbard G, Gray E, Hatzis N, et al. "Collateral damages": preparing residents for coping with patient suicide. Acad Psychiatry. 2013;37(6):429–30.
38. Prabhakar D, Balon R, Anzia JM, Gabbard GO, Lomax JW, Bandstra BS, et al. Helping psychiatry residents cope with patient suicide. Acad Psychiatry. 2014;38(5):593–7.

16 Understanding Risk Factors and Warning Signs for Suicide: A Primer for Preventing Suicide in Physicians

Ruby C. Castilla-Puentes

Introduction

Suicide among physicians has been a largely unacknowledged phenomenon for decades, obscured by secrecy and shame. Physicians die by their own hands at a rate much higher than that of the general population. Of all professions, the medical profession consistently remains near the top of occupations with the highest risk of death by suicide. Exact numbers are not known. Although it is impossible to estimate with accuracy because of inaccurate cause of death reporting and coding, the number most frequently used in the United States is approximately 400 physicians/year (or perhaps a doctor daily). Female physicians' suicide rate is about 130% higher than the general female population. For male physicians, the suicide rate is about 40% higher than that of the general male population. Because of their greater knowledge of and better access to lethal means, physicians have a far higher suicide completion rate than the general population. Estimates of successful completion of suicide range from 1.4 to 2.3 times the rate achieved in the general population. Although female physicians attempt suicide far less often than their counterparts in the general population, their completion rate equals that of male physicians and, thus, far exceeds that of the general population (2.5–4 times the rate by some estimates).

Among physicians, risk for suicide increases when mental health conditions go unaddressed, and self-medication occurs as a way to address anxiety, insomnia, or other distressing symptoms. Although self-medicating, mainly with prescription medications, may reduce some symptoms, the underlying health problem is not effectively treated. This can lead to a tragic outcome. Following two key objectives: (1) to identify at-risk physicians and (2) to refer them to appropriate care this

R. C. Castilla-Puentes, M.D. Dr.P.H., M.B.A.
Board of Directors American Society of Hispanic Psychiatry,
Medical Safety at Johnson and Johnson, Philadelphia, PA, USA

Dornsife School of Public Health, Drexel University, Philadelphia, PA, USA
e-mail: RCastil4@its.jnj.com

T. Falcone, J. Timmons-Mitchell (eds.), *Suicide Prevention*,
https://doi.org/10.1007/978-3-319-74391-2_16

chapter will discuss how to identify warning signs for physician suicide and how to approach colleagues that are displaying signs of risks for suicide. In this chapter, suicidal behavior includes suicide plans, attempts, and completed suicides.

Differentiating Between Risk Factors and Warning Signs

Risk factors are characteristics that make it more likely that individuals will consider, attempt, or die by suicide. Risk factors for completed suicide are typically examined by psychological autopsy, a process that reconstructs factors that contribute to suicide via interviews with key informants. Unfortunately, few psychological autopsy studies have been undertaken for physician suicides. In Finland during a 12-month period, a study found that all physicians who died by suicide had a mood disorder and that, sadly, none had received adequate diagnosis or treatment for their mood disorder [1]. In the United States, a similar study of physicians found that in addition to mood disorders, substance use problems, financial problems, a tendency to overwork, career dissatisfaction, and professional and personal losses were also identified risk factors [2, 3] (see Table 16.1).

Risk factors are often confused with warning signs of suicide, and frequently suicide prevention efforts mix the two. But the two are vastly different. Warning signs indicate an immediate risk of suicide, whereas risk factors indicate someone is at heightened risk for suicide but indicate little or nothing about immediate risk [4]. Warning signs are only applicable to individuals, whereas risk and protective factors are found in individuals and communities. Being able to tell the difference between a risk factor and a warning sign is important in communications about suicide risk. The warning signs help people know what actions they can take *right now* to help someone at immediate risk for suicide. Instead, risk factors help people understand what might need to change within *an individual or a community* in order to decrease suicide risk over time [5]. Although risk factors generally contribute to long-term risk, immediate stressors, also called warning signs, may create the final impetus for the suicidal act. Warning signs may include relationship problems or

Table 16.1 Risk factors for physician suicide

Sex: Male or female
Race: White
Marital status: Divorced, separated, or single
Mood disorders: Psychiatric conditions or history (especially depression, bipolar disorders, anxiety)
Alcohol or other substance abuse
Access to lethal means
Previous self-harm or suicide attempts
Excessive risk taking (especially high-stakes gambler, thrill seeker, involved in extreme high-risk sports and activities)
Burnout, personality with characteristics of perfectionism, competitiveness, and to blame for clinical errors

Table 16.2 Warning signs for physician suicide

Pain, recent diagnosis of chronic or debilitating medical condition, and worsening medical prognosis
Lack of trust, recent relationship problems or breakups, separation or divorce; currently having marital disruption
Recent acute depressive episode, depression or depressive symptoms, or any new psychiatric diagnosis. Acute verbal and nonverbal indicators of increase in the severity of mood or psychiatric symptoms (e.g., lack of eye contact, anxiety, hallucinations and unusual beliefs, agitation, speed of speech)
Increase in the alcohol or drug consumption
Self-medication, request for medications or substances with lethal outcomes (e.g., anesthetics, sedatives, etc.)
Changes of mental state at time of self-harm or suicide attempt or threat (alcohol or drug intake, social situation, relationship changes, bereavements)
Financial hardships, legal difficulties, public humiliation or shame
Professional issues, change in status, threats to status, autonomy, security, financial stability, increased work demands
Plans for others after death: suicide notes, changes to will, consequences
Wish to be dead. Feelings of hopelessness. Regret/remorse over current/previous attempt
Expectation about outcome of self-harming behavior or suicide attempt/threat
Specific plans. Other self-harming behaviors

breakups, financial hardships, legal difficulties, public humiliation or shame, worsening medical prognosis, and other stressful events [6]. The warning signs for physician suicide are listed in Table 16.2.

Although there has been considerable criticism of the physician suicide data (largely because death certificates and other traditional sources of information have proven unreliable and, in many cases, it is difficult to determine if death is a result of suicide or an accident), in general, it is accepted that physician suicide rate ranges between 28 and 40 per 100,000, compared with the overall rate in the general population of 12.3 per 100,000 [7].

The risk factors for physician suicide described in Table 16.1 are discussed in detail in the following section. The warning signs for physician suicide listed in Table 16.2 are also described in detail in the subsequent section.

Risk Factors for Physician Suicide

Suicide results from a complex interplay of risk factors that are biological, psychological, and social in nature [8]. The major risk factors are mental disorders and substance use disorders. More than 90% of those who die by suicide have at least one of these disorders, most frequently depression (as major depressive disorder or bipolar disorder) and/or alcohol abuse. The risk is much greater when both are present. Since most people with these disorders do not die by suicide, additional risk factors are also at play, including stressful events and predisposing factors (e.g., impulsivity). Although contradictory evidence exists about differences in suicide rates among specialties, the fact that physicians complete suicide at a higher rate that the general population seems clear. The fact that overall mortality from other causes of death is lower for physicians (than the general population) while the suicide rate is doubled raises serious concern [9].

Sex: Male or Female

A review of studies of suicide in physicians found higher rates of suicide in physicians compared with the general population. The relative risks ranged from 1.1 to 3.4 in male physicians and from 2.5 to 5.7 in female physicians [10].

More reliable data regarding the mental health of male physicians comes from a landmark prospective study performed by Vaillant et al. [11]. Although the sample a group of 268 male Harvard sophomores is not an overall representation of physicians, the data are enlightening. This study followed this group over a period of 30 years. Of this sample, 47 men attended medical school and 46 men graduated. When these 47 men were compared with 79 controls, the physicians were significantly more likely than the controls to have relatively poor marriages, to use drugs and alcohol heavily, and to obtain psychotherapy. In addition 17% of the 47 physicians were hospitalized for psychiatric illness, 34% underwent psychotherapy, and 34% abused drugs. A closer examination of the early histories of these physicians revealed that these difficulties were strongly associated with life adjustment before medical school, such as childhood instability and adolescent adjustment problems. The study also found that physicians were more likely than controls to show traits of dependency, pessimism, passivity, and self-doubt. The authors concluded that problems are more likely to develop when physicians ask themselves to give more than they have been given.

Female physicians have lower rates of suicide attempts than do other females in a nationally representative study [12]. Other studies examined physician deaths and determined that the suicide rate among female physicians was between two and four times that of women in the general population [13, 14]. It is important to note that, in the general population, the rate of completed suicide among men is approximately three times the completed suicide rate of women; thus, male and female physicians die by suicide at close to the same rate.

Depression has been well studied more in female physicians than in male physicians. Community studies in which female professionals were interviewed and evaluated for a lifetime history of depression found that 51% of female physicians had a history of depression. Among physicians, psychiatrists had the highest rates, with 73% reporting a history of depression compared with 46% of other female physicians [15].

The sources of stress on women physicians include problems related to minority status and discrimination; lack of role models, mentors, or sponsors; and role strain. These stressors are not found exclusively in women (e.g., those from other ethnic groups, disabled individuals, and those of non-heterosexual orientation may also suffer from these types of stressors), but they are important aspects of what women face which can explain the increased risk for suicide [16]. A psychological theory proposes that self-esteem for women is predicated on establishing mutually satisfying, reciprocal relationships [17]. These relationships are characterized by mutual support and empathy, which enhance the growth and development of each party in the relationship. This reliance on connections with others is incompatible with the identity traditionally associated with medical practice: competitive, detached, and self-contained. A survey of more than 300 physicians (more than 80% male) found that while empathy and compassion were characteristics valued by physicians, they were characteristics identified as least likely to be associated with promotion and career advancement [18]. This adds a level of stress for women in the medical profession. The career, itself, is incongruent with personal identity.

An additional factor may be that women experience role strain because of the women's role and everyday demands. Evidence suggests that work-family conflict may exert a special stress on women physicians. Studies found that in heterosexual marriages between two physicians, wives were more likely to make accommodations in their career based on consideration of effects on spouses and children [19]. In a study of the relationship of family responsibilities and sex to academic productivity, approximately 2000 members at academic medical centers were evaluated. Investigators found men and women faculty without children had equivalent career accomplishments. Among faculty with children, this variable (having dependent children) had a much more deleterious effect on the women's career and seemed to account for much of the slowed career progression of women physicians in academia [20]. Finally, physician surveys find that female physicians are more likely than men to work part time, particularly if they have children [21]. In summary, it is also possible that part of the increased suicide rate found in women physicians is explained by the aforementioned facts and that these women make better informed attempts than other women, because they have full knowledge of the requirements for lethality.

Race: White

The largest US study of white, male physician deaths in 28 states found that, compared with white, male professionals, physicians' proportionate mortality ratio was higher for suicide than for all other leading causes of death. In the general population, the male suicide rate is more than four times higher than that in females, whereas in physicians the female rate is as high as the male rate [22].

Marital Status

Marital problems, separation, or divorce can certainly contribute to depressive symptoms, which can increase the likelihood of suicidality. Although marriage is considered to be an effective defense to emotional distress, this does not seem to be true for women physicians [23]. Marital problems are common, perhaps in part because of the tendency of physicians to postpone addressing marital problems and to avoid conflict in general [24].

Mood Disorders: Depression

Suicide risk is increased by a factor of at least 10 across a range of psychiatric diagnoses, and an estimated 47–74% of suicides are directly attributable to mental disorders [25]. In general, physicians are notoriously reluctant to seek treatment for any personal illness. Research suggests that one in three physicians have no regular source of medical care [26]. This is especially true in the case of potential mental illness. Depression is at least as common in the medical profession as in the general population, affecting an estimated 12% of males and up to 19.5% of females [27].

Because of the stigma associated with depression, which seems to be greatly magnified among medical practitioners, self-reporting likely underestimates the prevalence of the disease in medical populations. Indeed, although physicians seem to have generally heeded their own advice about avoiding common risk factors for early mortality, they are reluctant to address depression, a significant cause of morbidity and mortality that disproportionately affects them. A study revealed that although 1 in 16 had experienced suicidal ideation in the past 12 months, only 26% had sought any mental help. In addition, there was a strong correlation between depressive symptoms, with the incidence of suicidal ideation. More than 60% of those with suicidal ideation indicated they were reluctant to seek help due to concern that it could affect their medical license [28]. Other studies reveal that this concern about regulatory intervention is a very common concern hampering help seeking for mental health issues [29]. Reports of physician suicide data relative to nonphysician victims revealed a significant lower prevalence of antidepressant medication in the blood of physician victims, which is an objective indication of the truth that physicians do not receive mental health care in proportion to their need [23]. In addition, physicians who attempt suicide (usually with drugs) are more likely than nonphysicians to succeed in killing themselves, which may partly account for the increased rate of death by suicide.

Alcohol or Other Substance Abuse

Approximately 10–12% of physicians develop a substance use disorder during their careers, a rate similar to or exceeding that of the general population [30]. Although physicians' elevated social status brings many rewards, it also has an isolating effect when they are confronted with a disease such as addiction, which has a social stigma. This isolation can lead to tragic consequences, both in delaying the recognition of and in intervening in the disease condition, as well as in the attendant risk of death by overdose or suicide [31]. Further causes for delay in diagnosis include fear on the part of the physician that disclosure of an addictive illness might cause loss not only of prestige but also of his or her license to practice medicine and thus livelihood. Additionally, in an effort to protect the family or practice workers from economic collapse by the loss of the physician's job and income, a physician's family members and colleagues will often participate in a "conspiracy of silence" [32].

In a 5-year longitudinal cohort study of 904 physicians, researchers found that 87% of whom were male and 50% reported abuse of multiple substances. Alcohol was the primary drug of abuse in almost a half of physicians. Opioids were identified in 36%, stimulants in 8%, and other substances in 6%; almost 14% reported a history of intravenous drug use and 17% previous treatment for addiction [33]. The authors found that certain specialties, such as anesthesiology, emergency medicine, and psychiatry, appeared to be overrepresented in these programs relative to their numerical representation in the national physician pool. Indeed, other investigators have suggested that these specialties seem to have a disproportionate propensity toward addiction [34].

Evaluation of physicians with alcohol or other substance abuse disorders is difficult and requires a multidisciplinary team with vast experience working with this population [35]. The intellect, the potential to develop exceptional rationalization, denial, and resistance techniques make the recognition of their disease difficult [36]. During the initial evaluation, most physicians will deny having a problem. Although a detailed substance use history is essential to the diagnosis, it can be remarkably difficult to obtain. Therefore, collateral information from friends, family, coworkers, and pharmacies is required to gather documentation to support the diagnostic evaluation, and the evaluating program will typically require signed releases from the physician undergoing evaluation to obtain this vital information. Both a complete medical history and a physical examination are necessary because addicted individuals have often neglected their health. A family evaluation gathers information about the individual's functioning and determines how the family has been affected. Co-occurring psychiatric illness, i.e., substance use disorder combined with a major depressive disorder, bipolar affective disorder, or anxiety or panic disorder, is common in the addicted physician and can undermine recovery from addiction; thus, psychiatric and psychological evaluations are needed [37].

Access to Lethal Means

The most common means of suicide by physicians are lethal medication overdoses and firearms [38]. With regard to knowledge and access to lethal means, there is no doubt that physicians understand the physiology of death and have more access to lethal means than the general population, as evidenced by their higher success rate at dying by suicide. A high ratio of suicide completions to attempts may result from physicians' greater knowledge of toxicology and access to lethal drugs, since overdoses of medications and firearms are the two most common methods of suicide [3]. The literature suggests that certain specialists, such as psychiatrists and anesthesiologists (due to the access to lethal means), are at increased suicide risk [39].

Previous Self-Harm or Suicide Attempts

Suicide is associated with multiple risk factors, but similar to the general population, in physicians, the strongest predictor is prior history of suicide attempts. An individual who has made a previous suicide attempt is nearly six times more likely to make another attempt [40]. There is some suggestion that women physicians make fewer suicide attempts than other women, but, because they have the knowledge and access to medications, they are more likely to die by suicide [41].

Excessive Risk Taking (Especially High-Stakes Gambler, Thrill Seeker, and Involved in Extreme High-Risk Activities)

The practice of medicine brings with it unique risks, timelines, stresses, intense emotions around issues of suffering, fear, sexuality, mortality, problem patients who can be demanding, and extensive uncertainty due to the limits of medical knowledge. Physicians often struggle during training and in later years to harden themselves to these issues involved in extreme high-risk activities [42]. Physicians respond to the stresses of high-risk activities in a variety of ways. Some have problems with depression, substance abuse, and marital conflict; others may not have overt psychiatric illness but display other signs of psychologic impairment including self-harm or suicide behaviors [42]. Authors have reviewed many problems that residents have during training, including the almost universal experience of episodic cognitive impairment, chronic anger, pervasive cynicism, and family discord [43]. Such signs of distress certainly merit examination of the process of medical training to prevent impulsive and nonadaptive behaviors in practicing physicians [44].

Personality with Characteristics of Perfectionism, Competitiveness, and to Blame for Clinical Errors

Using a longitudinal, prospective design, investigators look for personality antecedents of burnout [45]. The short version of the Minnesota Multiphasic Personality Inventory (MMPI) was administered to 440 physicians, before entering medical school, and then were surveyed an average of 25 years later. Low self-esteem, feelings of inadequacy, dysphoria and obsessive worry, passivity, social anxiety, and withdrawal from others were correlated with significantly higher burnout scores.

Perfectionism and the competitiveness engendered in medical training were identified as key reasons for experiencing distress about clinical errors. Studies on evaluating the impact of clinical mistakes found physicians experienced great distress over making mistakes. Although they recognized the ubiquity of mistakes in clinical practice, they however believed they could not disclose the mistakes to colleagues and experienced a lack of support from colleagues in addressing these concerns [46]. Perfectionism may lead to conscientiousness during medical school and to a thorough clinical practice, but it may also raise an unforgiving attitude when mistakes inevitably occur. Fear of legal consequences exacerbates distress about clinical errors.

Further supporting the concept of physicians' predisposition to impairment, in a report of psychiatrically hospitalized physicians, investigators reinforce the theory that the personality of impaired physicians seems to predispose them to problems when attempting to cope with occupational stresses [47]. The premorbid personality of impaired physicians was characterized as obsessive (e.g., overzealous), with a difficulty to relax or acknowledge personal limits or vulnerabilities. In addition, the importance of genetic vulnerability was studied making special note of the difference in prevalence of depression in first-degree relatives among depressed and non-depressed women professionals [48]. The study was replicated in a study of depressed interns, indicating that 50% of the depressed interns had at least one first-degree relative with depression [49].

Warning Signs for Physician Suicide

Pain, Recent Diagnosis of Chronic or Debilitating Medical Condition, and Worsening Medical Prognosis

Physicians are demonstrably poor at recognizing depression in patients, let alone themselves. Furthermore, they are notoriously reluctant to seek treatment for any personal illness. Research suggests that one in three physicians has no regular source of medical care [50]. To some extent, physicians' reluctance to reach out is self-imposed. They may feel an obligation to appear healthy, perhaps as evidence of their ability to heal others. Inquiring about another physician's health can shatter this mutual myth of invulnerability, and volunteering support or assistance unasked may seem like an affront to a colleague's self-sufficiency. Thus, the concerned colleague or partner may say nothing, while wondering privately if the colleague has become impaired.

Similar to the general population, in physicians, depression is a common comorbidity with chronic pain. The true prevalence of depression in chronic pain varies with the population sampled (e.g., physicians, students, community, primary care, pain clinics, sports medicine, orthopedic clinics). A recent literature review examining the prevalence of depression and pain found that mean prevalence rates of concomitant major depression in pain patients were 52% in pain clinics, 38% in psychiatric clinics, 56% in orthopedic or rheumatology clinics, 85% in dental clinics addressing chronic facial pain, 13% in gynecologic clinics focusing on chronic pelvic pain, 18% in population-based settings, and 27% in primary care clinics [51]. The authors identified several studies revealing a strong association between depression and pain, demonstrating that pain patients are more likely to be depressed than patients without pain and that the presence of pain may obscure the detection and treatment of depression, thus placing these vulnerable patients at heightened risk for suicide [52]. Similarly, a systematic review revealed that risk of successful suicide was doubled in chronic pain patients relative to non-pain controls. General risk factors for suicide in chronic pain patients included family history of suicide, previous suicide attempt, gender (female), and presence of comorbid depression. Pain-specific risk factors included location and type of pain, high pain intensity, long pain duration, and presence of co-occurring insomnia [53].

Pain catastrophizing has been conceptualized as an exaggerated, negative focus on pain that can contribute to depression, pain intensity, and disability [54]. In a sample of approximately 1500 patients with chronic pain, 32% reported some degree of recent suicidal ideation [55]. Magnitude of depression and pain catastrophizing predicted the occurrence and degree of suicidal ideation with poor pain coping skills being strongly associated with suicide, independent of depression, and pain severity. Targeting improved sleep and pain coping skills may reduce the incidence of suicidal ideation and attempts.

Increasing literature shows that a subset of pain patients experience suicidal ideation. In physicians, concern is regarding fatal self-prescription opioid overdose to control chronic pain. Clinicians should be cognizant of the presence of depression and the risk of suicide, particularly when physicians have access to large doses of potentially lethal medications, such as opioids or benzodiazepines [56].

Lack of Trust, Recent Relationship Problems or Breakups, Separation or Divorce, and Currently Having Marital Disruption

Difficulty with trust may also be part of the problem. Although physicians are accustomed to hearing and protecting the confidences of others, it may be hard for them to let their guard down and really believe that they can trust another [57]. Divorce rates among physicians have been reported to be 10–20% higher than those in the general population [58]. Moreover, those couples that include a physician who remain married reported marriages that are unhappy. They may postpone the pleasures of life that others enjoy. This psychology of postponement may be related to the personality traits that are widely suggested as being key ingredients in professional success. Many physicians place work above all else, and it has been speculated that this may serve the purpose for them of helping to avoid intimacy, thus placing pressure on familiar relationships [59]. Self-denial also occurs and interferes with the work-life balance. Physicians become masters at delayed gratification. Many physicians spend years coping with the high level of demand required in medicine, often harboring the expectation that later they will be rewarded with a happy, more balanced life. This interferes with family relationships. The goal-oriented approach leads to neglecting alternative sources of gratification or self-esteem; thus, physicians may not have a way to find a meaningful balance between work and other life activities.

Recent Acute Depressive Episode, Depression or Depressive Symptoms, or Any New Psychiatric Diagnosis

Published reports of physician depression are very difficult to find. Physicians find it embarrassing to share their experience of mental illness with others and know that doing so is somewhat risky. Recent cases of resident and physician suicides have triggered the need of sharing of experiences of depression by physicians. This suggests that either the incidence of depression is rising or that the medical community is beginning to admit and address the extent of the problem [60]. In addition, depression often coexists with medical illness particularly in patients older than 60 years, the group at highest risk for suicide. After the illness has been acknowledged, treatment of the depressed physician poses unique challenges. Physicians tend to be treated as "special patients," by their colleagues, which can ultimately erode the quality of their care; for example, a physician may write a prescription for antidepressants for a physician friend without performing the extensive evaluation that is usually conducted on depressed patients. Because physicians are often reluctant to seek help, many come to treatment only when they are no longer able to practice [61].

Another phenomenon that may play a role in physician depression and suicide is that everyone likes to be considered special, and with fellow physicians, doctors often enjoy special treatment when they do seek help [62]. However, the very fact that they are doctors themselves may cause other doctors to be less aggressive in their treatment. Physicians may be more reluctant to go for help and admit their own problems if they believe they have been labeled by others as strong and healthy. Difficulty setting appropriate limits is another characteristic hypothesized to be common among physicians. There is a common expectation that physicians must be available whenever needed, and this can lead to a sense of obligation that makes it difficult to set limits without great guilt. Medical training observes few time boundaries; long hours are assumed to be part of the medical training. Professional identity often internalizes this assumption, so that setting limits is perceived as lacking in professional commitment.

The fact that 35% of physicians do not have a regular source of health care, which is associated with less use of preventive medical services, supports the observation that the medical profession does not encourage physicians to admit health vulnerabilities or seek help [26]. Physicians' use of mental health services also appears low, but there is virtually no information on patterns of seeking help. Medical students have particularly low rates of seeking help, with only 22% of those who had screened positive for depression using mental health services [63]. Reports support that only 42% of depressed students with suicidal ideation received treatment. The most frequently cited barriers to care included lack of time (48%), lack of confidentiality (37%), stigma (30%), cost (28%), and fear of documentation on academic record (24%). Concerns about confidentiality and career prospects may weigh more heavily for students, residents, and young practicing physicians [64].

Increase in the Alcohol or Drug Consumption

There is a strong and well-identified link between suicide and both substance abuse and depression [65]. It has been estimated that 40% of physician suicides are associated with alcoholism and 20% with drug abuse. An association between mood disorders, substance abuse, and suicide among physicians has been described. Substance abuse probably has received more attention than suicide or depression as a problem within medicine, and reported prevalence rates vary widely. Recent data suggest that the prevalence of alcoholism and illicit drug abuse by physicians is similar to that among the general population, but physicians may be at increased risk for prescription drug abuse. The availability of addictive agents may play a role in the increased rates of drug addiction among physicians. Physicians also have the opportunity to self-medicate and otherwise treat themselves rather than entrust their care to others, and this may have terrible consequences. Also, physicians are more knowledgeable about the lethal doses of various medications, so this may play a role in the increased rates of successful suicide.

Self-Medication and Request for Substances with Lethal Outcomes (e.g., Anesthetics, Sedatives, etc.)

One report indicates that physicians do not follow schedules for routine medical care for themselves and their families and prescribe medication for themselves rather than seek consultation from a practitioner [66]. This erroneous mentality may also play a role in the increased rates of psychosocial distress within medicine's ranks. Doctors are commonly expected to be strong and support others, but many doctors believe that it is not acceptable to reveal their own weaknesses and vulnerabilities to others. A physician whose thought processes are clouded by depression and the anticipated consequences of seeking treatment for it may believe that self-treatment is the only safe option. However, the potentially devastating effects initiated by a physician's self-reporting of depression may delay or impede appropriate treatment. Because many states require reporting by other licensed physicians of a physician who may be suffering from a potentially impairing condition, physicians can be reluctant to use their own names when seeking treatment, utilizing their insurance coverage, or even seeking antidepressant treatment from colleagues. Evidence suggests that even if physicians are treated for suicidality, the quality of treatment, paradoxically, may be compromised because of collegial relationships and deference from the treating clinician who may give more freedom to the physician-patient to control the focus of therapy and to self-medicate [67]. Most physicians treat themselves, at least on occasion. This is especially likely when the physician believes that the consequences of seeking treatment may subject him or her to stigma, shame, or worse. In addition, some physicians self-medicate with antidepressants, a practice that should be strongly discouraged. The depressed physician may decide to leave treatment prematurely. Even if a physician accepts somatic therapies, many have difficulty appreciating that stress-reducing lifestyle changes may be equally important in maintaining emotional health. Too often, attempts at self-treatment are unsuccessful. Failure to obtain consultation and treatment for depression needlessly and significantly increases the risk of physician suicide.

Professional Issues, Change in Status, Threats to Status, Autonomy, Security, Financial Stability, and Increased Work Demands

The stresses associated to the practice of medicine are well known. Physicians are subject to long hours, the need to make rapid and important decisions, exposure to unpleasant and emotionally taxing illnesses, and the need to absorb large quantities of new and complicated information. The sleep deprivation can lead to depression as well as cognitive impairment and irritability [68]. Individuals respond to stress in different ways based on genetic predilection, personality makeup, coping skills, and external supports. Most physicians are highly resilient individuals and thrive even in a stressful environment. Researches conducted a mail survey to assess professional stress among family physicians. They reported a significant correlation among perceived stress in medical practice and depression [69]. Although only 3% of respondents reported clinical depression, almost 33% of the total sample experienced symptoms within a subclinical range. Physicians who become psychiatrically impaired are often found to be predisposed to depression before entering medical training.

More recent studies found that physicians experienced stress with a changing set of problems, in particular paperwork and administrative hassles, loss of autonomy, and excessive professional demands [70]. Additionally clinical faculty and academic physicians have reported stressors such as long working hours, little vacation time, and conflicts between work and personal life [71]. Although stressors may be changing, there is no evidence that links them to the elevated suicide rate among physicians. Nor is there evidence that physicians are subject to more occupational stress than other professionals. Rather, recent research indicates that stressful events thought to precipitate suicide are themselves often precipitated by the behavior of patients with affective disorders. Even when suicidal patients do not engender stressful events, their experience of being intensely affected by them is often a function of their preexisting depression [72].

Financial Hardships, Legal Difficulties, Public Humiliation, or Shame

Physicians with psychiatric disorders often encounter overt or covert discrimination in medical licensing, hospital privileges, health insurance, and/or malpractice insurance [73]. Since 1983, the American Psychiatric Association expressed concern that licensing board questions focused on diagnosis or treatment of mental illness would deter physicians from seeking help [74]. It is logical to infer that physicians' concern about disclosure of mental health records is widespread, although studies are lacking. Breaches of confidentiality also are believed to harm openness between the physician (as patient) and the treating clinician and may result in needless disclosures to coworkers. Those concerns, coupled with professional attitudes that broadly discourage admission of health vulnerabilities, are likely the driving forces behind physicians' disinclination to seek mental health care. Considering that identities of many physicians are closely tied to their professional image makes them more vulnerable to distress when problems arise at work.

Summary and Conclusions

Suicidal behavior is a complex problem with no single cause or absolute predictors. Risk factors for physician suicide are similar to those in the general public and include:

- Diagnoses of major depressive disorder, bipolar disorder, alcohol use disorder, anxiety disorder, and borderline personality disorder
- Prior suicide attempt
- Difficult childhood/troubled family of origin
- Family history of mood disorders or suicide
- History of sexual abuse
- Relationship problems or domestic violence
- Multiple current stressors, including for physicians
- Being named as defendant in a lawsuit
- General job problems (e.g., concerns about job security, increased work demands)
- License restriction
- Financial problems
- Professional isolation

The identities of many physicians are closely tied to their professional image, making them more vulnerable to distress when problems arise at work. It is important for all physicians to be aware of the warning signs of suicide, which include:

- Increased substance (alcohol or drug) use
- Feeling or expressing that there is no reason for living or no sense of purpose in life
- Anxiety, agitation, difficulty sleeping, or sleeping all the time
- Feeling trapped, like there's no way out

- Hopelessness
- Withdrawal from friends, family, and society
- Rage, uncontrolled anger, and seeking revenge
- Acting reckless or engaging in risky activities, seemingly without thinking
- Mood changes
- Threatening to hurt or kill oneself or talking about wanting to hurt or kill oneself
- Looking for ways to kill oneself by seeking access to firearms, pills, or other means
- Talking or writing about death, dying, or suicide when these actions are unusual for the person

The first step in treating depression is recognizing it. A physician who is suffering from depression may not appear to be sad. Symptoms may include a marked irritability or apathy, weight changes as a result of decreased appetite, or carbohydrate, sugar cravings. The physician's quality of work may decline because of sleep problems, fatigue, or poor concentration, and the physician may fall behind on record keeping and other administrative duties. Attempts to compensate for low productivity may result in working excessive hours or going on rounds at unusual times. Physicians who are depressed may be unusually self-critical of their patient care and unable to forgive themselves if a problem occurs. The depressed physician may withdraw from participating in once-enjoyable social activities and may exhibit an increased use of alcohol or drugs. Understanding risk factors and warning signs for suicide in physicians is the first step in the identification of those at high risk. Prevention of suicide in doctors requires a range of strategies, including management of psychiatric disorder, measures to reduce occupational stress, and restriction of access to means of suicide when doctors are depressed. Not every suicide is preventable, but physicians at risk must be helped. This chapter was also created to encourage treatment of depression and prevention of suicide in physicians by improving professional attitudes and institutional policies to support physicians who seek help. Physicians cannot be separated from the knowledge, professional exposure, and the medications that make lethal self-harm possible. Prevention and intervention must, therefore, be directed at the behavioral health factors producing the depression and despair leading to the desire to die. Physicians must be included in community-wide prevention programs to reduce the incidence of suicide among adults. Like their patients, physicians would benefit from greater familiarity with suicide's risk and protective factors, danger and warning signs, myths and misconceptions, sources of help, and learning how to seek help.

References

1. Lindeman S, Heinanen H, Vaisanen E, Lonnqvist J. Suicide among medical doctors: psychological autopsy data on seven cases. Arch Suicide Res. 1998;4:135–41.
2. American Medical Association Council on Scientific Affairs. Physician mortality and suicide: results and implications of the AMA-APA pilot study. Conn Med. 1986;50:37–43.

3. Center C, Davis M, Detre T, Ford DE, Hansbrough W, Hendin H, et al. Confronting depression and suicide in physicians: a consensus statement. JAMA. 2003;289(23):3161–6. https://doi.org/10.1001/jama.289.23.3161.
4. Rudd MD, Berman AL, Joiner TE, Nock MK, Silverman MM, Mandrusiak M, et al. Warning signs for suicide: theory, research, and clinical applications. Suicide Life Threat Behav. 2006;36(3):255–62.
5. Suicide Prevention Resource Center, Rodgers P. Understanding risk and protective factors for suicide: a primer for preventing suicide. Education Development Center: Newton; 2011.
6. Hampton T. Experts address risk of physician suicide. JAMA. 2005;294(10):1189–91.
7. Hawton K. Suicide in doctors while under fitness to practise investigation. BMJ. 2015;350:h813.
8. Goldsmith SK, Pellmar TC, Kleinman AM, Bunney WE. Reducing suicide: a national imperative. Washington, DC: National Academies Press; 2002.
9. Samkoff JS, Hockenberry S, Simon LJ, Jones RL. Mortality of young physicians in the United States, 1980–1988. Acad Med. 1995;70(3):242–4.
10. Lindeman S, Laara E, Hakko H, Lonnqvist J. A systematic review on gender-specific suicide mortality in medical doctors. Br J Psychiatry. 1996;168:274–9.
11. Vaillant GE, Sobowale NC, McArthur C. Some psychological vulnerabilities of physicians. N Engl J Med. 1972;287:372–5.
12. Frank E, Dingle AD. Self-reported depression and suicide attempts among US women physicians. Am J Psychiatry. 1999;156:1887–94.
13. Craig AG, Pitts FN Jr. Suicide by physicians. Dis Nerv Syst. 1968;219:763–72.
14. Steppacher RC, Mausner JS. Suicide in male and female physicians. JAMA. 1974;228:323–8.
15. Weiner A, Marten S, Wochnick E, Davis MA, Fishman R, Clayton PJ. Psychiatric disorders among professional women. Arch Gen Psychiatry. 1979;36(2):169–73.
16. Robinson G. Stresses on women physicians: consequences and coping techniques. Depress Anxiety. 2003;17:180–9.
17. Miller JB. Toward a new psychology of women. Boston: Beacon Press; 1976.
18. Carmel S, Glick CS. Compassionate-empathic physicians: personality traits and social-organizational factors that enhance or inhibit this behavior pattern. Soc Sci Med. 1996;43:1253–61.
19. Johnson CA, Johnson BE, Liese BS. Dual doctor marriages: career development. Fam Med. 1992;24:205–8.
20. Carr PL, Ash AS, Friedman RH, Scaramucci A, Barnett RC, Szalacha LE, et al. Relation of family responsibilities and gender to the productivity and career satisfaction of medical faculty. Ann Intern Med. 1998;129(7):532–8.
21. Buddeberg-Fischer B, Stamm M, Buddeberg C, Bauer G, Hämmig O, Knecht M, et al. The impact of gender and parenthood on physicians' careers-professional and personal situation seven years after graduation. BMC Health Serv Res. 2010;10(1):40.
22. Silverman M. Physicians and suicide. In: Goldman LS, Myers M, Dickstein LJ, editors. The handbook of physician health: essential guide to understanding the health care needs of physicians. Chicago: American Medical Association; 2000.
23. Gold KJ, Sen A, Schwenk TL. Details on suicide among US physicians: data from the National Violent Death Reporting System. Gen Hosp Psychiatry. 2013;35(1):45–9.
24. Myers M. Doctors' marriages: a look at the problems and their solutions. 2nd ed. New York: Springer; 1994.
25. Swanson JW, McGinty EE, Fazel S, Mays VM. Mental illness and reduction of gun violence and suicide: bringing epidemiologic research to policy. Ann Epidemiol. 2015;25(5):366–76.
26. Gross CP, Mead LA, Ford DE, Klag MJ. Physician, heal thyself? Regular source of care and use of preventive health services among physicians. Arch Intern Med. 2000;160(21):3209–14.
27. Schernhammer ES, Colditz GA. Suicide rates among physicians: a quantitative and gender assessment (meta-analysis). Am J Psychiatry. 2004;161(12):2295–302.
28. Shanafelt TD, Balch CM, Dyrbye L, Bechamps G, Russell T, Satele D, et al. Special report: suicidal ideation among American surgeons. Arch Surg. 2011;146(1):54–62.
29. Gold KJ, Andrew LB, Goldman EB, Schwenk TL. "I would never want to have a mental health diagnosis on my record": a survey of female physicians on mental health diagnosis, treatment, and reporting. Gen Hosp Psychiatry. 2016;43:51–7.

30. Hughes PH, Brandenburg N, Baldwin DC Jr, Storr CL, Williams KM, Anthony JC, et al. Prevalence of substance use among US physicians. [published correction appears in JAMA. 1992;268(18):2518]. JAMA. 1992;267(17):2333–9.
31. Myers MF, Gabbard GO. The physician as patient: a clinical handbook for mental health professionals. Washington, DC: American Psychiatric Publishing; 2008.
32. Berge KH, Seppala MD, Schipper AM. Chemical dependency and the physician. Mayo Clin Proc. 2009;84(7):625–31.
33. McLellan AT, Skipper GS, Campbell M, DuPont RL. Five year outcomes in a cohort study of physicians treated for substance use disorders in the United States. BMJ. 2008;337:a2038.
34. Silverstein JH, Silva DA, Iberti TJ. Opioid addiction in anesthesiology. [published correction appears in anesthesiology. 1993;79(5):1160]. Anesthesiology. 1993;79(2):354–75.
35. Graham AW, Schultz TK, Mayo-Smith MF, Ries RK, Wilford BB. Principles of addiction medicine. 3rd ed. American Society of Addiction Medicine: Chevy Chase, MD; 2007.
36. Gastfriend DR. Physician substance abuse and recovery: what does it mean for physicians—and everyone else? [editorial]. JAMA. 2005;293(12):1513–5.
37. Domino KB, Hornbein TF, Polissar NL, Renner G, Johnson J, Alberti S, et al. Risk factors for relapse in health care professionals with substance use disorders. JAMA. 2005;293(12):1453–60.
38. Austin AE, van den Heuvel C, Byard RW. Physician suicide. J Forensic Sci. 2013;58(Suppl 1):S91–3.
39. Council on Scientific Affairs. Results and implications of the AMA-APA Physician Mortality Project, Stage II. JAMA. 1987;257:2949–53.
40. Chang B, Gitlin D, Patel R. The depressed patient and suicidal patient in the emergency department: evidence-based management and treatment strategies. Emerg Med Pract. 2011;13(9):1–23.
41. Arnetz BB, Hörte LG, Hedberg A, Theorell T, Allander E, Malker H. Suicide patterns among physicians related to other academics as well as to the general population. Acta Psychiatr Scand. 1987;75(2):139–43.
42. McCue J. The effects of stress on physicians and their medical practice. N Engl J Med. 1982;306:458–63.
43. Reuben DB. Psychologic effects of residency. South Med J. 1983;76:380–3.
44. Kirsling R, Kochar M. Suicide and the stress of residency training: a case report and review of the literature. Psychol Rep. 1989;64:951–9.
45. McCranie EW, Brandsma JM. Personality antecedents of burnout among middle-aged physicians. Behav Med. 1988;14(1):30–6.
46. Christensen JF, Levinson W, Dunn PM. Heart of darkness: the impact of perceived mistakes on physicians. J Gen Intern Med. 1992;7:424–31.
47. Jones R. A study of 100 physicians as psychiatric inpatients. Am J Psychiatry. 1977;134:1119–23.
48. Clayton PJ, Marten S, Davis MA, Wochnik E. Mood disorder in women professionals. J Affect Disord. 1980;2:37–46.
49. Valko RJ, Clayton PJ. Depression in internship. Dis Nerv Syst. 1975;36:26–9.
50. Miller M, Mcgowen R. The painful truth: physicians are not invincible. South Med J. 2000;93(10):966–73.
51. Bair MJ, Robinson RL, Katon W, Kroenke K. Depression and pain comorbidity: a literature review. Arch Intern Med. 2003;163(20):2433–45.
52. Kroenke K, Price RK. Symptoms in the community: prevalence, classification, and psychiatric comorbidity. Arch Intern Med. 1993;153(21):2474–80.
53. Tang NK, Crane C. Suicidality in chronic pain: a review of the prevalence, risk factors and psychological links. Psychol Med. 2006;36(05):575–86.
54. Turner JA, Jensen MP, Warms CA, Cardenas DD. Catastrophizing is associated with pain intensity, psychological distress, and pain-related disability among individuals with chronic pain after spinal cord injury. Pain. 2002;98(1):127–34.

55. Edwards RR, Smith MT, Kudel I, Haythornthwaite J. Pain-related catastrophizing as a risk factor for suicidal ideation in chronic pain. Pain. 2006;126(1–3):272–9.
56. Cheatle MD. Depression, chronic pain, and suicide by overdose: on the edge. Pain Med. 2011;12(s2):S43–8.
57. Verghese A. The tennis partner: a doctor's story of friendship and loss. New York: Harper Collins; 1998.
58. Sotile WM, Sotile MO. The medical marriage: a couple's survival guide. New York: Carol Publishing; 1996.
59. Gabbard GO, Menninger RW. The psychology of postponement in the medical marriage. JAMA. 1989;261:2378–81.
60. Carroll AE. Silence is the enemy for doctors who have depression. New York Times. 11 Jan 2016. https://www.nytimes.com/2016/01/12/upshot/silence-is-the-enemy-for-doctors-who-have-depression.html.
61. Bittker TE. Reaching out to the depressed physician. JAMA. 1976;236:1713–6.
62. Stoudemire A, Rhoads JM. When the doctor needs a doctor: special considerations for the physician-patient. Ann Intern Med. 1983;98:654–9.
63. Givens JL, Tjia J. Depressed medical students' use of mental health services and barriers to use. Acad Med. 2002;77:918–21.
64. Roberts LW, Hardee JT, Franchini G, Stidley CA, Siegler M. Medical students as patients: a pilot study of their health care needs, practices, and concerns. Acad Med. 1996;71:1225–32.
65. Simon W, Lumry GK. Suicide among physician patients. J Nerv Ment Dis. 1968;147:105–12.
66. Forsythe M, Calnan M, Wall B. Doctors as patients: postal survey examining consultants and general practitioners adherence to guidelines. BMJ. 1999;319:605–8.
67. Levine RE, Bryant SG. The depressed physician: a different kind of impairment. Hosp Physician. 2000;36(2):67–73.
68. Levin R. Beyond "the men of steel": the origins and significance of house staff training stress. Gen Hosp Psychiatry. 1988;10(2):114–21.
69. Friedman RC, Bigger JT, Kornfeld DS. The intern and sleep loss. N Engl J Med. 1971;285:201–3.
70. Kaiser Family Foundation. National survey of physicians, part III: doctors' opinions about their profession. 2002. http://www.kff.org/content/2002/20020426c/PhysicianSurveypartIII.pdf.
71. Linn LS, Yager J, Cope D, Leake B. Health status, job satisfaction, job stress, and life satisfaction among academic and clinical faculty. JAMA. 1985;254:2775–82.
72. Hendin H, Haas AP, Maltsberger JT, Lipschitz A, Weintraub K. Determination of precipitating events in the suicide of psychiatric patients. Suicide Life Threat Behav. 2003;33:111–9.
73. Miles SH. A challenge to licensing boards: the stigma of mental illness. JAMA. 1998;280(10):865.
74. American Psychiatric Association. Position statement on confidentiality of medical records: does the physician have a right to privacy concerning his or her own medical records? Am J Psychiatry. 1984;141(2):331.

Index

T. Falcone, J. Timmons-Mitchell (eds.), *Suicide Prevention*,
https://doi.org/10.1007/978-3-319-74391-2

N

Printed by Printforce, the Netherlands